FIRST AID FOR THE

USMLE STEP 2

A STUDENT TO 3rd Edition **STUDENT GUIDE**

Notice

FIRST AID FOR THE

USMLE STEP 2

A STUDENT TO 3rd Edition STUDENT GUIDE

TAO LE, MD
University of California, San Francisco, Class of 1996
Co-founder and Chief Medical Officer, Medsn

CHIRAG AMIN, MD
University of Miami, Class of 1996

VIKAS BHUSHAN, MD
University of California, San Francisco, Class of 1991
Co-founder and Chairman, Medsn

ESTHER CHOO, MD
Yale University, Class of 2001
Boston Medical Center
Resident in Emergency Medicine

McGraw-Hill
Medical Publishing Division

New York   Chicago   San Francisco   Lisbon   London   Madrid
Mexico City   Milan   New Delhi   San Juan   Seoul
Singapore   Sydney   Toronto

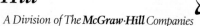

McGraw-Hill

A Division of The McGraw·Hill Companies

First Aid for the USMLE Step 2, Third Edition

Copyright © 2001 by The **McGraw-Hill Companies**, Inc. All rights reserved. Printed in the United States of America. Except as permitted under the United States Copyright Act of 1976, no part of this publication may be reproduced or distributed in any form or by any means, or stored in a data base or retrieval system, without the prior written permission of the publisher.

Previous editions copyright © 1999, 1996 by by Appleton & Lange.

3 4 5 6 7 8 9 0   VNHVNH   0 9 8 7 6 5 4 3 2

ISBN 0-07-137770-0

ISSN 1532-320X

This book was set in Goudy by Rainbow Graphics.
The editor was Catherine A. Johnson.
The production supervisor was Lisa Mendez.
Project management was provided by Rainbow Graphics.
Editorial services was provided by Andrea Fellows.
The interior designer was Elizabeth Sanders.
The index was prepared by Angie Wiley Indexing Services.

Von Hoffman Graphics was printer and binder.

This book is printed on acid-free paper.

INTERNATIONAL EDITION ISBN 0-07-112464-0
Copyright © 2001. Exclusive rights by The McGraw-Hill Companies, Inc., for manufacture and export. This book cannot be re-exported from the country to which it is consigned by McGraw-Hill. The International Edition is not available in North America.

To our families, friends, and loved ones, who endured
and assisted in the task of assembling this guide.

&

To the contributors to this and future editions, who took
time to share their knowledge, insight, and
humor for the benefit of students.

Contributors

ANTONY CHU
Contributing Author,
Exam Guide and Review Resources
Yale University, Class of 2002

ERIC HAZEN
Contributing Author, High-Yield Facts
Yale University, Class of 2002

JASON VIEDER, DO, MBA
Contributing Author, High-Yield Facts
Philadelphia College of Osteopathic Medicine,
Class of 2001

Associate Contributors

RYAN DAVIES, MD
Columbia Presbyterian Medical Center
Resident in General Surgery

AVERY S. GRAUER, MD
Yale-New Haven Hospital
Resident in Internal Medicine

KRISTY AHRLICH
Yale College
Class of 2003

Reviewers

VLADIMIR CORIC, MD
Fellow in Forensic Psychiatry
Yale-New Haven Hospital

BRAD HERSKOWITZ, MD
Chief Resident in Neurology
Yale-New Haven Hospital

ANWAR KHAN, MD
Fellow in Radiation Oncology
Yale-New Haven Hospital

MIKHAIL KOSIBOROD, MD
Fellow in Cardiology
Yale-New Haven Hospital

DANA LOO, MD
Staff Physician
Yale-New Haven Hospital

ALEX MAROTTA, MD
Resident in Pediatrics
Yale-New Haven Hospital

Contents

Color Illustration Section (16 pages) between pages 456 and 457

Preface

With the third edition of *First Aid for the USMLE Step 2*, we continue our commitment to providing students with the most useful and up-to-date preparation guide for the USMLE Step 2. The third edition represents a thorough revision in many ways and includes:

- A completely revised and updated exam preparation guide for the new computerized USMLE Step 2. Includes detailed analysis as well as all new study and test-taking strategies for the new computer-based testing (CBT) format.
- Revisions and new material based on student experience with the 2000 and 2001 administrations of the USMLE Step 2.
- Concise summaries of over 300 heavily tested clinical topics.
- A basic science primer for each medical subspecialty, focusing on clinically relevant high-yield basic science facts from the 2001 edition of *First Aid for the USMLE Step 1*.
- A "rapid review" that tests your knowledge of each topic.
- Boards-type clinical vignettes, with explanations, from McGraw-Hill's updated *PreTest*® series for the USMLE Step 2.
- A new collection of over 120 high-yield glossy photos similar to those appearing on the USMLE Step 2 exam.
- Useful reference links to prototypical clinical cases from the popular *Underground Clinical Vignette* series (S2S Medical Publishing).
- A completely revised, in-depth guide to clinical science review and sample examination books.

The third edition would not have been possible without the help of the many students and faculty members who contributed their feedback and suggestions. We invite students and faculty to continue sharing their thoughts and ideas to help us improve *First Aid for the USMLE Step 2*. (See How to Contribute, p. xv, and User Survey, p. xxiii.)

Santa Monica	Tao Le
Santa Monica	Chirag Amin
Los Angeles	Vikas Bhushan
New Haven	Esther Choo

June 2001

Acknowledgments

This has been a collaborative project from the start. We gratefully acknowledge the thoughtful comments, corrections, and advice of the many medical students, international medical graduates, and faculty who have supported the authors in the continuing development of *First Aid for the USMLE Step 2*.

For significant contributions to the third edition, we would like to thank Patricia Moore, Seth Goldbarg, Biren Modi, and Brian Lester.

Thanks to Melanie Nelson (NBME) for providing updated USMLE Step 2 information. For help obtaining information concerning review books, we thank Barnes & Noble bookstore (New York City). Thanks to Elizabeth Sanders and Ashley Pound for the interior design.

For support and encouragement throughout the process, we are grateful to the Choo family, Kelly Ray, Thao Pham, the residents of 44 Pearl Street in New Haven, and the Yale University School of Medicine Office of Student Affairs.

Thanks to our publisher, McGraw-Hill, for the valuable assistance of their staff. For enthusiasm, support, and commitment for this challenging project, thanks to our editor, Catherine Johnson. For outstanding editorial work, we thank Andrea Fellows. A special thanks to Jimmy and Bennie Sauls (Rainbow Graphics) for remarkable production work.

For contributions, corrections, and surveys we thank Ken Lin, Michael Fehm, Sarita Shah, Heston Lamar, Derrick Aipoalani, Gaurong Daftary, Wen-Yi Lee, Michael Torres, Asher Christensen, Margaret Brick, James Lee, Gennifer Lin, Fritz Beenan, Gary Warnick, Maya Salameh, Scott Swiger, and Dave Ziegman.

Our apologies if we accidentally omitted or misspelled your name.

Santa Monica	Tao Le
Santa Monica	Chirag Amin
Los Angeles	Vikas Bhushan
New Haven	Esther Choo

How to Contribute

This version of *First Aid for the USMLE Step 2* incorporates hundreds of contributions and changes suggested by faculty and student reviewers. We invite you to participate in this process. We also offer **paid internships** in medical education and publishing ranging from three months to one year (see next page for details).

Please send us your suggestions for:

- Study and test-taking strategies for the computerized USMLE Step 2
- New facts, mnemonics, diagrams, and illustrations
- High-yield topics that may reappear on future Step 2 exams
- Personal ratings and comments on review books that you have examined

For each entry incorporated into the next edition, you will receive $10 cash per entry, as well as personal acknowledgment in the next edition. Diagrams, tables, partial entries, updates, corrections, and study hints are also appreciated, and significant contributions will be compensated at the discretion of the authors. Also let us know about material in this edition that you feel is low yield and should be deleted.

The preferred way to submit entries, suggestions, or corrections is via electronic mail. Please include name, address, school affiliation, phone number, and e-mail address (if different from address of origin). If there are multiple entries, please consolidate into a single e-mail or file attachment. Please send submissions to:

firstaidteam@yahoo.com

Otherwise, please send entries, neatly written or typed or on disk (Microsoft Word), to: First Aid for the USMLE Step 2, 1015 Gayley Ave., #1113, Los Angeles, CA 90024, Attention: Contributions. Please use the contribution and survey forms on the following pages. Each form constitutes an entry. Attach additional pages as needed.

Internship Opportunities

The author team is pleased to offer part-time and full-time paid internships in medical education and publishing to motivated medical students and physicians. Internships may range from three months (e.g., a summer) up to a full year. Participants will have an opportunity to author, edit, and earn academic credit on a wide variety of projects, including the popular *First Aid* series. Writing/editing experience, familiarity with Microsoft Word, and Internet access are desired. For more information, e-mail a résumé or a short description of your experience along with a cover letter to the authors at their e-mail addresses above.

Note to Contributors

All entries become property of the authors and are subject to editing and reviewing. Please verify all data and spellings carefully. In the event that similar or duplicate entries are received, only the first entry received will be used. Include a reference to a standard textbook to facilitate verification of the fact. Please follow the style, punctuation, and format of this edition if possible.

Contribution Form 1

Contributor Name: _____

School/Affiliation: _____

Address: _____

_____

Telephone: _____

E-mail: _____

Topic:

Signs and Symptoms:

Diagnosis:

Management:

Notes, Diagrams, Tables, and Mnemonics:

Reference:

You will receive personal acknowledgment and $10 cash for each entry that is used in future editions.

Please seal with tape only.
No staples or paper clips.

-------------------------------- (fold here) --------------------------------

BUSINESS REPLY MAIL
FIRST-CLASS MAIL PERMIT NO. 74036 LOS ANGELES CA

POSTAGE WILL BE PAID BY ADDRESSEE

MSC 1113
FIRST AID FOR THE USMLE STEP 2
1015 GAYLEY AVE
LOS ANGELES CA 90024-8980

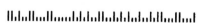

-------------------------------- (fold here) --------------------------------

Contribution Form II

Contributor Name: _____

School/Affiliation: _____

Address: _____

_____

Telephone: _____

E-mail: _____

Please place the clinical topic (e.g., ulcerative colitis) on the first line and the high-yield vignette or topic on the following two lines.

1. Subject: _____

   Vignette: _____

   _____

2. Subject: _____

   Vignette: _____

   _____

3. Subject: _____

   Vignette: _____

   _____

4. Subject: _____

   Vignette: _____

   _____

5. Subject: _____

   Vignette: _____

   _____

6. Subject: _____

   Vignette: _____

   _____

7. Subject: _____

   Vignette: _____

   _____

8. Subject: _____

   Vignette: _____

   _____

9. Subject: _____

   Vignette: _____

   _____

10. Subject: _____

    Vignette: _____

    _____

You will receive personal acknowledgment and $10 cash for each entry that is used in future editions.

Please seal with tape only.
No staples or paper clips.

--(fold here)--

BUSINESS REPLY MAIL
FIRST-CLASS MAIL PERMIT NO. 74036 LOS ANGELES CA

POSTAGE WILL BE PAID BY ADDRESSEE

MSC 1113
FIRST AID FOR THE USMLE STEP 2
1015 GAYLEY AVE
LOS ANGELES CA 90024-8980

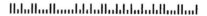

--(fold here)--

Contribution Form III

Contributor Name: _____

School/Affiliation: _____

Address: _____

_____

Telephone: _____

E-mail: _____

We welcome additional comments on review resources rated in Section III as well as reviews of resources not rated in Section III. Please fill out each review entry as completely as possible. Please do not leave "Comments" blank. Rate texts using the letter grading scale provided on p. 459, taking into consideration current ratings of other books on that subject.

1. ***Title/Author:*** _____   Days needed to read: _____

   Publisher/Series: _____   ISBN Number: _____

   Rating: _____   ***Comments:*** _____

   _____

   _____

2. ***Title/Author:*** _____   Days needed to read: _____

   Publisher/Series: _____   ISBN Number: _____

   Rating: _____   ***Comments:*** _____

   _____

   _____

3. ***Title/Author:*** _____   Days needed to read: _____

   Publisher/Series: _____   ISBN Number: _____

   Rating: _____   ***Comments:*** _____

   _____

   _____

4. ***Title/Author:*** _____   Days needed to read: _____

   Publisher/Series: _____   ISBN Number: _____

   Rating: _____   ***Comments:*** _____

   _____

   _____

5. ***Title/Author:*** _____   Days needed to read: _____

   Publisher/Series: _____   ISBN Number: _____

   Rating: _____   ***Comments:*** _____

   _____

   _____

You will receive personal acknowledgment and $10 cash for each entry that is used in future editions.

Please seal with tape only.
No staples or paper clips.

-------------------------------- (fold here) --------------------------------

BUSINESS REPLY MAIL
FIRST-CLASS MAIL PERMIT NO. 74036 LOS ANGELES CA

POSTAGE WILL BE PAID BY ADDRESSEE

MSC 1113
FIRST AID FOR THE USMLE STEP 2
1015 GAYLEY AVE
LOS ANGELES CA 90024-8980

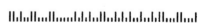

-------------------------------- (fold here) --------------------------------

User Survey

Contributor Name: _____

School/Affiliation: _____

Address: _____

_____

Telephone: _____

E-mail: _____

What student-to-student advice would you give someone preparing for the computerized USMLE Step 2?

What commercial review courses have you been enrolled in, and what were your overall assessments of the courses?

What would you change about the study and test-taking strategies listed in Section I: Guide to Efficient Exam Preparation?

Were there any high-yield facts, topics, or vignettes in Section II that you think were inaccurate or should be deleted? Which ones and why? What would you change or add?

What review resources for the USMLE Step 2 are not covered in Section III? Would you change the rating of any of the review resources in Section III? If so, which one(s) and why?

What other suggestions do you have for improving *First Aid for the USMLE Step 2*? Any other comments or suggestions? What did you dislike most about the book? What did you like most?

You will receive personal acknowledgment and $10 cash for each entry that is used in future editions.

Please seal with tape only.
No staples or paper clips.

--------------------------------- (fold here) ---------------------------------

BUSINESS REPLY MAIL
FIRST-CLASS MAIL PERMIT NO. 74036 LOS ANGELES CA

POSTAGE WILL BE PAID BY ADDRESSEE

MSC 1113
FIRST AID FOR THE USMLE STEP 2
1015 GAYLEY AVE
LOS ANGELES CA 90024-8980

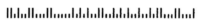

--------------------------------- (fold here) ---------------------------------

Guide to Efficient Exam Preparation

The goal of Step 2 is to examine your ability to apply your knowledge of medical facts to actual situations that you may encounter as a resident.

INTRODUCTION

For many U.S. medical graduates, the United States Medical Licensing Examination (USMLE) Step 2 is often looked upon as an afterthought, shoved somewhere in between residency applications, "away" rotations, and matching. Nevertheless, the clinical approach of the questions allows you to pull together your clinical experience on the wards with the numerous "factoids" and classical disease presentations that you have memorized over the years.

USMLE STEP 2—THE CBT BASICS

The USMLE Step 2 is the second of three examinations that you must pass in order to become a licensed physician in the United States.

The computerized Step 2 exam is a one-day (nine-hour, 400-question) multiple-choice exam. It includes test questions in internal medicine, obstetrics and gynecology, pediatrics, preventive medicine, psychiatry, and surgery.

The computer-based test (CBT) is administered by Prometric, Inc.®, a subsidiary of Thomson Learning. Prometric test centers, also known as Sylvan Technology Centers (STCs), offer Step 2 testing year-round. In most test centers, the exam will be offered Monday through Saturday. Weekly schedules can vary, however, at international test centers. For the most up-to-date information refer to www.usmle.org.

How Will the CBT Be Structured?

- **Test Format.** The CBT format consists of 400 questions given in one day, with eight question "blocks" of 50 questions timed at 60 minutes each (Fig. 1). During the time allotted to complete each block, the examinee will be able to answer test questions in any order as well as to review responses and change answers. Once the allotted block time has expired, however, further review of test questions or changing of answers within that block will not be possible. Expect to spend nine hours at the test center.

- **Test blocks.** As noted above, the CBT exam is divided into 60-minute blocks. These blocks were designed to reduce eye strain and fatigue during the exam. Once an examinee finishes a particular block, he or she must click on a screen icon to continue to the next block. Examinees will not be able to go back and change answers from any previous block.

Testing Conditions: What Will the CBT Be Like?

Because of the unique environment of the CBT, it's important that you familiarize yourself ahead of time with your test-day conditions. Familiarizing yourself with the testing interface before the exam can add to your break time! This is because a 15-minute tutorial, offered on exam day, may be skipped if you are already familiar with the exam procedures and the testing interface (CD-ROM, see below). The 15 minutes are added to your allotted break time (should you choose to skip the tutorial).

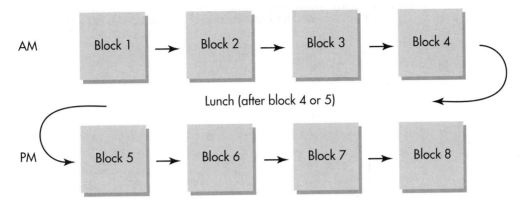

FIGURE 1. Schematic of CBT Exam

For security reasons, examinees will not be allowed to bring any personal electronic equipment into the testing area. This includes digital watches, watches with computer communication and/or memory capability, cellular telephones, and electronic paging devices. Food and beverages are prohibited. The testing centers are monitored by audio and video surveillance equipment.

The following information is based on software previews from the National Board of Medical Examiners (NBME). Check the USMLE website (http://www.usmle.org) or with your medical school for updates.

The typical question screen (Fig. 2) has a question followed by a number of choices on which an examinee can click, along with navigational buttons at the bottom of the screen. There is also a button that allows the examinee to mark the question for review. A countdown timer occupies the upper right-hand corner of the screen. If the question happens to be longer than the screen (very rare), a scroll bar will appear on the right, allowing the examinee to see the rest of the question. Regardless of whether the examinee clicks on

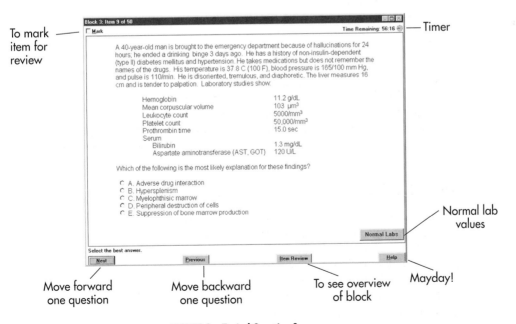

FIGURE 2. Typical Question Screen

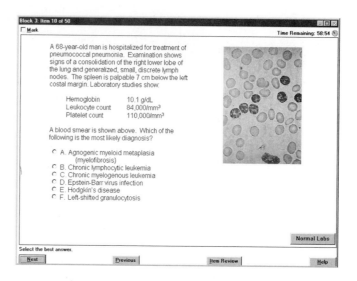

FIGURE 3.   Question Screen with Illustration

an answer or leaves it blank, he or she must click the "Next>>" button in order to advance to the next question.

Some questions contain figures or color illustrations (Fig. 3). These are typically situated to the right of the question. Although the contrast and brightness of the screen can be adjusted, there are no other ways to manipulate the picture (e.g., zooming or panning).

The examinee can also call up a window displaying normal lab values (Fig. 4). However, if he or she does not click on "Tile" in the normal-values screen, the normal-values window will often obscure the question. In addition, the examinee will have to scroll down for most laboratory values.

There exists an option to mark a question for review at a later time. Clicking "Item Review" at the bottom of the screen will access a screen (Fig. 5) showing an over-

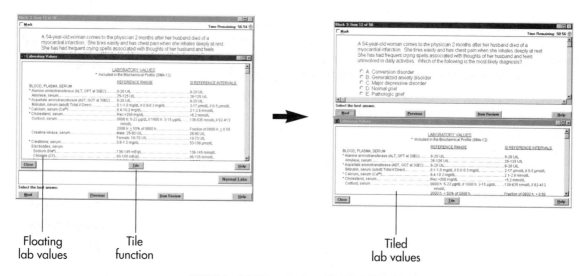

Floating lab values

Tile function

Tiled lab values

FIGURE 4.   Lab Values Screen—Floating and Tiled

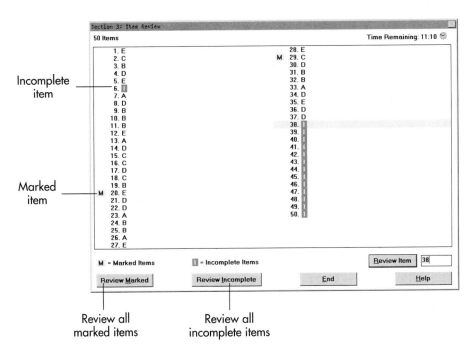

FIGURE 5. Item Review Screen

view of the block, allowing the examinee to pinpoint questions marked for review as well as unanswered questions. This also serves as a quick way of navigating to any question in the block, even unmarked, completed questions.

What Does the CBT Format Mean for Me?

The significance of the CBT format to you depends on the requirements of your school and your level of computer knowledge. If you hate computers and freak out whenever you see one, you might want to face your fears as soon as possible. Spend some time playing with a Windows-based system and pointing and clicking icons or buttons with a mouse. These are the absolute basics, and you won't want to waste valuable exam time figuring them out on test day. Your test taking will proceed by pointing and clicking, essentially without the use of the keyboard.

For those who feel they would benefit, USMLE offers an opportunity to take a simulated test, or "CBT Practice Session at a Prometric center." Students are eligible to take the three and one-half-hour practice session after they have received their fluorescent orange scheduling permit (see below).

The same USMLE Step 1 sample test items (150 questions) available on the CD or USMLE website, www.usmle.org, are used at these sessions. *No new items will be presented.* The session is divided into three one-hour blocks of 50 test items each and costs about $42. The student receives a printed percent-correct score after completing the session. No explanations of questions are provided.

You may register for a practice session online at www.usmle.org.

Keyboard shortcuts:
A–E—Letter choices.
Enter or Alt–N—Move to
next question.
Alt–P—Move back one
question.
Alt–T—Countdown timers
for current session and
overall test.

Ctrl-Alt-Delete are the
keys of death during
the exam. Don't touch
them!

How Do I Register to Take the Exam?

Starting with the 2001 USMLE application cycle, registration packets with printed materials are no longer provided to medical schools. Your medical school should have a supply of the 2001 CD, which contains electronic files of all the printed materials, such as the 2001 USMLE Bulletin of Information. Step 2 applications, which are not on the CD, may be printed from the USMLE website.

The preliminary registration process for the USMLE Step 2 is essentially unchanged, which is to say that students are required to complete registration forms and send exam fees to the NBME. The application allows applicants to select one of 12 overlapping three-month blocks in which to be tested (e.g., June/July/August, July/August/September). The application includes a photo ID form that must be certified by an official at your medical school to verify your enrollment. After the NBME processes your application, it will send you a bright orange slip of paper called a scheduling permit.

The scheduling permit you receive from the NBME will contain your USMLE identification number, the eligibility period in which you may take the exam, and two unique numbers. One of these is known as your "scheduling number." You will need this number to make your exam appointment with Sylvan. The other number is known as the "Candidate Identification Number," or CIN. Examinees must enter their CIN at the Sylvan workstation in order to access their exam. Sylvan has no access to the codes and will not be able to supply these numbers. **Do not lose your permit!** You will not be allowed to take the boards unless you present this permit along with an unexpired, government-issued photo identification with your signature (such as a driver's license or passport). Make sure the name on your photo ID exactly matches the name appearing on your scheduling permit.

Because the exam is scheduled on a "first-come, first-serve" basis, call Sylvan as soon as you receive your scheduling permit!

Once you receive your scheduling permit, you must call the Sylvan toll-free number to arrange a time to take the exam. Although requests for taking the exam may be completed more than six months before the test date, examinees will not receive their scheduling permits earlier than six months before the eligibility period. The eligibility period is the three-month period you have chosen to take the exam. Because exam scheduling is given on a "first-come, first-serve" basis, it is recommended that you telephone Sylvan as soon as you have received your permit. Be sure to consult www.usmle.org for further details.

When Should I Register for the Exam?

Although there are no deadlines for registering for Step 2, you should plan to register at least nine months ahead of your desired test date. This will ensure that you will get either your STC of choice or one within a 50-mile radius of your first choice. You should also be able to schedule a date within two weeks of your desired test date.

Because of the limited number of computers available, only a certain number of examinees will be able to take the computer exam on any given day. Of course, precisely how difficult it will be to schedule an exam will depend on the location of the STC and on the number of test takers (both U.S. students and IMGs) in the region. Some areas may have more test takers than available STCs.

Choose your three-month eligibility period carefully. If you need to reschedule outside your initial three-month period, you must submit a new application along with another $385 application fee. If space is available, you may reschedule up to five days before your test date.

Where Can I Take the Exam?

There are two general locations available for taking the new computerized exam:

- **Sylvan Testing Centers.** If you register early, you can take the exam at your preferred site or at the next-closest testing center within a 50-mile radius. Note that there is a difference between Sylvan Learning Centers (SLCs) and Sylvan Testing Centers (STCs). Sylvan Testing Centers are add-on centers to Sylvan Learning Centers. The USMLE will be offered only at SLCs with an STC.

- **Medical schools.** The NBME is authorizing a limited number of medical schools to serve as non-Sylvan testing centers. This means that some medical schools will choose to dedicate some of their own computer resources for the administration of the computer exam. Owing to costs and limited resources, these sites will be limited and may only test their own students. Check with your student affairs office to see if your school is administering the USMLE.

Your testing location is arranged with Prometric when you call for your test date (after you receive your scheduling permit). For a list of Prometric locations nearest you, contact www.prometric.com.

How Long Will I Have to Wait Before I Get My Scores?

The USMLE reports scores three to four weeks after the examinee's test date. During peak times, score reports may take up to six weeks. Official information concerning the time required for score reporting is posted on the USMLE website: www.usmle.org.

What Did Other Students Like/Dislike About the CBT Format?

Feedback from students about the CBT format has been overwhelmingly positive. Students note that the testing environment was not as stressful as imagined and add that they enjoyed the test's point-and-click simplicity. "It's nice to be able to work at your own pace and take breaks whenever you want," commented one student.

Among the complaints expressed, students were most concerned with image quality, eye strain, temperature extremes (heat/cold), and background noise at the Prometric center. Students noted that the quality of some images made it difficult to answer certain questions and that they would like to be able to enlarge images. Eye strain seemed to affect other test takers; taking a short break usually afforded relief. In addition, some students noted that the clicking of mice and keyboard chatter by other students bothered them. Earplugs (provided by the testing center) helped but didn't completely block all such sounds.

Beware of the awkward lab-values screen, background noise, variable image quality, and eye strain.

What About Time?

Time is of special interest on the CBT exam. Here's a breakdown of the exam schedule:

Tutorial	15 minutes
60-minute question blocks (50 questions per block)	8 hours
Break time (includes time for lunch)	45 minutes
Total test time	9 hours

The computer will keep track of how much time has elapsed. However, the computer will show you only how much time you have remaining in a given block. Therefore, it is up to you to determine if you are pacing yourself properly (at a rate of approximately one question per 60–72 seconds).

The computer will not warn you if you are spending more than your allotted time for a break. Thus, taking long breaks between early question blocks or for lunch may mean that you will not be able to take breaks later in the day. You should budget your time so that you can take a short break when you need it but still have time to eat.

Be especially careful not to waste too much time in between blocks (you should keep track of how much time elapses from when you finish a block of questions to when you start the next block). After you finish one question block, you'll need to click the mouse when you are ready to proceed to the next block of questions.

It should be noted that the 45-minute break time is the minimum break time for the day. You can gain extra break time (but not time for the question blocks) by skipping the tutorial or by finishing a block ahead of the allotted time.

Since digital watches are not allowed, get used to keeping track of break time with an analog watch.

For security reasons, digital watches are not allowed. This means that only analog watches are permitted. You should therefore get used to timing yourself with an analog watch so that you know exactly how much time you have left. Some analog watches come with a bevel that helps keep track of 60-minute periods. This may be useful for keeping track of break time.

If I Freak Out and Leave, What Happens to My Score?

Your scheduling permit shows a Candidate Identification Number (CIN) that you will enter onto the computer screen to start your exam. Entering the CIN is the same as breaking the seal on a test book, and you are considered to have started the exam. However, no score will be reported if you do not complete the exam. In fact, if you leave at any time from the start of the test to the last block, no score will be reported. However, the fact that you started but did not complete the exam will appear on your USMLE score transcript.

The exam ends when all blocks are completed or time has expired. As you leave the testing center, you will receive a written test-completion notice to document your completion of the exam.

In order to receive an official score, you must finish the entire exam. This means that you must start and either finish or run out of time for each block of the exam. Again, if you do not complete all the blocks, your exam will be documented as an incomplete attempt, and no score will be reported.

What Types of Questions Are Asked?

- Almost all questions are case-based. Some are two to three sentences in length, while others are two to three paragraphs long and contain laboratory data. Very often, a substantial amount of extraneous information is given, making for dense, slow reading. Also, it is common for a clinical scenario to be given followed by a question that could be answered without your having actually read the case. It is your job to determine which information is superfluous and which is pertinent to the case at hand.

- Questions often describe clinical findings instead of naming eponyms (e.g., they cite "audible hip click" instead of "positive Ortolani's sign"), so it is important to know what each sign and "keyword" actually represents.

- Subject areas vary randomly from question to question, although groups of matching questions often have a unifying theme.

Almost all questions are case-based.

Most questions have a single best answer, and there have been no negatively phrased questions on recent exams. Some questions are matching sets that call for multiple responses—the number to select is specified at the end of each question. The questions usually describe clinical situations, which require that you identify a diagnosis, the underlying pathophysiology of the disease being described, the next appropriate step in management, interpretation of laboratory findings, potential for prevention, or overall prognosis. The part of the vignette that actually asks the question—the stem—is usually at the end of the scenario. From student experience, there are a few stems that are consistently addressed throughout the exam:

- What is the most likely diagnosis? (40%)
- Which of the following is the most appropriate initial step in management? (20%)
- Which of the following is the most appropriate next step in management? (20%)
- Which of the following is the most likely cause of . . . ? (5%)
- Which of the following is the most likely pathogen . . . ? (3%)
- Which of the following would most likely prevent . . . ? (2%)
- Other (10%)

How Is the Test Scored?

Except for an initial delay, CBT scores should be mailed within two weeks. Like the Step 1 score report, it includes your pass/fail status, two numeric scores, and a performance profile by discipline and disease process (Figs. 6A and 6B). The first score is a three-digit scaled score based on a predefined proficiency standard as set by the September 1996 group of examinees. For recent examinations, the mean and standard deviation for first-time test takers from U.S. and Canadian medical schools were 210 and 23, respectively, with most scores falling between 140 and 260. In 2000, a score of 174 was required to pass. The second score scale, the two-digit score, defines 75 as the minimum passing score (equivalent to a score of 174 on the first scale). A score of 82 is equivalent to a score of 200 on the first scale.

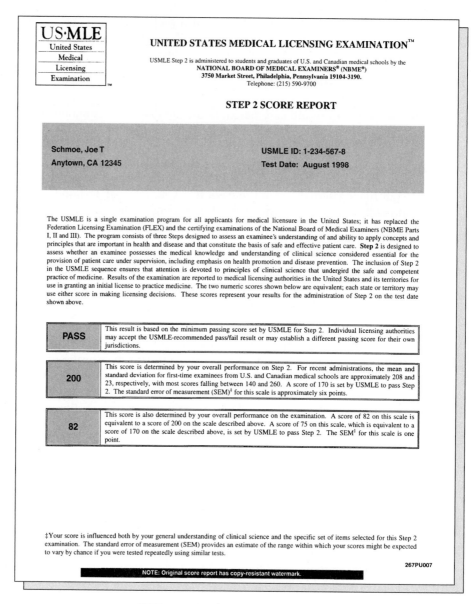

FIGURE 6A. Sample Score Report—Front Page

The overall pass rate for first-time NBME-registered examinees has ranged between 90% and 95% over the past few years. The pass rate for a specific group may be higher, reaching as high as 99% for first-time allopathic test takers. The overall pass rate for ECFMG-registered examinees rose in 1999–2000 (70%) when compared to 1998–1999 (59%) (see Table 1).

USMLE Publications

We strongly encourage students to use the free materials provided by the testing agencies and to study the following NBME publications.

Consider saving a block of questions from the sample test to take a few days before the exam.

- **USMLE 2001 Bulletin of Information.** This publication provides you with nuts-and-bolts details about the exam (included on www.usmle.org; free to all examinees).

INFORMATION PROVIDED FOR EXAMINEE USE ONLY
The Performance Profile below is provided solely for the benefit of the examinee.
These profiles are developed as assessment tools for examinees only and will not be reported or verified to any third party.

USMLE STEP 2 PERFORMANCE PROFILES

PHYSICIAN TASK PROFILE	Lower Performance	Borderline Performance	Higher Performance
Preventive Medicine & Health Maintenance			xxxxxxxxxx*
Understanding Mechanisms of Disease			xxxx*
Diagnosis			xxxxxx*
Principles of Management			xxxxxxxxxx*

NORMAL CONDITIONS & DISEASE CATEGORY PROFILE

	Lower Performance	Borderline Performance	Higher Performance
Normal Growth & Development; Principles of Care			xxxxxxxxxxxxxxxxx*
Immunologic Disorders			xxxxxxxxxxx*
Diseases of Blood & Blood Forming Organs			xxxxxxxxxxx*
Mental Disorders			xxxxxxxxxxx*
Diseases of the Nervous System & Special Senses			xxxxxxxxxxx*
Cardiovascular Disorders		xxxxxxxxxxxxxxxx	
Diseases of the Respiratory System			xxxxxxxxxxxxx*
Nutritional & Digestive Disorders			xxxxxxxxxxx*
Gynecologic Disorders			xxxxxxxxxxxx*
Renal, Urinary & Male Reproductive Systems			xxxxxxxxxxx*
Disorders of Pregnancy, Childbirth & Puerperium		xxxxxxxxxxxxxxxxxxxxx	
Musculoskeletal, Skin & Connective Tissue Diseases			xxxxxxxxx*
Endocrine & Metabolic Disorders			xxxxxxxxxxxxx*

DISCIPLINE PROFILE

	Lower Performance	Borderline Performance	Higher Performance
Medicine			xxx*
Obstetrics & Gynecology			xxxxxxxxxxx*
Pediatrics			xxxxxxxx*
Psychiatry			xxxxxxxxxxx*
Surgery			xx*

The above Performance Profile is provided to aid in self-assessment. The shaded area defines a borderline level of performance for each content area; borderline performance is comparable to a HIGH FAIL / LOW PASS on the total test.

Performance bands indicate areas of relative strength and weakness. Some performance bands are wider than others. The width of a performance band reflects the precision of measurement: narrower bands indicate greater precision. An asterisk indicates that your performance band extends beyond the displayed portion of the scale. Small differences in the location of bands should not be over interpreted. If two bands overlap, the performance in the associated areas should not be interpreted as significantly different.

This profile should not be compared to those from other Step 2 administrations.

Additional information concerning the topics covered in each content area can be found in the *USMLE Step 2 General Instructions, Content Description, and Sample Items.*

007PU267

FIGURE 6B. Sample Score Report—Back Page

- **Step 2 Computer-Based Content and Sample Test Questions.** This is a hard copy of test questions and test content also found on the CD-ROM.
- **USMLE website (http://www.usmle.org).** In addition to allowing you to become familiar with the CBT format, the sample items provide the only questions direct from the test makers. Student feedback varies as to the similarity of these questions to those on the actual exam. Consider taking one block of questions, allowing yourself one minute per question to approximate the pacing of the "real thing."

Adaptive Testing: The Next Generation

Eventually, the NBME may implement computer-adaptive sequential testing (CAST) in order to customize "the difficulty of the [USMLE] to the proficiency of each examinee across various stages of the examination." Essentially, this means that an "adaptive" exam will eventually use your perfor-

TABLE 1. Passing Rates for 1999–2000 USMLE Step 2

	1999–2000	
	No. Tested	Passing (%)
NBME-registered Allopathic		
First-time takers	16,279	98%
Repeaters	1,127	66%
NBME total	**17,406**	93%
Osteopathic		
First-time takers	175	92%
Repeaters	8	40%
Osteopathic total	**183**	90%
ECFMG*-registered Examinees		
First-time takers	6,027	70%
Repeaters	3,172	41%
ECFMG total	**9,199**	60%
Total U.S./Canadian	**17,589**	93%

*Educational Commission for Foreign Medical Graduates.
Adapted from http://www.nbme.org/annualreport/2000.

mance on a block of questions to determine the difficulty of the block that follows. This will allow the exam to accurately assess your proficiency using fewer questions. Unlike most standardized exams you've seen, this means that all questions will not be created equal (i.e., they will not be worth the same).

When the NBME field-tested a CAST version of Step 1, its exam algorithm (Fig. 7) selected an easy, moderate, or difficult block of 60 new items based on the examinee's answers to the previous block. Highly proficient examinees tended to get progressively harder test materials, whereas less proficient examinees tended to get progressively easier test materials.

CAST implementation has been delayed indefinitely.

Under CAST, the difficulty of the items is directly factored into each examinee's final score. The NBME claims that "this process of customizing the test difficulty to each examinee's proficiency increases the overall accuracy of the scores and any related pass/fail decisions." The NBME adds, however, that although some examinees may receive more difficult blocks of questions, " . . . the score you achieve will not be affected by the difficulty of the question blocks selected for you." The NBME states that "every examinee will be tested on equivalent content."

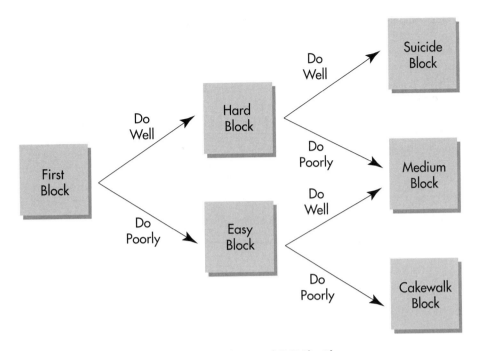

FIGURE 7. Simplified Schematic of CAST Algorithm

When will the new computerized USMLE be an "adaptive" exam? No one knows. After an initial CBT trial period, the NBME plans to change the exam to a CAST format, but implementation has been delayed indefinitely.

DEFINING YOUR GOAL

Arguably the first and most important thing to do in your Step 2 preparation is to define how well you want to do on the USMLE Step 2 exam. Your goals will ultimately determine the extent of preparation that will be necessary. The amount of time spent in preparation for this exam varies widely among medical students, ranging anywhere from several months to two days (as in the jokingly stated adage "two weeks for Step 1, two days for Step 2, and a number-2 pencil for Step 3") to no preparation at all. Possible goals include:

- **"Simply passing."** This goal may be sufficient for the majority of U.S. medical students. This may apply to you if you are entering a less competitive specialty.

- **Beating the mean.** Beating the mean (207 for recent exam administrations) signifies an ability to integrate your clinical and factual knowledge to an extent that is superior to that of your peers. Others redefine this goal as achieving a score one standard deviation above the mean (230). This is also the so-called "magic number" that many students have aimed for on the USMLE Step 1, as it supposedly represents the score that one must receive in order to be strongly considered by the more competitive residency programs (Fig. 8). Highly competitive residency programs may use your Step 1 and Step 2 (if available) scores as a screening tool or as selection criteria (Fig. 9). IMGs should aim to beat the mean, as USMLE scores are likely to be a selection factor even for less competitive U.S. residency programs. For additional discussion of

Less Competitive	More Competitive	Most Competitive
Pediatrics	Emergency Medicine	Dermatology
Family Practice	OB/GYN	ENT
Internal Medicine	Radiology	Orthopedics
Anesthesiology	General Surgery	Ophthalmology
Psychiatry		

FIGURE 8. Competitive Specialties

the residency application process and the USMLE Step 2, please refer to *First Aid for the Match* (ISBN 0838526071).

■ **Acing the exam.** Perhaps you are one of those individuals for whom nothing less than the best will do—and for whom excelling on standardized exams is a source of pride and satisfaction. For you, the USMLE Step 2 will represent the culmination of several years of exams as well as a final opportunity as a medical student to excel at what you do best. An exceptional score on the USMLE Step 2 might also represent a way to "make up" for a less-than-satisfactory score on Step 1, especially if taken in the fall, so that it can be seen by residency programs and used to strengthen your application.

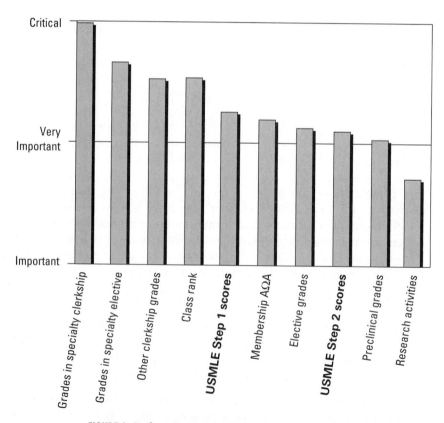

FIGURE 9. Academic Factors Important to Residency Directors

- **Evaluating your clinical knowledge.** This is a commendable goal that can be used as an addendum to any of the other goals mentioned in this section. In many ways, this should be the ultimate rationale for taking the exam, since it is technically the reason the exam was designed in the first place. Specifically, the case-based nature of the USMLE Step 2 differs significantly from the more fact-based Step 1 exam in that it more thoroughly examines your ability to recognize classic clinical presentations, deal with acute emergent situations, and go through the step-by-step thought processes involved in the treatment of particular diseases. In short, this exam will allow you to assess your ability to apply your vast collection of medical facts to the situations you are likely to encounter during your residency.

- **Preparing for internship.** Making the transition to internship can be challenging. Studying for the USMLE Step 2 is an excellent way to review and consolidate all of the information that has slowly but surely been fading from memory during your third year. Use the Step 2 preparation as an opportunity to gear up for internship, especially if you are taking the exam in the spring.

Step 2 is an opportunity to consolidate your clinical knowledge and prepare for internship.

When to Take the Exam

With CBT, you now have a wide variety of options regarding when to take Step 2. Here are a few factors to consider:

- The nature of your objectives as defined above.

- The specialty in which you are applying. Some competitive residency programs may request your Step 2 scores. Ask your adviser or the residency director at your school if this applies to you. If you already have a strong application, then taking Step 2 in the fall could potentially hurt you if you do poorly. However, if you need to shore up your application in a strong field, consider taking the exam (and truly preparing for it) in the fall.

- At many medical schools, passing the USMLE Step 2 is a prerequisite for graduation. This would be another reason to take the exam in the fall or winter. Should you fail, the CBT will allow you to retake the exam 60 days after your last exam date.

- **Proximity to clerkships.** Many students feel that the core clerkship material is fresher in their minds early in the fourth year, making a good argument for taking Step 2 earlier in the fall. Many students organize their rotation schedules such that they have numerous electives and a relatively "light" clinical load during their fourth year. Such students often discover that much of the clinical information they learned on their core rotations has faded. On the other hand, preparation for the USMLE Step 2 is also an excellent tool for review before internship.

- **The extent to which you seek a stress-free fourth year.** If you think it's very likely that you'll pass, you may want to take the exam later so that you don't have to worry about the possibility that your score will affect your match possibilities. On the other hand, taking the USMLE Step 2 exam early gets it out of the way, allowing for a stress-free fourth year without the specter of an exam looming over you.

- **The nature of your schedule.** Some students like to plan the test around a clerkship or vacation month in which they have some free time—or at least not when they are on their toughest fourth-year clerkship. It would be counterproductive to take the exam at the same time that you have scheduled a subinternship in your planned specialty, since you will want to concentrate on performing well on the rotation for a good evaluation and, possibly, a letter of recommendation.

STUDY RESOURCES

Quality and Cost Considerations

Although there is an ever-increasing number of USMLE Step 2 review books and software on the market, the quality of the material is highly variable (see Section III, Database of Review Resources). Some common problems are as follows:

- Certain review books are too detailed to be reviewed in a reasonable amount of time or cover subtopics not emphasized on the exam (e.g., a 400-page anesthesiology book).

- Many sample question books were originally written years ago and have not been updated to reflect trends on the revised USMLE Step 2.

- Many sample question books use poorly written questions or contain factual errors in the explanations.

- Explanations for sample questions range from nonexistent to overly detailed.

- Software for boards review is of highly variable quality, may be difficult to install, and may be fraught with bugs.

Clinical Review Books

If a given review book is not working for you, stop using it no matter how highly rated it may be.

Most review books are the products of considerable effort by experienced educators. There are many such books, so you must choose which ones to buy on the basis of their relative merits. Although recommendations from other medical students are useful, many students simply recommend whatever books they used without having compared them to other books on the same subject. In a similar fashion, some students blindly advocate one publisher's series without considering the broad range of quality encountered within most series. Weigh different opinions against each other, read the reviews and ratings in Section III of this guide, and examine the books closely in the bookstore. You are investing not only money but also your limited study time. Do not worry about finding the "perfect" book, as many subjects simply do not have one. The best review book for you reflects the way you like to learn.

There are two types of review books: books that are stand-alone titles and books that are part of a series. Books in a series generally have the same style, and you must decide if that style is helpful for you. However, a given style is not optimal for every subject.

Find out which books are up to date. Some new editions represent major improvements, whereas others contain only cursory changes. You should take into consideration how a book reflects the format of the USMLE Step 2. Some may not have been updated adequately to reflect the changing question style and format of the current USMLE Step 2.

Texts and Notes

Unless you are planning an all-out offensive against Step 2 (and actually have the time), avoid standard texts in preparing for it. Many textbooks are too detailed for high-yield boards review. Even popular handbooks like the *Washington Manual* can be a chore to read, as they were designed for directed reading and reference rather than for cover-to-cover perusal. When using texts or notes, engage in active learning by making tables, diagrams, new mnemonics, and conceptual associations whenever possible. If you already have your own mnemonics, then do not bother trying to memorize those of someone else. Supplement incomplete or unclear material with reference to other appropriate textbooks. Keep a good medical dictionary on hand to sort out definitions.

Commercial Courses

Commercial preparation courses can be helpful for some students, but they are expensive and require significant time commitment. They are often effective in organizing study material for students who feel overwhelmed by the sheer volume of material involved in preparing for Step 2. Note, however, that multiweek courses may be quite intense and may thus leave limited time for independent study. Note also that some commercial courses are designed for first-time test takers while others focus on students who are repeating the examination. Still other courses focus on IMGs, who must take all three Steps in a limited amount of time.

Practice Tests

Taking practice tests provides valuable information about strengths and weaknesses in your fund of knowledge and test-taking skills. Some students use practice examinations simply as a means of breaking up the monotony of studying and adding variety to their study schedule. Other students study almost entirely from practice tests. Students report that many practice tests have questions that are, on average, shorter and less clinically oriented than the current USMLE Step 2. Step 2 questions demand fast reading skills and application of clinical facts in a problem-solving format. Approach sample examinations critically, and do not waste time with low-quality questions until you have exhausted better sources.

Use practice tests to identify concepts and areas of weakness, not just facts that you missed.

After taking a practice test, try to identify concepts and areas of weakness, not just the facts that you missed. Use the experience to motivate your study and prioritize what areas need the most work.

Use quality practice examinations to improve your test-taking skills. This is especially important to help familiarize yourself with the style of the USMLE Step 2. Analyze your ability to pace yourself so that you have enough time to complete each block comfortably. Practice examinations are also a good means of training yourself to concentrate for long periods of time under appropriate time pressure. Analyze the pattern of your responses to questions to determine if you have made systematic errors in answering questions. Common mistakes are reading too much into the question, second-guessing your initial impression, and misinterpreting the question.

By now, you are probably familiar with USMLE exams and most likely have worked out some of your own strategies. However, the clinical vignette style of USMLE Step 2 may be unfamiliar to you. Using student experience from recent Step 2 exams, here are a few strategies that may be helpful.

Planning

If you are unfortunate enough to be on a difficult rotation at the time of the USMLE Step 2, you will need to plan ahead and start studying earlier. A demanding call schedule may leave you chronically tired. Ask your resident early if you can take a couple of call nights off in order to catch up on some rest just before the exam. Regardless of what rotation you are on, make sure to give your resident and the attending advance warning of exam dates. This will allow them to make adjustments in the call schedule for you, as well as to arrange for coverage of your patients if you are on a subinternship.

Things to Bring with You to the Exam

Don't forget your scheduling permit and a photo ID that includes your signature. You will **not** be admitted to the exam if you fail to bring your permit, and Sylvan will charge a rescheduling fee. A watch is useful to help you pace yourself, although digital timers are not allowed. It may also be nice to have some snacks on hand for a little "sugar rush." They will need to be stored in a locker until you take a break. In addition, it might be a good idea to bring your lunch, because break time is limited. Also consider bringing fluids, but not too much; you don't want to waste valuable time running to the bathroom. Should you need earplugs, they will be provided at the STC. Finally, consider layering clothing to deal with temperature variations at the testing center.

Pacing

Pacing is key with lengthy clinical vignettes.

You have 60 minutes per block in which to complete 50 questions. The test is quite fast-paced. Many scenarios are lengthy and time-consuming to read. Many students report feeling pressed for time before they find a rhythm, so keep close track of time using the clock in the corner of the screen and possibly your analog watch. With CBT, examinees report that the most efficient use of time is to answer questions in order. You may, however, return to any problematic question within the same block.

Difficult Questions

Do not waste valuable time on difficult or impossible questions.

The cruel reality of the USMLE Step 2 exam is that no matter how much you study, there will still be questions you won't be able to answer. Plan for these. If you recognize that a question is not solvable in a reasonable period of time, do not waste time on it. Move on after making an educated guess; you will not be penalized for wrong answers. Remember, each USMLE exam contains 10–20% experimental questions that will not count toward your score. Don't let tough questions throw you.

Images

Many of the questions can be answered without the picture.

Don't be afraid of questions that include imaging, which may arise with topics such as radiology, dermatology, and ophthalmology. Most questions will be basic and will include common diagnoses. A quick review, however, can be helpful. Use the high-yield glossy section of this book and consider using short glossy segments of textbooks such as the one found in Harrison's. Try reading the clinical scenario, question, and answers prior to studying the x-ray or picture. If all else fails, pick the most common diagnosis. It is helpful to know the normal radiographic appearance of hands, feet, chest, and pelvis in order to recognize gross abnormalities that may be given on the exam.

Guessing

There is **no penalty** for wrong answers. Thus, no test block should be left with unanswered questions. A hunch is better than a random guess. We suggest selecting an answer you recognize over one that is totally unfamiliar. If you have studied a subject and do not recognize a particular option, then it is more likely a distractor than a correct answer.

Finding the "Meat" of the Question

Many of the clinical vignettes in Step 2 are painfully long and contain a significant amount of information. If you think you may be pressed for time, consider reading the stem of the question first and skimming the answers prior to reading the vignette. Sometimes, after reading the stem and answers, you might be able to seek out key pieces of information in the vignette to help you answer the question. A word of caution, however: Do not overlook details in tricky or tough questions. If you have time, it might indeed be worthwhile to read each vignette carefully to avoid making errors. Try the "meat of the question" technique on the sample items. It may not be useful for everyone.

Changing Your Answer

The conventional wisdom regarding "reconsidering" answers is not to change answers that you have already marked unless there is a convincing and logical reason to do so. In other words, when in doubt, go with your first hunch.

Other Tidbits

Other helpful hints include the following:

- Note the age and race of the patient in each clinical scenario. In most questions, ethnicity is not given. When it is given, the ethnicity of the patient is often relevant. For example, African-American heritage contributes to the epidemiology, pathophysiology, prognosis, outcome, and even treatment of some diseases. Know these well (see high-yield facts), especially for more common diagnoses.

- Some of the questions that many students felt were the most difficult involved choosing the "most important initial step" or the "next step in management" of a disease. It can be difficult to prioritize treatment options, so pay close attention to management strategies as you study. Students who took the Step 2 exam noted that treatment and management issues are often more important than differentials.

- Be able to recognize key factors that distinguish major diagnoses.

- Consider completing an emergency medicine rotation prior to taking Step 2. Questions about acute patient management (e.g., trauma) in an emergency setting are common.

National Board of Medical Examiners (NBME)
Department of Licensing Examination Services
3750 Market Street
Philadelphia, PA 19104-3190
(215) 590-9700
http://www.nbme.org

Educational Commission for Foreign Medical Graduates (ECFMG)
3624 Market Street, Fourth Floor
Philadelphia, PA 19104-2685
(215) 386-5900 or (202) 293-9320
Fax: (215) 386-9196
http://www.ecfmg.org

Federation of State Medical Boards (FSMB)
400 Fuller Wiser Road, Suite 300
Euless, TX 76039-3855
(817) 571-2949
Fax: (817) 868-4099
http://www.fsmb.org

USMLE Secretariat
3750 Market Street
Philadelphia, PA 19104-3190
(215) 590-9600
http://www.usmle.org

Many figures in this chapter are reproduced, with permission, from the National Board of Medical Examiners.

First Aid for the International Medical Graduate

International Medical Graduate (IMG) is the term now used to describe any student or graduate of a non-U.S. or non-Canadian medical school, regardless of whether he or she is a U.S. citizen. The old term "Foreign Medical Graduate" (FMG) was replaced because it was misleading when applied to U.S. citizens attending medical schools outside the United States.

THE IMG'S STEPS TO LICENSURE IN THE UNITED STATES

If you are an IMG, you must go through the following steps (not necessarily in this order) to become licensed to practice in the United States. You must complete these steps even if you are already a practicing physician and have completed a residency program in your own country:

- Complete the basic sciences program of your medical school (equivalent to the first two years of U.S. medical school).
- Take the USMLE Step 1. You can do this while still in school or after graduating, but in either case your medical school must certify that you completed the basic sciences part of your school's curriculum before taking the USMLE Step 1.
- Complete the clinical clerkship program of your medical school (equivalent to the third and fourth years of U.S. medical school).
- Take the USMLE Step 2. If you are still in medical school, your school must certify that you are within one year of graduating for you to be allowed to take Step 2.
- Take the Test of English as a Foreign Language (TOEFL) recognized by the Educational Commission for Foreign Medical Graduates (ECFMG).
- Graduate with your medical degree.
- Obtain an ECFMG certificate; to do this, candidates must accomplish the following:
  —pass Step 1 and Step 2
  —pass TOEFL or the ECFMG English Test
  —pass the Clinical Skills Assessment (CSA) if the above three requirements were not met as of June 30, 1998
  —have medical credentials verified by the ECFMG
- Then, to receive the ECFMG certificate, you send the ECFMG a copy of your degree, which they will verify with your medical school. You may have to wait eight weeks or more for the certificate. You must have the certificate if you wish to obtain a position in an accredited residency program; some programs do not allow you to apply unless you already have this certificate.
- Apply for residency positions in your field of interest, either directly or through the National Residency Matching Program ("the Match"). To be entered into the Match, you need to have passed all the examinations necessary for ECFMG certification (i.e., Step 1, Step 2, CSA, and the English test) by a certain deadline. If you do not pass these exams by the deadline, you will be withdrawn from the Match.
- Obtain a visa that will allow you to enter and work in the United States if you are not already a U.S. citizen or green-card holder (permanent resident).
- If required for IMGs by the state in which your residency is located, obtain an educational/training/limited medical license. Your residency program may assist you with this application. Note that medical licensing is the prerogative of each individual state, not of the federal government, and that states vary with respect to their laws about licensing (although all 50 states recognize the USMLE).

- Take USMLE Step 3 during your residency, and then obtain a full medical license. Note that as an IMG you will not be able to take Step 3 and obtain an independent license until you have completed one, two, or three years of residency, depending on which state you live in (except in the 11 states that allow IMGs to take Step 3 at the beginning of residency). However, if you live in a state that requires two or three years of residency as a prerequisite to taking Step 3, you can take Step 3 and then obtain a license in another state. Once you have a license in any state, you are permitted to practice in federal institutions such as VA hospitals and Indian Health Service facilities in any state. This can open the door to "moonlighting" opportunities. For details on individual state rules, write to the licensing board in the state in question or contact the Federation of State Medical Boards (FSMB; see below).
- Complete your residency and then take the appropriate specialty board exams in order to become board certified (e.g., in internal medicine or surgery). If you already have a specialty certification in your home country (e.g., in surgery or cardiology), some specialty boards may grant you six months' or one year's credit toward your total residency time.
- Currently, many residency programs are accepting applications through ERAS (Electronic Residency Application Service). For more information, see *First Aid for the Match* or contact:
  ECFMG ERAS program
  P.O. Box 13467
  Philadelphia, PA 19101-3467
  (215) 386-5900
  http://www.ecfmg.org/erasinfo.htm

Timing of the USMLE

For an IMG, the timing of a complete application is critical. It is extremely important that you send in your application early if you are to garner the maximum number of interview calls. A rough guide would be to complete all exam requirements by June of the year in which you wish to apply. This would translate into sending both your score sheets and your ECFMG certificate, which is imperative for an interview call, by this date.

Many IMGs also benefit from taking the USMLE Step 1 before Step 2 because a sizable portion of the Step 2 exam tests fundamental concepts of basic sciences. It should be added, however, that it is up to each candidate to arrive at his or her own time frame and to avoid procrastinating about taking these crucial tests.

USMLE STEP 1 AND THE IMG

The USMLE Step 1 is often the first—and, for most IMGs, the most challenging—hurdle to overcome. The USMLE is a standardized licensing system that gives IMGs a level playing field; it is the same exam series taken by U.S. graduates, even though it is administered by the ECFMG rather than by the National Board of Medical Examiners (NBME). This means that pass marks for IMGs for both Step 1 and Step 2 are determined by a statistical process that is based on the scores of U.S. medical students in 1991. In general, to pass Step 1, you will probably have to score higher than the bottom 8–10% of U.S. and Canadian graduates. In 1998, however, only 62% of ECFMG candidates passed

Developing good test-taking strategy is especially critical for the IMG.

Step 1 on their first attempt, compared with 94% of U.S. and Canadian medical students and graduates.

Of note, 1994–1995 data showed that USFMGs (U.S. citizens attending non-U.S. medical schools) performed 0.4 SD lower than IMGs (non-U.S. citizens attending non-U.S. medical schools). Although their overall scores were lower, USFMGs performed better than IMGs on behavioral sciences.

A good Step 1 score is key to a strong IMG application.

In general, students from non-U.S. medical schools perform worst in behavioral science and biochemistry (1.9 and 1.5 SDs below U.S. students) and comparatively better in gross anatomy and pathology (0.7 and 0.9 SD below U.S. students). Although they are derived from 1994–1995, these data may help you focus your studying efforts.

As an IMG, you must to do your best on Step 1. Few if any students feel totally prepared to take Step 1, but IMGs in particular require serious study and preparation to reach their full potential on this exam. A poor score on Step 1 is a distinct disadvantage when applying for most residencies. Remember that if you pass Step 1, you cannot retake it to try to improve your score. Your goal should thus be to beat the mean, because you can then assert confidently that you have done better than average for U.S. students. Good Step 1 scores will lend credibility to your residency application.

Do commercial review courses help improve your scores? Reports vary, and such courses can be expensive. Many IMGs decide to try the USMLE on their own first and then consider a review course only if they fail. Just keep in mind that many states require that you pass the USMLE within three attempts. (For more information on review courses, see Section III.)

USMLE STEP 2 AND THE IMG

There is a big difference between textbook learning of a language and actually being immersed in the culture that goes with it.

In the past, the Step 2 examination had a reputation for being much easier than Step 1, but this is not necessarily the case for IMGs or U.S. medical students. In August 1999–2000, 70% of ECFMG candidates passed Step 2 on the first attempt, compared with 95% of U.S. and Canadian candidates. Also note that because this is a clinical sciences exam, cultural and geographic considerations play a greater role than is the case with Step 1. For example, if your medical education gave you a lot of exposure to malaria, brucellosis, and malnutrition but little to alcohol withdrawal, child abuse, and cholesterol screening, you must do some work to familiarize yourself with topics that are more heavily emphasized in U.S. medicine. You must also have a basic understanding of the legal and social aspects of U.S. medicine, because you will be asked questions about communicating with and advising patients.

The English Language Test

Native English-speaking IMGs are also required to take the English-language test.

If you did not pass the ECFMG English test by March 3, 1999, you will be required to pass the Test of English as a Foreign Language (TOEFL) to fulfill the English-language proficiency requirement for ECFMG certification. The administration date of a submitted TOEFL must be after March 3, 1999, to meet the requirement. A passing performance on the ECFMG English test taken prior to March 3, 1999, however, will continue to be accepted. For more information, check online at http://www.ecfmg.org/2001ib/ibelpt.html or www.toefl.org.

Clinical Skills Assessment

Starting in June 1998, the ECFMG introduced the Clinical Skills Assessment (CSA), an interactive test with role-playing "patients," in an effort to level the disparities that existed among the more than 1400 medical schools worldwide in both curricula and educational standards. The goal of the CSA is to ensure that IMGs can gather and interpret histories, perform physical examinations, and communicate in the English language at a level comparable to that of U.S. graduates.

The CSA simulates clinical encounters that are common in clinics, doctors' offices, and emergency departments. The test is standardized, which means that "standardized patients" (SPs)—i.e., laypeople who have been extensively trained to simulate various clinical problems—give the same responses to all candidates participating in the assessment. For quality assurance purposes, a videotape records all clinical encounters. Eleven cases are presented to the IMG that are mixed in terms of age, sex, ethnicity, organ system, and discipline. The five main areas emphasized are:

- Eye, ear, nose, throat, and musculoskeletal system
- General symptoms
- Cardiopulmonary system
- GI and GU systems
- Neuropsychiatry

Candidates are scored on only 10 of the 11 patient encounters. The non-scored encounter is added for research purposes, with results applied to future administration of the CSA.

Test Administration. Before entering a room to interact with an SP, you are given an opportunity to review preliminary information. This information, which is posted on the door of each room, includes the following:

- Patient characteristics (name, age, sex)
- Chief complaint and vitals (temperature, respiratory rate, pulse, BP)

After entering the room, you are given 15 minutes (with a warning bell sounded at 10 minutes) to perform the clinical encounter, which should include introducing yourself, obtaining an appropriate history, performing a focused clinical exam, formulating a differential diagnosis, and planning a diagnostic workup. You are expected to answer any questions the SP might ask as well as to discuss the diagnoses being considered and to advise the SP about his or her follow-up plans. After you leave the room, you have 10 minutes to write a patient note (PN).

"Do's and Don'ts." Ground rules for the clinical encounter are:

- Candidates are not permitted to perform rectal, pelvic/genital, or female breast exams. If a candidate feels that such examinations are warranted, he or she may suggest that they be conducted as part of the diagnostic workup.
- Candidates are not allowed to reenter a room once they have left it. It is therefore recommended that they obtain all the information they need before ending the clinical encounter.
- Time is not on the candidate's side, so it is advisable to "home in" on relevant problems and to conduct a focused clinical exam. For example, if a 40-year-old diabetic and smoker presents with chest pain, candidates should rule out problems of cardiopulmonary, gastrointestinal, and

musculoskeletal origin to narrow the examination down to these systems. A CNS exam should therefore be the last one on the candidate's list in this particular example.

Scoring of the CSA. Your score will be based on the clinical encounter as a whole and on your overall communications skills.

- **Integrated Clinical Encounter (ICE) score.** The skills you demonstrate in the clinical encounter will be evaluated as follows:
    1. Although SPs will not evaluate your performance, they will document your ability to gather data pertinent to the clinical encounter. Specifically, SPs will note on checklists whether you successfully obtained relevant information or correctly performed the physical exam. Your final data gathering (DG) score represents an average of your performance with all ten SPs.
    2. Health care professionals will score your PN according to predefined criteria, with your final PN score representing the average of your individual PN scores over all ten clinical encounters. Your ICE score will then represent the sum of your DG and PN scores.

    $$ICE = DG + PN$$

- **Communication (COM) score.** In addition to assessing your data-gathering skills, SPs will evaluate your interpersonal skills (IPS) and your proficiency in spoken English. Your IPS will be assessed on the following four criteria: rapport, interviewing skills, personal manner, and counseling. Your overall COM score is the sum of your averaged IPS scores and your spoken English proficiency rating.

The grade you receive on the CSA is either a "pass" or a "fail." The "pass" grade indicates you have met the standards set by experts for the ICE and COM. CSA scores, like those of all ECFMG tests, are mailed in six to eight weeks.

Applying for CSA. Applicants seeking to take the CSA must complete the four-part application form (Form 706—pink form) in full and mail to the ECFMG along with a $1200 registration fee. By calling (215) 386-5900 (Monday through Friday, 8 a.m. to 5:30 p.m. EST), you can have an operator help you schedule your test date. It is advisable to have several preferred dates in mind (all within one year of your notification of registration). The operator will formally schedule you on a mutually acceptable day, and your admissions permit will then be mailed to you. Alternatively, you can schedule your CSA date through the Internet at www.ecfmg.org. There is no application deadline, since the CSA is administered throughout the year (except on major U.S. holidays).

After the ECFMG receives your fee and application form and determines that you are eligible to take the CSA, you must schedule your test date within four months and take the CSA within one year of the date indicated on your notification of registration.

Test Site Location. The CSA is administered at the following address:

ECFMG
3624 Market Street
CSA Center, 3rd Floor
Philadelphia, PA 19104-2685

If you are living outside the United States, you will need to apply for a visa that will allow you lawful entry into the United States in order to take the CSA. A B2 visa may be issued by a consulate. Documents that are recommended to facilitate this process include:

- The CSA admission permit and letter from ECFMG (explains why the applicant must enter the United States)
- Your medical diploma
- Transcripts from your medical school
- Your USMLE score sheets
- A sponsor letter or affidavit of support stating that you (if you are sponsoring yourself) or your sponsor will bear the expense of your trip and that you have sufficient funds to meet that expense
- An alien status affidavit

Preparing for the CSA. You can prepare for the CSA by addressing common outpatient clinical issues. To improve doctor–patient communication skills, you can try "acting out" dialog with friends or relatives. Since time will be a major factor, do not forget to time the encounter as if it were a real test by giving yourself 15 minutes for data gathering and 10 minutes for the patient note. The following volumes may also be of use to you in your preparation for the CSA:

- *Manual of Family Practice*, Robert Taylor (Lippincott Williams & Wilkins)
- *Family Practice Review: Problem-Oriented Approach*, R. Swanson (Mosby)

RESIDENCIES AND THE IMG

It is becoming harder for IMGs to obtain residencies in the United States given the rising concerns about an oversupply of physicians in the United States. Official bodies such as the Council on Graduate Medical Education (COGME) have recommended that the total number of residency slots be reduced from the current 144% of the number of U.S. graduates to 110%. Furthermore, changes introduced in the 1996 immigration law are likely to make it much harder for noncitizens or legal residents of the United States to remain in the country after completing a residency.

In the residency Match, U.S.-citizen IMG applications rose from 1700 in 1998 to 1821 in 1999 and 2169 in 2000, and the percentage of such IMGs accepted was 46%, 47%, and 51%, an increase from 43.5% in 1997 (Fig. 10). For non-U.S.-citizen IMGs, applications rose from 7957 in 1998 to 7977 in 1999 and fell to 6287 in 2000, while the percentage accepted fell to 31% and 32%, from 34.5% in 1997, and rose slightly to 38% in 2000. These percentages may drop

FIGURE 10. IMGs in the Match			
IMG Applicants	**1998**	**1999**	**2000**
U.S. IMG citizens	1700	1821	2169
% U.S. IMGs accepted	46%	47%	51%
Non-U.S. citizens	7957	7977	6287
% non-U.S. citizens accepted	31%	32%	38%

in the future, however, especially as some large hospitals that traditionally hire many IMGs (such as those in New York) cut back on their residency slots.

VISA OPTIONS FOR THE IMG

As an IMG, you need a visa to work or train in the United States unless you are a U.S. citizen or a permanent resident (i.e, hold a green card). Two types of visas enable you to accept a residency appointment in the United States: J1 and H1B. Most sponsoring residency programs (SRPs) prefer a J1 visa. Above all, this is because SRPs are authorized by the U.S. Immigration and Naturalization Service (INS) to issue a Form IAP 66 directly to an IMG, whereas they have to go through considerable paperwork and an application to the Immigration and Labor Department to apply to the INS for an H1B visa on behalf of an IMG.

The J1 Visa. Also known as the Exchange Visitor Program, the J1 visa was introduced to give IMGs in diverse specialties the chance to use their training experience in the United States to improve conditions in their home countries. As mentioned above, the INS authorizes most SRPs to issue Form IAP 66 in the same manner that I20's are issued to regular international students in the United States.

To enable an SRP to issue an IAP 66, you must obtain a certificate from the ECFMG indicating that you are eligible to participate in a residency program in the United States. First, however, you must ask the Ministry of Health in your country to issue a statement indicating that your country needs physicians with the skills you propose to acquire by joining a U.S. residency program. This statement, which must bear the seal of your country's government and must be signed by a duly designated government official, is intended to satisfy the U.S. Secretary of Health and Human Services that there is such a need. The Health Ministry in your country should send this statement to the ECFMG (or they may allow you to mail it to the ECFMG).

How can you find out if the government of your country will issue such a statement? In many countries, the Ministry of Health maintains a list of medical specialties in which there is a need for further training abroad. You can also consult seniors in your medical school. A word of caution: If you are applying for a residency in internal medicine and internists are not in short supply in your country, it may help to indicate an intention to pursue a subspecialty after completing your residency training.

The text of your statement of need should read as follows:

Name of applicant for visa: _____. There currently exists in _____ (your country) a need for qualified medical practitioners in the specialty of _____. (Name of applicant for visa) has filed a written assurance with the government of this country that he/she will return to _____ (your country) upon completion of training in the United States and intends to enter the practice of medicine in the specialty for which training is being sought.

Stamp (or seal and signature) of issuing official of named country.
Dated _____

To facilitate the issuing of such a statement by the Ministry of Health in your country, you should submit a certified copy of the agreement or contract from your SRP in the United States. The agreement or contract must be signed by you and the residency program official responsible for the training.

Armed with Form IAP 66, you should go to the U.S. consulate nearest to the residential address indicated in your passport. As for other nonimmigrant visas, you must show that you have a genuine nonimmigrant intent to return to your home country. You must also show that all your expenses will be paid.

When you enter the United States, bring your Form IAP 66 along with your visa. You are usually admitted to the United States for the length of the J1 program, designated as "D/S," or duration of status. The duration of your program is indicated on the IAP 66.

Duration of Participation. The duration of a resident's participation in a program of graduate medical education or training is limited to the time normally required to complete such a program. If you would like to get an idea of the typical training time for the various medical subspecialties, you may consult the *Directory of Medical Specialties*, published by Marquis Who's Who for the American Board of Medical Specialties. The authority charged with determining the duration of time required by an individual IMG is the United States Information Agency (USIA). This may change, however, because the USIA is likely to be merged into the State Department.

The maximum amount of time for participation in a training program is ordinarily limited to seven years unless the IMG has demonstrated to the satisfaction of the USIA director that his or her home country has an exceptional need for the specialty in which he or she will receive further training. The USIA director may grant an extension of stay in the event that an IMG needs to repeat a year of clinical medical training or needs time for training or education to enable him or her to take an exam required for board certification.

Requirements After Entry into the United States. Each year, all IMGs participating in a residency program on a J1 visa must furnish the Attorney General of the United States with an affidavit (Form I-644) attesting that they are in good standing in the program of graduate medical education or training in which they are participating and that they will return to their home countries upon completion of the education or training for which they came to the United States.

Restrictions Under the J1 Visa. Not later than two years after the date of entry into the United States, an IMG participating in a residency program on a J1 visa is allowed one opportunity to change his or her designated program of graduate medical education or training if his or her director approves that change.

The J1 visa includes a condition called the "two-year foreign residence requirement." The relevant section of the Immigration and Nationality Act states:

> "Any exchange visitor physician coming to the United States on or after January 10, 1977, for the purpose of receiving graduate medical education or training is automatically subject to the two-year home-country physical presence requirement of section 212(e) of the Immigration and Nationality Act, as amended. Such physicians

are not eligible to be considered for section 212(e) waivers on the basis of 'No Objection' statements issued by their governments."

The law thus requires that a J1 visa holder, upon completion of the training program, leave the United States and reside in his or her home country for a period of at least two years. Currently there is pressure from the American Medical Association to extend this period to five years.

An IMG on a J1 visa is ordinarily not allowed to change from J1 to most other types of visas or (in most cases) to change from J1 to permanent residence while in the United States until he or she has fulfilled the "foreign residence requirement." The purpose of the foreign residence requirement is to ensure that an IMG uses the training he or she obtained in the United States for the benefit of his or her home country. The U.S. government may, however, waive the two-year foreign residence requirement under the following circumstances:

- If you as an IMG can demonstrate a "well-founded fear of persecution" if forced to return to your country;
- If you as an IMG can prove that returning to your country would result in "exceptional hardship" to you or to members of your immediate family who are U.S. citizens or permanent residents; or
- If you are sponsored by an "interested governmental agency."

Applying for a J1 Visa Waiver. IMGs who have sought a waiver based on the last alternative have found it beneficial to approach the following potentially "interested government agencies":

- **The Department of Health and Human Services (HHS).** HHS's considerations for a waiver have been as follows: (1) the program or activity in which the IMG is engaged is "of high priority and of national or international significance in an area of interest" to HHS (merely providing medical services in a medically underserved area would not be sufficient); (2) the IMG must be an "integral" part of the program or activity "so that the loss of his/her services would necessitate discontinuance of the program or a major phase of it"; and (3) the IMG "must possess outstanding qualifications, training, and experience well beyond the usually expected accomplishments at the graduate, postgraduate, and residency levels and must clearly demonstrate the capability to make original and significant contributions to the program."

  In practice, HHS is more likely to recommend waivers for IMGs engaged in research than for those who treat patients. HHS waiver applications should be mailed to Joyce E. Jones, Executive Secretary, Exchange Visitor Review Board, Room 627-H, Hubert H. Humphrey Building, Department of Health and Human Services, 200 Independence Avenue, S.W., Washington, D.C. 20201.

- **The Veterans Administration (VA).** With over 170 health care facilities located in various parts of the United States, the VA is a major employer of physicians in this country. In addition, many VA hospitals are affiliated with university medical centers. Unlike HHS, the VA sponsors IMGs working not only in research but also in patient care (regardless of specialty) and in teaching. The waiver applicant may engage in teaching and research in conjunction with clinical duties. The VA's latest guidelines (issued on June 22, 1994) provide that it will act as an interested government agency only when the loss of the IMG's services would necessitate the discontinuance of a program or a major phase of it and when recruitment efforts have failed to locate a U.S. physician to fill the position.

The procedure for obtaining a VA sponsorship for a J1 waiver is as follows: (1) the IMG should deal directly with the Human Resources Department at the local VA facility; and (2) the facility must request that the VA's chief medical director sponsor the IMG for a waiver. The waiver request should include the following documentation: (1) a letter from the director of the local facility describing the program, the IMG's immigration status, the health care needs of the facility, and the facility's recruitment efforts; (2) recruitment efforts, including copies of all job advertisements run within the preceding year; and (3) copies of the IMG's licenses, test results, board certifications, IAP 66 forms, etc.

The VA contact person in Washington, D.C., should be contacted by the local medical facility rather than by IMGs or their attorneys.

- **The Appalachian Regional Commission (ARC).** The ARC sponsors physicians in certain places in the eastern and southern United States, namely, in the states of Alabama, Georgia, Kentucky, Maryland, Mississippi, New York, North Carolina, Ohio, Pennsylvania, South Carolina, Tennessee, Virginia, and West Virginia. Since 1992, the ARC has sponsored approximately 200 primary care IMGs annually in counties within its jurisdiction that have been designated as Health Professional Shortage Areas (HPSA) by HHS.

  In accordance with its February 1994 revision of its J1 waiver policies, the ARC requires that waiver requests be submitted initially to the ARC contact person in the state of intended employment. If the state concurs, a letter from the state's governor recommending the waiver must be addressed to Jesse J. White, Jr., the federal co-chairman of the ARC. The waiver request should include the following: (1) a letter from the facility to Mr. White stating the proposed dates of employment, the IMG's medical specialty, the address of the practice location, an assertion that the IMG will practice primary care for at least 40 hours per week in the HPSA, and details as to why the facility needs the services of the IMG; (2) a J1 Visa Data Sheet; (3) the ARC federal co-chairman's J1 Visa Waiver Policy and the J1 Visa Waiver Policy Affidavit and Agreement with the notarized signature of the IMG; (4) a contract of at least two years' duration; (5) evidence of the IMG's qualifications, including a résumé, medical diplomas and licenses, and IAP 66 forms; and (6) evidence of recruitment efforts within the preceding six months. Copies of advertisements, copies of résumés received, and reasons for rejection must also be included. The ARC will not sponsor IMGs who have been out of status for six months or longer.

  Requests for ARC waivers are processed in Washington, D.C., by Laura Dean Greathouse, ARC, 1666 Connecticut Avenue, N.W., Washington, D.C. 20235. ARC is usually able to forward a letter confirming that a waiver has been recommended to the USIA to the requesting facility or attorney within 30 days of the request.

- **The Department of Agriculture (USDA).** The USDA sponsors physicians who practice in family medicine, general surgery, pediatrics, obstetrics and gynecology, emergency medicine, internal medicine, and general psychiatry in rural areas. The USDA does not sponsor physicians to practice in areas located within the jurisdiction of the ARC.

For an area to be deemed "rural," the county in which the health care facility is located must have a population of less than 20,000 according to the last census. Also, the facility must be located in a health professional shortage area (HPSA). The IMG must sign a contract with a health care facility for a minimum period of three years. An IMG whose immigration status has lapsed for six months or more will not be considered for sponsorship by the USDA.

Since August 1994, USDA has required that each request for a waiver be supported by a letter of concurrence ("no objection") from the Department of Health in the state of intended employment. A few states (e.g., Georgia, Mississippi, New York, and Ohio) require that the USDA waiver request and accompanying documentation be submitted directly to them. If they concur with the request, they forward the entire packet together with a no-objection letter to the USDA.

USDA waiver requests should be mailed to Linda Seckel, Program Manager, J1 Visa Residency Waiver Program, Bldg. 005, Room 320, BARC-West, 10300 Baltimore Blvd., Beltsville, MD 20705-2350. The current processing time is approximately four months.

- **State Departments of Public Health.** There is no application form for a state-sponsored J1 waiver. However, USIA regulations specify that an application must include the following documents: (1) a letter from the State Department of Public Health identifying the physician and specifying that it would be in the public interest to grant him a J1 waiver; (2) an employment contract that is valid for a minimum of three years and that states the name and address of the facility that will employ the physician and the geographic areas in which he or she will practice medicine; (3) evidence that these geographic areas are located within HPSAs; (4) a statement by the physician agreeing to the contractual requirements; (5) copies of all IAP 66 forms; and (6) a completed USIA Data Sheet. Applications are numbered in the order in which they are received, since only 20 physicians per year may be granted waivers in a particular state. Individual states may choose to participate or not to participate in this program. Participating states include Alabama, Alaska, Arkansas, Arizona, Delaware, Florida, Georgia, Illinois, Indiana, Iowa, Kentucky, Maine, Massachusetts, Michigan, Minnesota, Mississippi, Missouri, Nebraska, Nevada, New Hampshire, New Mexico, New York, North Carolina, North Dakota, Ohio, Oklahoma, Pennsylvania, Rhode Island, South Carolina, Vermont, and Washington. Undecided states include California, Connecticut, New Jersey, Virginia, and Wyoming. Nonparticipating states include Hawaii, Idaho, Kansas, Louisiana, Montana, Oregon, South Dakota, Tennessee, Texas, and Utah.

The H1B Visa. Since 1991, the law has allowed medical residency programs to sponsor foreign-born medical residents for H1B visas. There are no restrictions to changing the H1B visa to any other kind of visa, including permanent resident status (green card), through employer sponsorship or through close relatives who are U.S. citizens or permanent residents. There was an overall ceiling of 65,000 H1B visas for professionals in all categories until mid-1998, when the number was raised to 95,000. It is advisable for SRPs to apply for H1B visas as soon as possible in the official year (beginning October 1), when the new quota officially opens up.

H1B visas are intended for "professionals" in a "specialty occupation." This means that an IMG intending to pursue a residency program in the United

States with an H1B visa needs to clear all three USMLE Steps before becoming eligible for the H1B. The ECFMG administers Step 1 and 2. Step 3 is conducted by the individual states. You will need to contact the FSMB or the medical board of the state where you intend to take the Step 3 for details.

USMLE STEP 3 AND THE IMG

Basic eligibility requirements for USMLE Step 3 are as follows:

- Obtain the MD degree (or its equivalent) or a DO degree by the application deadline.
- Pass both USMLE Step 1 and Step 2 (or the equivalents). Applicants must receive notice of a passing score by the application deadline.
- Graduates of foreign medical schools should be ECFMG certified or successfully complete a "fifth pathway" program (at a date no later than the application deadline).
- Apply to the following states, which do not have postgraduate training as an eligibility requirement:

  1. **California**
     Medical Board of California
     1426 Howe Ave., Suite 54
     Sacramento, CA 95825-3236
     www.medbd.ca.gov
     Phone: (916) 263-2389; Fax: (916) 263-2387
     Licensure inquiries: (916) 263-2499; (916) 263-2344

  2. **Connecticut**
     Connecticut Department of Public Health
     P.O. Box 340308
     Hartford, CT 06134-0308
     Phone: (860) 509-7579; Fax: (860) 509-8457
     Step 3 inquiries: FSMB at (817) 571-2949

  3. **Louisiana**
     Louisiana State Board of Medical Examiners
     P.O. Box 30250
     New Orleans, LA 70190-0250
     Phone: (504) 524-6763; Fax: (504) 568-8893

  4. **Maryland**
     Maryland Board of Physician Quality Assurance
     P.O. Box 2571
     Baltimore, MD 21215-0095
     Phone: (410) 764-4777; Fax: (410) 764-2478
     Step 3 inquiries: (800) 877-3926

  5. **Nebraska***
     Nebraska Department of Health
     P.O. Box 94986
     Lincoln, NE 68509-4986
     www.hhs.state.ne.us
     Phone: (402) 471-2118; Fax: (402) 471-3577
     Step 3 inquiries: FSMB at (817) 571-2949

*Nebraska requires that IMGs obtain a "valid indefinitely" ECFMG certificate.

6. **Nevada**
Nevada State Board of Medical Examiners
P.O. Box 7238
Reno, NV 89510
(702) 688-2559; Fax: (702) 688-2321
Step 3 inquiries: FSMB at (817) 571-2949

7. **New York**
New York State Board of Medicine
Cultural Education Center, Room 3023
Empire State Plaza
Albany, NY 12230
www.nysed.gov.opnme.html
Phone: (518) 474-3841; Fax: (518) 473-6995

8. **Rhode Island**
Rhode Island Board of Medical Licensure and Discipline
Department of Health
Cannon Building, Room 205
Three Capitol Hill
Providence, RI 02908-5097
Phone: (401) 277-3855; Fax: (401) 277-2158
Step 3 inquiries: FSMB at (817) 571-2949

9. **South Dakota**
South Dakota State Board of Medical and Osteopathic Examiners
1323 S. Minnesota Ave.
Sioux Falls, SD 57105
Phone: (605) 334-8343; Fax: (605) 336-0270
Step 3 inquiries: FSMB at (817) 571-2949

10. **Tennessee**
Tennessee Board of Medical Examiners
425 5th Avenue North
1st Floor, Cordell Hull Building
Nashville, TN 37247-1010
www.state.tn.us/health/downloads/dwnindex.htp
Phone: (615) 532-4384; Fax: (615) 532-5369
Step 3 inquiries: FSMB at (817) 571-2949

11. **Utah**
Utah Department of Commerce
Division of Occupational & Professional Licensure
P.O. Box 146741
Salt Lake City, UT 84114-6741
Phone: (801) 530-6628; Fax: (801) 530-6511

12. **West Virginia**
West Virginia Board of Medicine
101 Dee Dr.
Charleston, WV 25311
Phone (304) 558-2921; Fax: (304) 723-2877

H1B Application. An application for an H1B visa is not filed by the intending immigrating professional but by his or her employment sponsor—in your case, by the SRP in the United States. If an SRP is willing to do so, you will be told about it at the time of your interview for the residency program.

Before filing an H1B application with the INS, an SRP must file an application with the U.S. Labor Department affirming that the SRP will pay at least the normal salary for your job that a U.S. professional would earn. After receiving approval from the Labor Department, your SRP should be ready to file the H1B application with the INS. The SRP's supporting letter is the most important part of the H1B application package; it must describe the job duties to make it clear that the physician is needed in a "specialty occupation" (resident) under the prevalent legal definition of that term.

Most SRPs prefer to issue an IAP 66 for a J1 visa rather than filing papers for an H1B visa, because of the burden of paperwork and the attorney costs involved in securing approval of an H1B visa application. Even so, a sizable number of SRPs are willing to go through the trouble, particularly if an IMG is an excellent candidate or if the SRP concerned finds it difficult to fill all the available residency slots (although this is becoming rarer with continuing cuts in residency slots). If an SRP is unwilling to file for an H1B visa because of attorney costs, you could suggest that you would be willing to bear the burden of such costs. The entire process of getting an H1B visa can take anywhere from 10 to 20 weeks.

Although an H1B visa can be stamped by any U.S. consulate abroad, it is advisable to have it stamped at the U.S. consulate where you first applied for a visitor visa to travel to the United States for interviews.

Summary. Despite some significant obstacles, a number of viable methods are available to IMGs who seek to pursue a residency program or eventually practice medicine in the United States.

There is no doubt that the best alternative for IMGs is to obtain H1B visas to pursue their medical residencies. However, in cases where an IMG joins a residency program with a J1 visa, there are some possibilities of obtaining waivers of the two-year foreign residency requirement, particularly for those who are willing to make a commitment to perform primary care medicine in medically underserved areas.

RESOURCES FOR THE IMG

- ECFMG
  3624 Market Street, Fourth Floor
  Philadelphia, PA 19104-2685
  (215) 386-5900 or (202) 293-9320
  Fax: (215) 387-9963
  http://www.ecfmg.org

  The ECFMG telephone number is answered only between 9:00 a.m. and 12:30 p.m. and between 1:30 p.m. and 5:00 p.m. Monday through Friday EST. The ECFMG often takes a long time to answer the phone, which is frequently busy at peak times of the year, and then gives you a long voice-mail message, so it is better to write or fax early than to rely on a last-minute phone call. Do not contact the NBME, as all IMG exam matters are conducted by the ECFMG. The ECFMG also publishes the *Handbook for Foreign Medical Graduates and Information Booklet* on ECFMG certification and the USMLE program, which gives details on the dates and locations of forthcoming USMLE, CSA, and English tests for IMGs together with application forms. It is free of charge and is also available from the public affairs offices of U.S. embassies and consulates worldwide, as well as from Overseas Educational Advisory Centers. Single copies of the handbook may also be ordered by calling (215) 386-5900, preferably on weekends or between 6 p.m. and 6 a.m. Philadelphia time, or by faxing to (215) 387-9963. Requests for multiple copies must be made by fax or mail on organizational letterhead. The full text of the booklet is also available on the ECFMG's website at http://www.ecfmg.org.

- Federation of State Medical Boards
  400 Fuller Wiser Road, Suite 300
  Euless, TX 76039-3855
  (817) 868-4000
  Fax: (817) 868-4099

The FSMB publishes Exchange, Section I, which gives detailed information on examination and licensing requirements in all U.S. jurisdictions. The 1999–2000 edition costs $30. (Texas residents must add 7.75% state sales tax.) To obtain publications, write to Federation Publications at the above address. All orders must be prepaid by a personal check drawn on a U.S. bank, a cashier's check, or a money order payable to the Federation. Foreign orders must be accompanied by an international money order or the equivalent, payable in U.S. dollars through a U.S. bank or a U.S. affiliate of a foreign bank. Step 3 inquiries may also be made with the contact information above. The FSMB has a home page at http://www.fsmb.org.

- United States Information Agency
  301 4th Street, S.W.
  Washington, D.C. 20547
  (202) 619-4700
  http://www.ecfmg.org/evspusia.htm

This website summarizes the agency's policy regarding various program administration issues arising from the pursuit of graduate medical education or training in the United States by foreign medical graduates under the aegis of the Exchange Visitor Program.

- The Internet newsgroups misc.education.medical and bit.listserv.medforum can be valuable forums through which to exchange information on licensing exams, residency applications, and the like.
- Immigration information for IMGs is available from the sites of Siskind, Susser, Haas & Devine, a firm of attorneys specializing in immigration law:

    http://www.visalaw.com/~gsiskind/95feb/2feb95.html

- Another source of immigration information can be found on the website of the law offices of Carl Shusterman, a Los Angeles lawyer specializing in medical immigration law:

    http://shusterman.com

- International Medical Placement Ltd., a U.S. company specializing in recruiting foreign physicians to work in the United States, has a site at http://www.intlmedicalplacement.com. This site includes ordering information for several publications by FMSG, Inc., including USMLE Study Guides and residency matching information, as well as details on USMLE lecture courses offered by the author of these publications, Stanley Zaslau. The site also has information on seminars held by the company in foreign countries for physicians who are thinking of moving to the United States.

- *The International Medical Graduates' Guide to U.S. Medicine: Negotiating the Maze* by Louise B. Ball (199 pages; ISBN 1883620163) can be obtained from:

Galen Press
P.O. Box 64400
Tucson, AZ 85728-4400
(800) 442-5369 (United States and Canada) or (520) 577-8363
Fax: (520) 520-6459

Price: $28.95 plus $3.00 shipping and handling, add $2.95 for priority mail (U.S. dollars); Arizona residents add 7% sales tax.

This book has a lot of detailed information and is particularly strong on the intricacies of immigration law as it applies to foreign-citizen IMGs who wish to practice in the United States—although this is a rapidly changing field, and some of the information is probably out of date already. Also note that much of the book's contents may be relevant only to some IMGs, as many chapters are geared toward specific problems or situations (e.g., how to sponsor a relative, how a small American town may try to sponsor a foreign physician, how a U.S. faculty member can sponsor a foreign clinical research fellow), and there is considerable duplication across chapters.

Bottom line: Great for foreign citizens who need help in understanding how to "negotiate the maze" of medical immigration regulations, but not necessarily high yield for many other IMGs.

FIRST AID FOR THE STUDENT WITH A DISABILITY

The USMLE provides accommodations for students with documented disabilities. The basis for such accommodations is the Americans with Disabilities Act (ADA) of 1990. The ADA defines a disability as "a significant limitation in one or more major life activities." This includes both "observable/physical" disabilities (e.g., blindness, hearing loss, narcolepsy) and "hidden/mental disabilities" (e.g., attention deficit hyperactivity disorder, chronic fatigue syndrome, learning disabilities).

To provide appropriate support, the administrators of the USMLE must be informed of both the nature and the severity of an examinee's disability. Such documentation is required for an examinee to receive testing accommodations. Accommodations include extra time on tests, low-stimulation environments, extra or extended breaks, and zoom text.

Who Can Apply for Accommodations?

Students or graduates of a school in the United States or Canada that is accredited by the Liaison Committee for Medical Education (LCME) or the AOA may apply for test accommodations directly from the National Board. Requests are granted only if they meet the ADA definition of a disability. If you are a disabled student or a disabled graduate of a foreign medical school, you must contact the ECFMG (see next page).

Who Is Not Eligible for Accommodations?

Individuals who do not meet the ADA definition of disabled are not eligible for test accommodations. Difficulties not eligible for test accommodations include test anxiety, slow reading without an identified underlying cognitive deficit, English as a second language, or learning difficulties that have not been diagnosed as a medically recognized disability.

Understanding the Need for Documentation

Although most learning-disabled medical students are all too familiar with the often-exhausting process of providing documentation of their disability, you should realize that **applying for USMLE accommodation is different from these previous experiences.** This is because the National Board determines whether an individual is disabled solely on the basis of the guidelines set by the ADA.

Getting the Information

The first step in applying for USMLE special accommodations is to contact the NBME and obtain a guidelines and questionnaire booklet. This can be obtained by calling or writing to:

Testing Coordinator
Office of Test Accommodations
National Board of Medical Examiners
3750 Market Street
Philadelphia, PA 19104-3190
(215) 590-9700

Internet access to this information is also available at **www.ecfmg.org/ada intro.html.** This information is also relevant for IMGs, since the information is the same as that sent by the ECFMG.

Foreign graduates should contact the ECFMG to obtain information on special accommodations by calling or writing to:

ECFMG
3624 Market Street, 4th Floor
Philadelphia, PA 19104-2685
(215) 386-5900

When you get this information, take some time to read it carefully. The guidelines are clear and explicit about what you need to do to obtain accommodations.

Applying for Accommodations

Although the accommodation guidelines cited above are fairly self-explanatory, here are some key points to keep in mind:

- **Produce a history.** Send the National Board extensive past records. Since almost all learning disabilities are present from birth, sending even the earliest records of your disability is invaluable in an assessment. Even if you were diagnosed at a late age, a "paper trail" of your learning disability should still be evident. Grade-school reports, tutor-ing letters, job reports, previous physician notes, report cards, teacher comments, medication history, and other documents will go a long way toward providing significant evidence of your learning disability.

- **Send your "official" documentation.** Most individuals who were diag-nosed with a learning disability were tested with a specific battery of tests (an extensive list of these tests is given in the guidelines). Contact the physician who administered these tests and have the results sent to you. If you cannot locate that physician, obtain the documentation from the educational institutions you attended (college, high school, etc.). Verify that both the administering physician's clinical impressions and the results of your specific tests are included in your submitted material.

Reevaluating Your Disability

You might want to have your disability reevaluated for the USMLE. As stated previously, obtaining accommodations for the USMLE is different from any other process, as you are being evaluated solely on the basis of how well you meet the criteria specified by the ADA. Your evaluator should have this in mind when he or she performs the assessment. Sharing the information in the guidelines and questionnaire booklet with your evaluator will ensure that he or she is aware of this.

The purpose of a reevaluation is twofold. First of all, it is meant to produce further proof of the disability. In addition, it is meant to determine the need for accommodation based on the level of current functioning.

Reevaluation is not for everyone. An evaluation represents a considerable time commitment and is difficult to schedule during the hectic second year. An evaluation is also expensive, usually costing anywhere from $500 to $2000. Furthermore, since such a reevaluation is not being ordered for a strictly "medical reason" and since it is investigating a "previous condition," your insurance company may not cover it.

If you do decide to get reevaluated, the following is highly recommended:

- **Choose an expert.** You're in medical school. Use it! Most of the leading experts on learning disabilities are associated with medical school fac-ulty. Ask around for the leading expert on learning disabilities affiliated with your medical school, and use that physician as your evaluator. Make sure you stress to the evaluator that he or she is functioning as an independent evaluator and not as a school advocate. Using someone at your school is also desirable from a cost perspective; a faculty member may charge you a lowered evaluation fee.
- **Undergo some testing.** If you have undergone previous cognitive test-ing, this step is probably not that important. However, you might want to undergo some basic tests that assess your current level of cognitive functioning. A purely clinical evaluation is commonly limited in both scope and ability. **If you have never undergone a full evaluation, a comprehensive diagnostic battery is essential.** Make sure that your evaluator is not just looking at one or two sessions or subtests but at the entire gestalt.
- **Share your previous history with the evaluator.** Even though the USMLE reviewer will examine your documentation, your evaluator

should also have access to your medical history. In that way, he or she can highlight or emphasize certain aspects of your record.

■ **Ask for a differential diagnosis.** Evaluators should offer a differential, not just a single diagnosis. Once the differential has been made, evidence for or against any alternative diagnosis should be presented.

Finally, it is highly advisable that you talk from the heart. Part of the application is an essay you write about your disability. This is your opportunity to shine. If you have problems with writing, just speak from your soul. No one else but you can truly describe your learning disability; view this as an opportunity to share your difficulties with a receptive audience.

The Accommodations

As previously mentioned, a wide variety of accommodations exist for the USMLE. By far the most commonly requested and granted accommodation is for extra time. The ADA requires that individuals with a disability be provided with "equal access" to the testing program. Therefore, the purpose of accommodations is to "cancel" the effect of the disability, not to provide extra help in passing an examination.

Because the same types of impairments often vary in severity and frequently restrict different people to different degrees or in different ways, each request is considered individually to determine the effect of the impairment on the life of the applicant and whether a particular accommodation is even appropriate for that person.

The following additional material is excerpted from the NBME World Wide Web site (http://www.nbme.org/testacco.htm) and is copyright 1996 by The Federation of State Medical Boards of the United States, Inc., and the National Board of Medical Examiners.

If I am requesting an accommodation from the NBME on Step 1 or Step 2, when should I send in my request and documentation?

Mail your request and supporting documentation for test accommodations directly to the NBME Office of Test Accommodations at the *same time* you submit your Step 1 application. Don't submit your test accommodations request with your application.

Can my evaluator or my medical school send in my request for test accommodations?

No. A request for accommodations, by law, must be initiated by the person with a disability. Also, to protect your confidentiality, the NBME does not provide information concerning your request to third parties.

How does the NBME determine what is an appropriate accommodation for USMLE?

As part of the documentation, the examinee's evaluator should recommend appropriate accommodations to ease the impact of the impairment on the testing activity. Professional consultants in learning disabilities, attention deficit and hyperactivity disorder (ADHD), and various other psychiatric and physical conditions review the documentation and recommendations of evaluators to help match the type of assistance with the demonstrated need. The NBME consults with the examinee to determine what accommodations have been effectively used in the past.

If I apply for test accommodations on USMLE, does my disability evaluation have to be up to date?

For someone with a continuing history of accommodation, which would likely include high school and college as well as medical school, current testing is usually not necessary if objective documentation of the past accommodations is provided. However, the impact of the disability may change over time, and new testing may be necessary to demonstrate the current level of impairment and resulting need for accommodation. You will be advised if updated testing is needed.

What are some reasons my request for accommodations might not be approved?

- Insufficient documentation of a need for accommodation. Conditions such as learning disabilities and ADHD are permanent and lifelong. A diagnosis requires an objective history of chronic symptoms from childhood to adulthood as well as evidence of significant impairment currently.
- Lack of presence of a moderate to severe level of impairment attributable to the disorder.
- The identified difficulty is not considered to be a disability under the law, i.e., slow reading without evidence of an underlying language-processing disorder; language difficulties as a result of English as a second language.

Once my request for accommodations has been approved, do I need to arrange for accommodations the next time I register for a Step?

An examinee with a disability must request accommodations at the time of registration. NBME examinees must send a letter requesting accommodations to the Office of Test Accommodations. A repeated request must state whether any change in the accommodations is required, and if so, documentation of the needed change must be provided.

Accommodations are not granted automatically even if they were approved for previous Step administrations.

Miscellaneous Suggestions

- **Get your information to the USMLE early.** The earlier your information is received, the more time the USMLE will have for evaluating and considering your case. They will also have time to ask you for additional material should this prove necessary.

- **Use your winter holiday.** It is a lot easier to get this material ready for the USMLE when you are not in school. It is also immeasurably easier to be evaluated when you are not facing the pressures of the second year.

Database of High-Yield Facts

"There comes a time when for every addition of knowledge you forget something that you knew before. It is of the highest importance, therefore, not to have useless facts elbowing out the useful ones."
—Arthur Conan Doyle, "A Study in Scarlet"

"Never regard study as a duty, but as the enviable opportunity to learn."
—Albert Einstein

"Live as if you were to die tomorrow. Learn as if you were to live forever."
—Gandhi

Cardiovascular

Dermatology

Endocrinology

Epidemiology
   and Preventive Medicine

Ethics

Gastrointestinal

Hematology/Oncology

Infectious Disease

Musculoskeletal

Neurology

Obstetrics

Gynecology

Pediatrics

Psychiatry

Pulmonary

Renal

Selected Topics
   in Emergency Medicine

The third edition of *First Aid for the USMLE Step 2* contains a revised and expanded database of clinical material that student authors and faculty have identified as high yield for boards review. The facts are organized according to subject matter, whether medical specialty (e.g., Cardiovascular, Renal) or high-yield topics (e.g., Ethics) in medicine. Each subject is then divided into smaller subsections of related facts. Individual facts are generally presented in a logical approach, from basic definitions and epidemiology to **History/Physical Exam, Differential, Evaluation,** and **Treatment.** Lists, mnemonics, and tables are used when helpful in forming key associations.

The content is mostly useful for reviewing material already learned. This section is not ideal for learning complex or highly conceptual material for the first time. At the beginning of many sections we list supplementary high-yield review material from *First Aid for the USMLE Step 1* to jog your memory about important basic science concepts.

Black-and-white images appear throughout the text. In some cases, reference is made to the "clinical image" section at the end of Section II, which contains full-color glossy plates of histology and patient pathology by topic.

Selected topics have embedded references to the eight titles in the *Underground Clinical Vignettes* (UCV) *Step 2* series (S2S Medical Publishing). These annotations link the high-yield fact to a corresponding vignette, illustrating how that fact may appear in a Step 2 clinical scenario. The following annotation, for example, refers to cases 23 and 45 from *UCV Pediatrics:* **UCV** *Ped.23, 45*

UCV REFERENCE LEGEND	
UCV Title	**Abbreviation**
Emergency Medicine, 2nd ed.	EM
Internal Medicine, Vol. 1, 2nd ed.	IM1
Internal Medicine, Vol. 2, 2nd ed.	IM2
Neurology, 2nd ed.	Neuro
Obstetrics and Gynecology, 2nd ed.	OB
Pediatrics, 2nd ed.	Ped
Psychiatry, 2nd ed.	Psych
Surgery, 2nd ed.	Surg

At the end of each section we have a "review," which includes:

- A "rapid review" of common clues, facts, and associations.
- Boards-type clinical case scenarios extracted from the McGraw-Hill *PreTest* series. Multiple-choice question-and-answer explanations are provided.

The Database of High-Yield Facts is not comprehensive. Use it to complement your core study material and not as your primary study source. The facts and notes have been condensed and edited to emphasize the essential material. Work with the material, add your own notes and mnemonics, and recognize that not all memory techniques work for all students.

We update Section II biannually to keep current with new trends in boards content as well as to expand our database of high-yield information. However, we must note that inevitably many other very high-yield entries and topics are not yet included in our database.

We actively encourage medical students and faculty to submit entries and mnemonics so that we may enhance the database for future students. We also solicit recommendations of alternate tools for study that may be useful in preparing for the examination, such as diagrams, charts, and computer-based tutorials (see How to Contribute, page xv).

Disclaimer

The entries in this section reflect student opinions of what is high yield. Owing to the diverse sources of material, no attempt has been made to trace or reference the origins of entries individually. We have regarded mnemonics as essentially in the public domain. All errors and omissions will be gladly corrected if brought to the attention of the authors, either through the publisher or directly by e-mail.

Cardiovascular

Coronary artery anatomy

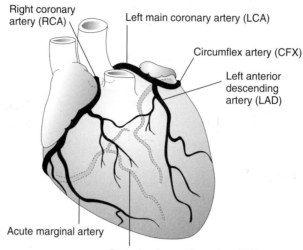

Right coronary artery (RCA)

Left main coronary artery (LCA)

Circumflex artery (CFX)

Left anterior descending artery (LAD)

Acute marginal artery

Posterior descending artery (PD)

(Redrawn, with permission, from Ganong WF, *Review of Medical Physiology*, 19th ed., Stamford, CT: Appleton & Lange, 1999: p. 592.)

In the majority of cases, the SA and AV nodes are supplied by the RCA. Eighty percent of the time, the RCA supplies the inferior portion of the left ventricle via the PD artery (= right dominant).

Coronary artery occlusion occurs most commonly in the LAD, which supplies the anterior interventricular septum.

Coronary arteries fill during diastole.

Diagnosis of MI

In the first six hours, EKG is the gold standard.

Cardiac troponin I is used within the first four hours up to seven to ten days; more specific than other protein markers.

CK-MB is test of choice in the first 24 hours post-MI.

LDH_1 (former test of choice) is also elevated from two to seven days post-MI.

AST is nonspecific and can be found in cardiac, liver, and skeletal muscle cells.

EKG changes can include ST elevation (transmural ischemia) and Q waves (transmural infarct).

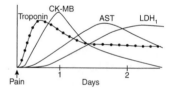

Troponin — CK-MB — AST — LDH₁

Pain   1   Days   2

HIGH-YIELD FACTS

Cardiovascular

Cardiac cycle

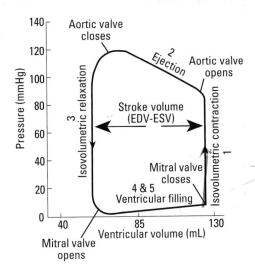

Phases:

1. Isovolumetric contraction—period between mitral valve closure and aortic valve opening; period of highest oxygen consumption
2. Systolic ejection—period between aortic valve opening and closing
3. Isovolumetric relaxation—period between aortic valve closing and mitral valve opening
4. Rapid filling—period just after mitral valve opening
5. Slow filling—period just before mitral valve closure

Sounds:

S1—mitral and tricuspid valve closure
S2—aortic and pulmonary valve closure
S3—end of rapid ventricular filling
S4—high atrial pressure/stiff ventricle

S3 is associated with dilated CHF
S4 ("atrial kick") is associated with a hypertrophic ventricle

a wave: **a**trial contraction
c wave: RV contraction (tricuspid valve bulging into atrium)
v wave: increased atrial pressure due to filling against closed tricuspid valve

Jugular venous distention is seen in right heart failure.

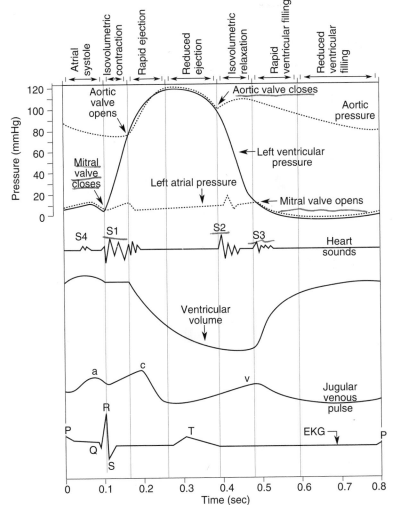

(Adapted, with permission, from Ganong WF, *Review of Medical Physiology*, 19th ed., Stamford, CT: Appleton & Lange, 1999: p. 541.)

HIGH-YIELD FACTS

Cardiovascular

Heart murmurs

a) Aortic stenosis — Crescendo–decrescendo systolic ejection murmur, with LV >> aortic pressure during systole.

b) Aortic regurgitation — High-pitched "blowing" diastolic murmur. Wide pulse pressure.

c) Mitral stenosis — Rumbling late diastolic murmurs. LA >> LV pressure during diastole. Opening snap.

d) Mitral regurgitation — High-pitched "blowing" holosystolic murmur. *Pan*

e) Mitral prolapse — Systolic murmur with midsystolic click. Most frequent valvular lesion, especially in young women.

f) VSD — Holosystolic murmur.

g) PDA *patent ductus Arteriosis* — Continuous machine-like murmur. / *pansystolic*

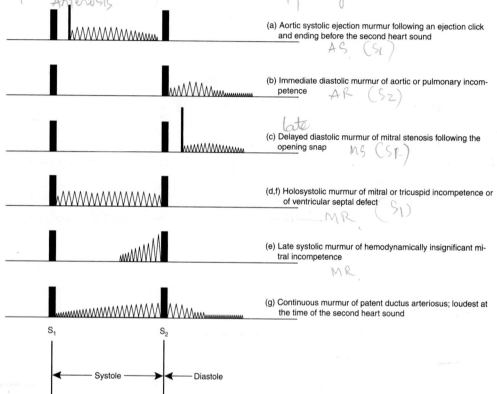

(a) Aortic systolic ejection murmur following an ejection click and ending before the second heart sound *AS (S₁)*

(b) Immediate diastolic murmur of aortic or pulmonary incompetence *AR (S₂)*

(c) Delayed diastolic murmur of mitral stenosis following the opening snap *late* *MS (SF)*

(d,f) Holosystolic murmur of mitral or tricuspid incompetence or of ventricular septal defect *MR (S₁)*

(e) Late systolic murmur of hemodynamically insignificant mitral incompetence *MR*

(g) Continuous murmur of patent ductus arteriosus; loudest at the time of the second heart sound

S₁   S₂

←— Systole —→ ←— Diastole

(Modified, with permission, from Wood P: *Diseases of the Heart and Circulation*, 3rd ed., Philadelphia, PA: Lippincott, 1968.)

Cardiac output (CO)

Cardiac output = (stroke volume) × (heart rate)

Fick principle:

$$CO = \frac{\text{rate of O}_2 \text{ consumption}}{\text{arterial O}_2 \text{ content} - \text{venous O}_2 \text{ content}}$$

$$\frac{\text{Mean arterial}}{\text{pressure}} = \left(\frac{\text{cardiac}}{\text{output}}\right) \times \left(\frac{\text{total peripheral}}{\text{resistance}}\right)$$

Similar to Ohm's law:

voltage = (current) × (resistance)

MAP = diastolic + ⅓ pulse pressure

Pulse pressure = systolic – diastolic

Pulse pressure ≈ stroke volume

During exercise, CO increases initially as a result of an increase in SV. After prolonged exercise CO increases as a result of an increase in HR.

If HR is too high, diastolic filling is incomplete and CO drops (e.g., ventricular tachycardia).

Cardiac output variables

Stroke volume affected by **C**ontractility, **A**fterload, and **P**reload.

Contractility (and SV) increased with:
1. Catecholamines (increased activity of Ca^{2+} pump in sarcoplasmic reticulum)
2. Increased intracellular calcium
3. Decreased extracellular sodium
4. Digitalis (increased intracellular Na^+, resulting in increased Ca^{2+})

Contractility (and SV) decreased with:
1. Beta-1 blockade
2. Heart failure

3. Acidosis
4. Hypoxia/hypercapnea

SV **CAP**

Stroke volume increases in anxiety, exercise, and pregnancy.

A failing heart has decreased stroke volume.

Myocardial O_2 demand is increased by:
Increased afterload ($\propto$ diastolic BP)
Increased contractility
Increased heart rate
Increased heart size (increased wall tension)

Myocardial action potential

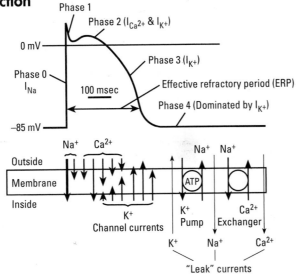

Occurs in atrial and ventricular myocytes and Purkinje fibers.

Phase 0 = rapid upstroke—voltage-gated Na^+ channels open.

Phase 1 = initial repolarization—inactivation of voltage-gated Na^+ channels. Voltage-gated K^+ channels begin to open.

Phase 2 = plateau—Ca^{2+} influx through voltage-gated Ca^{2+} channels balances K^+ efflux. Ca^{2+} influx triggers myocyte contraction.

Phase 3 = rapid repolarization—massive K^+ efflux due to opening of voltage-gated slow K^+ channels and closure of voltage-gated Ca^{2+} channels.

Phase 4 = resting potential—high K^+ permeability through K^+ channels.

Electrocardiogram

P wave—atrial depolarization.

P-R interval—conduction delay through AV node (normally < 200 msec).

QRS complex—ventricular depolarization (normally < 120 msec).

Q-T interval—mechanical contraction of the ventricles.

T wave—ventricular repolarization.

Atrial repolarization is masked by QRS complex.

ST segment—isoelectric, ventricles depolarized

U wave—caused by hypokalemia

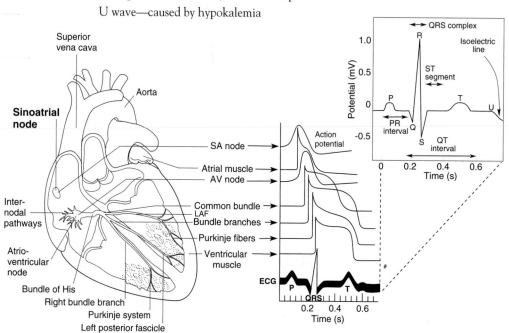

SA node "pacemaker" inherent dominance with slow phase of upstroke
AV node - 100-msec delay - atrioventricular delay

(Adapted, with permission, from Ganong WF, *Review of Medical Physiology*, 19th ed., Stamford, CT: Appleton & Lange, 1999: p. 522.)

Anti-anginal therapy

Goal: Reduction of myocardial O_2 consumption (MVO_2) by decreasing one or more of the determinants of MVO_2: end diastolic volume, blood pressure, heart rate, contractility, ejection time.

Component	Nitrates	Beta Blockers	Nitrates + Beta Blockers
End diastolic volume	↓	↑	No effect or ↓
Blood pressure	↓	↓	↓
Contractility	↑ (reflex response)	↓	Little/no effect
Heart rate	↑ (reflex response)	↓	↓
Ejection time	↓	↑	Little/no effect
MVO_2	↓	↓	↓↓

Calcium channel blockers:
- **N**ifedipine is similar to **N**itrates in effect
- Verapamil is similar to beta-blockers in effect

Lipid-lowering agents

Drug	Effect on LDL "Bad Cholesterol"	Effect on HDL "Good Cholesterol"	Effect on Triglycerides	Side Effects/Problems
Bile acid resins (cholestyramine, colestipol)	↓↓	No effect	Slight ↑	Patients hate it—tastes bad and causes GI discomfort
HMG-CoA reductase inhibitors (lovastatin, pravastatin, simvastatin, atorvastatin)	↓↓↓	↑	↓	Expensive Reversible ↑ LFTs Myositis
Niacin	↓↓	↑↑	↓	Red, flushed face that is ↓ by aspirin or long-term use
Lipoprotein lipase stimulators (gemfibrozil, clofibrate)	↓	↑	↓↓↓	Myositis, ↑ LFTs
Probucol	↓	↓	No effect	↓ HDL

(handwritten: Constipation!/gas)

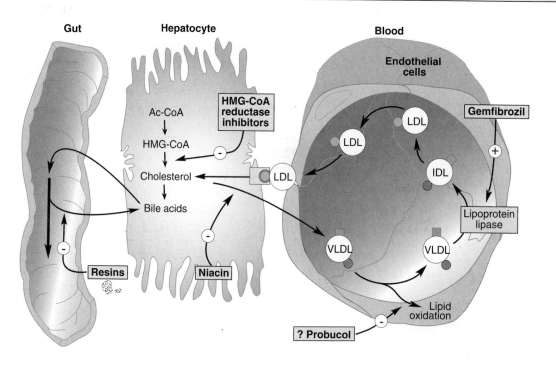

(Adapted, with permission, from Katzung BG and Trevor AJ, *Examination & Board Review: Pharmacology,* 5th ed., Stamford, CT: Appleton & Lange, 1998: p. 267.)

Abnormalities of cardiac rhythm can be asymptomatic, symptomatic, or lethal. The following tables review the major arrhythmias, their etiologies, signs/symptoms, EKG findings, and treatments. (See Tables 2.1–1 to 2.1–3.)

TABLE 2.1–1. Heart Block

Type	Etiology	Signs/Symptoms	EKG Findings	Treatment
Primary heart block	Occurs in normal individuals Increased vagal tone	Asymptomatic	PR interval > 0.2 second	None necessary
Secondary heart block (Mobitz type I)	**Drug effect** (beta blockade, digoxin, calcium channel blockers) Increased vagal tone	Usually asymptomatic	Increasing PR interval until a dropped beat occurs (Wenckebach); PR then resets.	Stop offending drug
Secondary heart block (Mobitz type II)	**Diseased infranodal conduction system**	Symptoms are rare	Unexpected dropped beat without change in PR interval	Ventricular pacemaker
Tertiary heart block (complete heart block)	No electrical communication between the atria and ventricles	Syncope, dizziness, acute heart failure, hypotension, cannon A waves	**No relationship between P waves and QRS complexes**	Ventricular pacemaker

[handwritten margin note: Sinc with Atropine θ of MI]

TABLE 2.1–2. Supraventricular Arrhythmias

Type	Etiology	Signs/Symptoms	EKG Findings	Treatment
Atrial fibrillation *[handwritten: D2.]*	Pulmonary disease Ischemia Rheumatic heart disease Anemia/atrial myxoma Thyrotoxicosis Ethanol Sepsis	Asymptomatic Shortness of breath, chest pain, palpitations Irregularly irregular pulse	Wavy baseline without discernible P waves Variable and irregular QRS response	**Anticoagulation Rate control** (Ca²⁺ channel blockers, beta-blockers, digoxin) Cardioversion (electrical, pharmacologic)
Atrial flutter *[handwritten: NL]*	Rapid fire of an ectopic beat in atria (250–350 bpm) Associated with CAD, CHF, COPD, valvulopathy, and pericarditis	Asymptomatic or palpitations, syncope, lightheadedness	Regular rhythm "Sawtooth" appearance of P waves	Rate control Cardioversion (electrical, pharmacologic)

[handwritten margin notes: ↓ erate; Fx ↑ adenosin stress test. —↓ dobutamin Echo.]

TABLE 2.1–2. Arrhythmias (continued)

HIGH-YIELD FACTS

Cardiovascular

Type	Etiology	Signs/ Symptoms	EKG Findings	Treatment
Multifocal atrial tachycardia (MAT)	Multiple atrial pacemakers or re-entrant pathways COPD	May be asymptomatic	Three or more varying P-wave morphologies Rate > 100	Treat underlying disorder Verapamil
Paroxysmal supraventricular tachycardia (SVT)	Rapid arrhythmia arising from atria or AV junction Usually secondary to reentry (e.g., WPW)	Palpitations, lightheadedness, angina, syncope	Rate 150–250 **Normal QRS** P waves may be present or hidden in T waves	Carotid massage Valsalva maneuver Adenosine ✳ Verapamil Cardioversion Radiofrequency catheter ablation

UCV *IM1.12*

TABLE 2.1–3. Ventricular Arrhythmias

Type	Etiology	Signs/ Symptoms	EKG Findings	Treatment
Premature ventricular contraction (PVC)	Ectopic beats arising from ventricular foci Common and often benign Causes include hypoxia, electrolyte abnormalities, hyperthyroidism	Usually asymptomatic **Palpitations, syncope**	Early, wide QRS complexes that are not preceded by a P wave PVCs are followed by a compensatory pause	No treatment needed if asymptomatic Treat underlying cause Beta-blockers or others antiarrhythmics in symptomatic patients
Ventricular tachycardia (VT)	**Associated with CAD/MI**	Asymptomatic Skipped beats Hemodynamic instability syncope	**Three or more consecutive PVCs** Wide QRSs in a regular rapid rhythm AV dissociation	**Antiarrhythmics** (lidocaine, procainamide, bretylium) If hemodynamically unstable, treat as VF
Ventricular fibrillation (VF)	Associated with CAD/MI	Syncope, hypotension, pulselessness	**Totally erratic tracing**	**Immediate electrical cardioversion** CPR Lidocaine and/or epinephrine

A. Ventricular Tachycardia

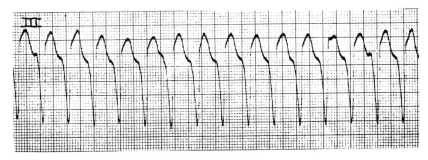

B. Ventricular Fibrillation

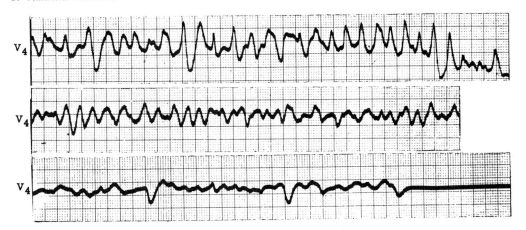

Ventricular tachycardia and ventricular fibrillation. Note the regular, wide-complex rhythm characteristic of ventricular tachycardia in contrast to the erratic tracing typically seen in ventricular fibrillation.

FIGURE 2.1–1. (A) Ventricular tachycardia. Wide QRS beats with no discernible P waves. **(B) Ventricular fibrillation.**
(Reproduced, with permission, from Saunders CE, *Current Emergency Diagnosis & Treatment,* 4th ed., Stamford, CT: Appleton & Lange, 1992: p. 515, Fig. 29–30; p. 517, Fig. 29–34.)

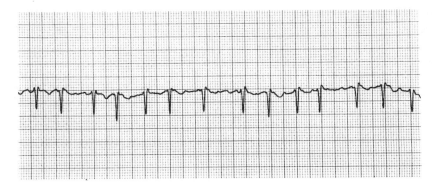

FIGURE 2.1–2. Atrial fibrillation. Note the absence of P waves and irregularly irregular ventricular rhythm. (Reproduced, with permission, from Stobo J, *The Principles and Practice of Medicine,* 23rd ed., Stamford, CT: Appleton & Lange, 1996: p. 78, Fig. 1–9–3B.)

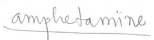
amphetamine

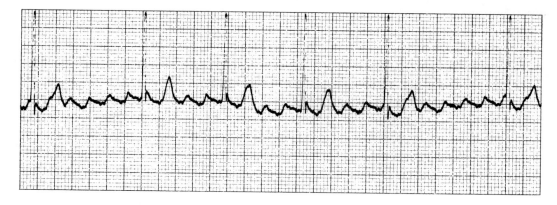

FIGURE 2.1–3. Atrial flutter. The "sawtooth" baseline of rapid but organized atrial activity (usually between 250 and 350 bpm) is characteristic. (Reproduced, with permission, from Ochs G, *Recognition and Interpretation of ECG Rhythms*, 3rd ed., Stamford, CT: Appleton & Lange, 1997: p. 34, Fig. 2–17.)

ANGINA PECTORIS

Episodes of <u>chest pain</u> due to **ischemic** cardiac disease (inadequate oxygen delivery to myocardium). Risk factors include age, hypercholesterolemia, diabetes, hypertension, family history, previous angina/MI, and tobacco, cocaine, and <u>amphetamine use</u>. Males are affected more frequently than females.

History

The classic triad involves **substernal chest pain** or pressure that is **precipitated by exertion** and **relieved by rest or nitrates.** Angina can radiate to the arms, jaw, and neck and can be associated with diaphoresis, nausea/emesis, or lightheadedness. Anginal symptoms can vary significantly among patients.

PE

Diaphoresis, elevated BP, tachycardia, and apical systolic murmur/gallop may be appreciated during an anginal episode.

Differential

MI, costochondritis, herpes zoster neuropathy, GERD (may also improve with nitrates), PUD, cholecystitis, pericarditis, aortic dissection, pulmonary embolus, pneumothorax, pneumonia, and pleurisy.

Evaluation

GERD and esophageal spasm may also improve with nitroglycerin.

EKG may show transient **ST-segment depression** (or elevation). Check **cardiac enzymes.** Risk-stratify by performing an **exercise stress test** or coronary **catheterization.**

Treatment

- Patients with suspected MI (according to clinical findings) must be admitted and monitored by EKG/telemetry until acute MI is ruled out by serial cardiac enzymes.

- Treat acute symptoms with sublingual **nitroglycerin, aspirin,** and **beta-blockers.** Start heparin drip in patients with EKG changes, multiple attacks, or unstable angina.
- If pain subsides, patients should be given nitrates (for further attacks), beta-blockers, and aspirin. Discuss **risk factor** (e.g., smoking, cholesterol, hypertension) **reduction.** Consider stress test.
- If pain increases in frequency, is unrelieved with nitroglycerin, or occurs at rest **(unstable angina),** proceed to **heparinization, angiography,** and possible **revascularization** (PTCA vs. CABG). Candidates for potential revascularization have symptoms of myocardial ischemia refractory to medical management, a positive stress test despite maximal medical regimen, or recurrent or persistent chest pain. Criteria for CABG include left main stenosis > 50%, three-vessel disease with reduced ejection fraction, and diabetic CAD.

MYOCARDIAL INFARCTION (MI)

MI occurs when occlusion or spasm of coronary vessels causes myocardial ischemia and tissue death. It is often secondary to acute thrombus formation on a ruptured atherosclerotic plaque. Risk factors include age, hypertension, hypercholesterolemia, a family history of early CAD, diabetes mellitus, and tobacco use. **Males** are affected more than females, and **postmenopausal females** are affected more than premenopausal females.

> **Risk factors for CAD—**
>
> **CAD HDL**
> **C**igarettes
> **A**ge and sex
> **D**iabetes mellitus
> **H**ypertension
> **D**eath from MI in family
> **L**DL high and **L**ow HDL

History

Patients present with acute-onset chest pain, often described as a pressure or tightness, that can **radiate to the left arm,** neck, or jaw. **Diaphoresis,** shortness of breath, lightheadedness, and nausea/vomiting may also be seen. Be alert to atypical presentations. MI may cause syncope. Elderly, diabetic, and postoperative patients are particularly likely to have "silent" MIs.

PE

Tachycardia, **new mitral regurgitation** (ruptured papillary muscle), low blood pressure (cardiogenic shock), and rales **(pulmonary edema).**

Differential

Angina, pulmonary embolism, aortic dissection, pneumothorax, pericarditis, GERD, costochondritis, herpes zoster, esophageal spasm, peptic ulcer, pneumonia, cholecystitis.

Evaluation

Evaluation should include **EKG** and **cardiac enzymes** (CK with CK-MB fraction, LDH, troponin I, troponin T). Diagnosis is based on a rise in cardiac enzymes and/or EKG changes (ST-segment elevation/depression or new LBBB; Figures 2.1–4 and 2.1–5) with an appropriate clinical presentation. MI is also associated with **arrhythmias,** including atrial fibrillation, supraventricular tachycardia, and ventricular arrhythmias. CXR may show signs of CHF.

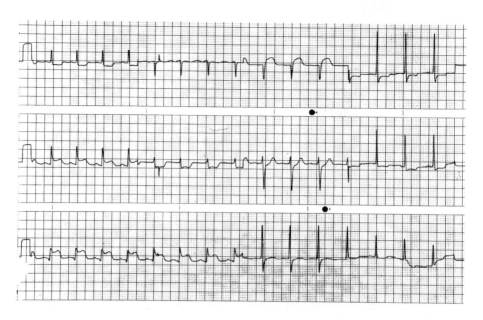

FIGURE 2.1–4. Inferior wall myocardial infarction. In this patient with acute chest pain, the EKG demonstrated acute ST elevation in leads II, III, and aVF with reciprocal ST depression and T-wave flattening in leads I, aVL, and V₄ to V₆. (Reproduced, with permission, from Stobo J, *The Principles and Practice of Medicine*, 23rd ed., Stamford, CT: Appleton & Lange, 1996: p. 20, Fig. 1–3–3A.)

Treatment MI

"Time is myocardium."

- **Acute management:** Give **oxygen, aspirin, beta-blockers** (hold in the presence of bradycardia, hypotension, or pulmonary edema), **nitroglycerin** (can cause hypotension), and **morphine** (for pain). Consider **thrombolysis** (if the patient presents within six hours of onset) with TPA, urokinase, or streptokinase or revascularization with **angioplasty.** If the patient is hypotensive, start IV fluids and stop nitroglycerin. Patients with suspected MI require hospital admission to a cardiac-monitored bed

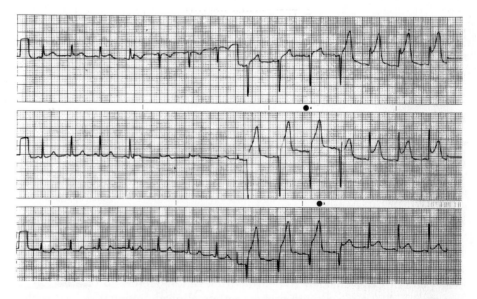

FIGURE 2.1–5. Anterior wall myocardial infarction. The patient presented with acute chest pain. EKG showed ST elevation in leads aVL and V₁ to V₆ and hyperacute T waves. (Reproduced, with permission, from Stobo J, *The Principles and Practice of Medicine*, 23rd ed., Stamford, CT: Appleton & Lange, 1996: p. 19, Fig. 1–3–2A.)

A.F ⟹ Arterial Embolism
M.S + Endocarditis ⟹ embolization (brain)
Endocarditis ⟹ pulmonary embolization

to watch for continuing ischemia and cardiac arrhythmias, especially in the first 24 hours post-MI.

- **Inpatient:** Treat with **aspirin, heparin, beta-blockers,** and **ACE inhibitors;** perform **stress test** and/or echo after five days to assess future risk. In the event of a positive stress test, perform **catheterization** to assess vessel patency. Consider PTCA or CABG for significant occlusions.
- **Long term:** Give **aspirin, beta-blockers, lipid-lowering agents,** and **ACE inhibitors** if tolerated (especially in patients with pulmonary edema). **Modify risk factors** by lowering cholesterol and BP, changing diet, and increasing exercise.

Complications

Complications following acute MI include reinfarction, LV wall rupture, pericarditis, **Dressler's syndrome** (autoimmune process with fever, pericarditis, and increased ESR occurring 2–4 weeks post-MI), papillary muscle rupture (with mitral regurgitation), aneurysmal dilatation of the left ventricle, and mural thrombi. **Lethal arrhythmia** is the most common cause of death following acute MI. More than six PVCs/min indicates a poor prognosis.

UCV EM.2

CONGESTIVE HEART FAILURE (CHF)

A condition in which cardiac output is unable to meet systemic demand. Risk factors include CAD, a family history of hypertrophic cardiomyopathy, hypertension, vascular heart disease, drug toxicity, alcohol abuse, and myocarditis. The most common cause of right-sided heart failure is left-sided failure.

History

Patients present with dyspnea on exertion (or at rest if severe), fatigue, lower extremity edema, **orthopnea, paroxysmal nocturnal dyspnea, nocturia,** and/or abdominal fullness.

PE

Physical exam may reveal sinus tachycardia and a laterally displaced PMI. Patients with right-sided failure may have elevated JVD **(jugular venous distention),** hepatomegaly, **hepatojugular reflex,** and bipedal **edema;** those with left-sided failure may have bilateral **basilar rales and S3** or S4 gallop.

Differential

MI, angina, pericarditis, nephrotic syndrome/renal failure, cirrhosis, pneumonia.

Causes of recurrent CHF—

FAILURE
Forgot medication
Arrhythmia/**A**nemia
Ischemia/**I**nfarct/
   Infection
Lifestyle (Na+ and
   fluid intake)
Upregulation (increased CO in
   pregnancy, hyperthyroidism)
Renal failure → fluid
   overload
Embolus (pulmonary)

Evaluation

Workup should include EKG, CXR (look for **cardiomegaly, cephalization of pulmonary vessels,** pleural effusions, vascular indistinctness, and prominent hila), and **echocardiography.** Diagnosis is based on the clinical picture and on an echocardiogram showing impaired cardiac function (hypertrophic or dilated cardiomyopathy may be observed). Rule out MI in acute exacerbations. If amyloid or viral myocarditis is suspected (e.g., in cases of previous viral prodrome or young age), a myocardial biopsy may be performed. Atrial fibrillation is common in CHF and increases the risk of embolization.

Treatment

- **Correct treatable causes** such as arrhythmias, alcohol-induced failure, LV dysfunction, thyroid disease, and valvular disease.
- **Acute:** If the patient has worsening dyspnea and other symptoms, diurese aggressively with a **loop diuretic** (such as furosemide) and a non-loop agent (monitor K^+ when using potassium-sparing agents). Use **ACE inhibitors** in all patients who can tolerate them. Patients may require hospital admission and may also require intubation. Dobutamine for inotropy (aka "dobutamine holiday") and nitroprusside for afterload reduction may be helpful.
- **Chronic:** Use **ACE inhibitors**/angiotensin receptor blockers (which have been shown to decrease mortality), **diuretics** (furosemide), and **digoxin.** Treat arrhythmias as they arise; limit dietary sodium and fluid intake. Use beta-blockers if tolerated. Consider **warfarin** for severe dilated cardiomyopathy, atrial fibrillation, or previous embolic episodes.
- Low-dose **spironolactone** has been shown to decrease risk of mortality by 30% when given with ACE inhibitors, digoxin, and diuretics in patients with **left systolic dysfunction.**
- Intractable CHF unresponsive to maximal medical therapy may require mechanical ventricular assist devices and cardiac transplantation.

UCV *IMI.4*

CARDIOMYOPATHIES

The cardiomyopathies are intrinsic diseases of the myocardium and are categorized as dilated, hypertrophic, and restrictive. Strictly speaking, they exclude impaired myocardial function attributable to ischemic, valvular, or hypertensive disease.

PRIMARY DILATED CARDIOMYOPATHY (balloon like heart)

Generally presents as CHF or dyspnea. **Left ventricular dilation** and **systolic dysfunction** must be present to make the diagnosis. The majority of cases are idiopathic, although known causes include alcohol, wet beriberi, coxsackievirus, cocaine, **doxorubicin,** and myocarditis as well as HIV and AZT. It comprises 90% of all cardiomyopathies.

> **The ABCD's of systolic dysfunction:**
>
> **A**lcohol
> **B**eriberi
> **C**oxsackie (B),
>   **C**ocaine
> **D**oxorubicin

History/PE

Classic signs of heart failure develop gradually. Examination may reveal cardiomegaly, the presence of an S3, and tricuspid and mitral regurgitation. Patients may present with fever if infectious causes are responsible.

Evaluation

Nonspecific ST-T changes, low-voltage QRS, sinus tachycardia, and ectopy may be seen on EKG. LBBB is also commonly found. Chest radiographs show an enlarged, **balloon-like heart** and pulmonary congestion. Echocardiography is diagnostic.

Treatment

All **alcohol usage should be stopped.** Therapies should be directed toward alleviating the symptoms of CHF (diuretics, ACE inhibitors, beta-blockers). Consider anticoagulation.

UCV *IM1.6*

HYPERTROPHIC CARDIOMYOPATHY → bootshape
IHSS   LVH

Also known as idiopathic hypertrophic subaortic stenosis, it is inherited as an autosomal-dominant trait in 50% of patients. Ventricular hypertrophy with a thickened septum results in decreased filling and diastolic dysfunction, while obstruction of the LV outflow tract results in systolic dysfunction. Obstruction is worsened as myocardial contractility is increased or as LV filling is decreased (Valsalva maneuvers, vasodilators). It is the most common cause of sudden death in young athletes.

History/PE

Syncope (after exertion), dyspnea, palpitations, and chest pain are the most common symptoms. Arrhythmias, atrial fibrillation, and elevated LA pressures are poor prognostic signs. Auscultation may reveal mitral regurgitation, a sustained apical impulse, an S4, and **systolic ejection murmur.** AS
— holosystolic (m)
└ Hypertrophic

Evaluation

EKG shows LVH and abnormal Q waves. CXR may show the classic "boot shape." Echocardiogram is diagnostic, showing thickened LV walls and dynamic obstruction of blood flow.

Treatment

Beta blockade is the initial treatment in symptomatic individuals. Calcium channel blockers (verapamil) are also helpful. Surgical options are dual-chamber pacing, partial excision of the myocardial septum, or an implantable defibrillator. Patients should avoid intense athletic competition and training.

UCV *IM1.7*

RESTRICTIVE CARDIOMYOPATHY

Characterized by **impaired diastolic filling** without significant contractile dysfunction. Caused by infiltrative disease (sarcoidosis, amyloidosis) or by scarring and fibrosis (endomyocardial fibrosis or radiation).

History/PE

Signs/symptoms of both left and right heart failure occur, but right heart symptoms (JVD, edema, and ascites) often predominate.

Evaluation

Differentiate from **constrictive pericarditis** because constrictive pericarditis is treatable. CT or MRI will show thickened pericardium in pericarditis. Biopsy is diagnostic.

Treatment

Treat the underlying cause and heart failure symptomatically (sodium restriction, diuretics for fluid overload).

PERICARDITIS

Inflammation of the pericardial sac, often with an effusion. Causes include viral infection, TB infection, SLE, uremia, drugs, and neoplasms. Pericarditis may also occur after MI, open heart surgery, or radiotherapy.

History

Patients may present with **pleuritic chest pain,** dyspnea, cough, and **fever.** Pain is often **positional** in nature, i.e., it worsens when the patient is supine and is relieved when the patient leans forward or with shallow breathing.

PE

Pericardial **friction rub** on auscultation (best heard with the patient leaning forward). In tamponade, **elevated CVP** and/or **pulsus paradoxus** (a fall in systolic BP > 10 mmHg on inspiration) may be seen.

Differential

Cardiac tamponade, heart failure, MI/angina, pneumonia, pneumothorax.

Evaluation

Obtain CXR, echocardiogram, and tests to rule out systemic causes. **Low-voltage, diffuse ST-segment elevation** or PR-segment depression on EKG (Figure 2.1–6) suggests the diagnosis. A pericardial effusion on echocardiography supports the diagnosis.

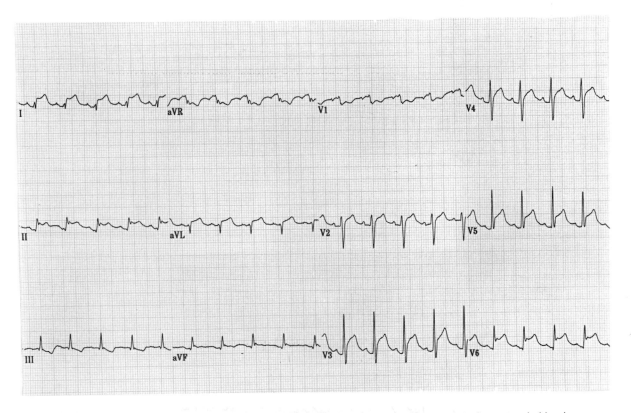

FIGURE 2.1–6. Pericarditis. There is characteristic ST elevation in all leads and PR depression in the precordial leads. (Reproduced, with permission, from Stobo J, *The Principles and Practice of Medicine*, 23rd ed., Stamford, CT: Appleton & Lange, 1996: p. 85, Fig. 1–10–1.)

Treatment

- Treat the underlying cause, e.g., **steroids**/immunosuppressants for SLE and aspirin/**NSAIDs** for viral pericarditis.
- Small effusions can be followed.
- If tamponade or a large effusion is present, **pericardiocentesis** is indicated with continuous drainage if necessary.

UCV *IM1.12*

CARDIAC TAMPONADE

Fluid in the pericardial sac resulting in compromised ventricular filling and decreased cardiac output. Cardiac tamponade is more closely related to the rate of fluid formation than to the size of the effusion. Risk factors include pericarditis and trauma (commonly stab wounds medial to the left nipple).

History

Patients present with severe chest pain, fatigue, dyspnea, tachycardia, and tachypnea that can rapidly lead to shock and death.

exudation: serum fibrin wbc from blood → into lesion or Inf. area

Tamponade should be suspected in any hemodynamically unstable patient who does not respond to initial resuscitative measures.

PE

cardiovascular pressure

Physical exam may reveal **Beck's triad** of **hypotension, distant heart sounds, and distended neck veins** (elevated CVP). Other common symptoms include a narrow pulse pressure, tachypnea, tachycardia, **pulsus paradoxus** (≥ 10 mmHg drop in BP with inspiration), and **Kussmaul's sign** (elevated CVP on inspiration).

Differential

Severe MI, tension pneumothorax.

Evaluation

Obtain an immediate **echocardiogram** if time permits. CXR may demonstrate an enlarged, globular heart. EKG may show decreased amplitude.

Treatment

Treat with urgent **pericardiocentesis** (the aspirate will be **nonclotting** blood); a pericardial window may be required. **Volume expansion** with aggressive IV fluids is also helpful.

UCV *EM.3*

ENDOCARDITIS

Inflammation of a heart valve, usually secondary to bacterial or other infectious causes. Risk factors include a history of rheumatic heart disease or **valvular heart disease** (including MVP), IV drug use, immunosuppression, and the presence of a **prosthetic heart valve.** Subacute bacterial endocarditis (SBE) is most commonly caused by **viridans streptococci,** while acute bacterial endocarditis (ABE) is most commonly caused by more virulent organisms such as *Staphylococcus aureus* (especially in IV drug users), *Streptococcus pneumoniae,* and *Streptococcus pyogenes* (see Table 2.1–4).

History

Endocarditis is a common cause of FUO.

In ABE, patients present rapidly with **high fever** and shaking chills. SBE is more insidious, presenting with low-grade fever that may last for weeks together with cough, shortness of breath, and/or **systemic symptoms** (weakness, fatigue, malaise). In a patient with a history of **valvular disease** or **IV drug use,** fever alone should raise suspicion of this diagnosis. Endocarditis is an intravascular infection that can seed other organs, so look for signs of lung, joint, and neurologic disease.

PE

Murmur (often regurgitant), **fever,** and/or joint tenderness. Small, tender nodules on finger and toe pads **(Osler's nodes),** small, peripheral hemorrhages *→palm* **(Janeway lesions),** subungual petechiae **(splinter hemorrhages),** and retinal *sole* hemorrhages **(Roth's spots)** may also be found. Endocarditis is usually left-

TABLE 2.1–4. Causes of Endocarditis

Acute	Subacute
Staphylococcus aureus (IVDA)	Streptococcus viridans
Streptococcus pneumoniae	Enterococcus
Neisseria gonorrhoeae	Staphylococcus epidermidis
strep - pyogenes	Fungi

Marantic	HACEK (culture-negative)	SLE
Cancer (mets seed valves)	*Haemophilus parainfluenzae*	Libman–Sacks
—poor prognosis; emboli	*Actinobacillus*	(autoantibody
→ cerebral infarcts	*Cardiobacterium*	to valve)
	Eikenella	
	Kingella	

sided (mitral, aortic) unless patients have a history of IV drug use, in which case it is more commonly right-sided. *Tricuspid*

Differential

Osteomyelitis, abscess, pneumonia, rheumatic fever, joint infection, prostatitis in males, STDs in females, and other causes of FUO.

Evaluation

Obtain at least **three sets of blood cultures** separated in time and location; multiple positive blood cultures revealing the same pathogen are considered strong evidence of bacterial endocarditis. Echocardiography can be used to look for vegetations, but a negative echo does not rule out the diagnosis. CXR may reveal **septic emboli** in right-sided endocarditis. Elevated ESR is common.

Treatment

- Treat empirically with **long-term antibiotic therapy,** usually for 28 days, with therapy initially given to cover gram-positive bugs and then tailored to specific organisms found on culture. Regimens with 14-day treatments include 14 days of an antistaphylococcal penicillin (e.g., nafcillin), with an aminoglycoside (e.g., gentamicin) added for the first five days for "augmentation."
- Always monitor for recurrence or relapse; treat relapses with longer courses of antibiotics.
- Give **antibiotic prophylaxis** (e.g., amoxicillin or erythromycin) **before dental work,** as patients now have valvular disease.
- Perform **valve replacement** in cases of worsening valvular function, systemic embolization, abscess formation, or development of conduction disturbances.

UCV IM1.8, IM2.1, 2

A sequela of **pharyngeal streptococcal infection.** Rheumatic fever is a systemic immune process that may result in rheumatic heart disease.

History/PE

- **Acute rheumatic fever:** Diagnosis is based on Jones criteria, which are divided into major and minor. Two major criteria or one major and two minor criteria are required for diagnosis. **Major criteria** include migratory polyarthritis, carditis (pericarditis, myocarditis), erythema marginatum, subcutaneous nodules, and chorea (Sydenham's). **Minor criteria** include fever, polyarthralgias, increased ESR, a history of rheumatic fever, antecedent strep infection, and a prolonged PR interval.
- **Rheumatic heart disease:** Valvular abnormalities secondary to rheumatic fever; most often **mitral stenosis** but can be mitral + aortic or mitral + aortic + tricuspid.

Differential

RA, SLE, endocarditis, osteomyelitis, Lyme disease, sickle cell disease.

Evaluation

antistreptolysin O

Elevated ESR and **positive ASO** antibody titers are seen. For rheumatic heart disease, perform echocardiography to assess valvular function.

Treatment

Bed rest, **salicylates, penicillin** or erythromycin; steroids if other treatments are not successful. The complications of this disease are the primary reason to treat streptococcal pharyngeal infections. Administer **antimicrobial prophylaxis** with amoxicillin (erythromycin if the patient is allergic to penicillin) during **medical/dental** procedures. Surgical replacement/repair of diseased valves may be required.

UCV *IM1.13, Ped.25*

Primary hypertension (high blood pressure due to an unidentified cause) **accounts for > 95% of all cases of hypertension.** High blood pressure is usually defined as a sustained increase in systolic BP > 140 and/or a diastolic BP > 90, typically based on **three readings separated in time** (Table 2.1–5). Risk factors for primary hypertension include a **family history** of hypertension or heart disease, a **high-sodium diet, smoking, obesity,** and **advanced age;** blacks are affected more frequently than whites.

History

Asymptomatic until complications develop.

Rheumatic fever, major criteria—

Joints (polyarthritis)
♡-heart (carditis)
Nodules (subcutaneous)
Erythema marginatum
Sydenham's chorea

Treat streptococcal pharyngeal infections to prevent rheumatic heart disease.

Primary (essential) hypertension is the most common cause of high blood pressure.

HIGH-YIELD FACTS

Cardiovascular

TABLE 2.1–5. Classification and Interpretation of Blood Pressure Measurements*

Category**	Systolic Blood Pressure (mmHg)	Diastolic Blood Pressure (mmHg)	Follow-up Recommended
Normal	< 130	< 85	Recheck in two years.
High normal	130–139	85–89	Recheck in one year.***
Hypertension			
Stage 1 (mild)	140–159	90–99	Confirm within two months.
Stage 2 (moderate)	160–179	100–109	Evaluate or refer within one month.
Stage 3 (severe)	180–209	110–119	Evaluate or refer within one week.
Stage 4 (very severe)	≥ 210	≥ 120	Evaluate or refer immediately.

* Reproduced from the sixth report of the Joint National Committee on Detection, Education, and Treatment of High Blood Pressure (JNCVI), *Arch Intern Med* 157:243, 1997.
** When systolic and diastolic pressures fall into different categories, the higher category should be selected to classify the individual's blood pressure.
*** Consider offering counseling about lifestyle modifications.

PE

Systolic BP > 140 and/or **diastolic BP > 90,** retinal changes (copper wires, AV nicking; see Clinical Image, plate 6), and sometimes a systolic click and/or loud S2. An S4 may also be auscultated.

Differential

Secondary hypertension (below), NSAIDs, pregnancy.

Evaluation

Perform tests for secondary causes if the patient's clinical picture is consistent with any type of secondary hypertension as well as periodic tests for complications of hypertension (EKG, BUN/creatinine).

Treatment

Begin with diet/lifestyle modification. **Diuretics** (inexpensive and particularly effective in African Americans) and **beta-blockers** (beneficial for patients with CAD) are good first-line agents. Other options are noted in Table 2.1–6.

Complications

CAD, kidney disease, **cerebrovascular disease,** aortic aneurysm, aortic dissection, LVH, CHF.

The best way to prevent stroke is to control hypertension.

TABLE 2.1–6. Selection of Antihypertensive Medications

	More Effective or Appropriate	Less Effective or Contraindicated
Coexisting conditions		
Prior MI	Beta-blocker, ACE inhibitor	Calcium channel blocker (with reduced ejection fraction)
Renal Dz	_Ace Inh._	
Angina pectoris	Beta-blocker, calcium channel blocker	Vasodilator (without concomitant beta-blocker)
CHF	Diuretic, ACE inhibitor, beta-blocker*	Calcium channel blocker (not amlodipine)
Diabetes mellitus	ACE inhibitor	Beta-blocker (if hypoglycemia occurs), diuretic (if glucose is high in type II diabetes)
Peripheral vascular disease		Beta-blocker (if there is rest pain or severe claudication)
Bronchospasm		Beta-blocker
BPH	Alpha-blocker	
Migraine	Beta-blocker, calcium channel blocker	
Gout		Diuretic
Osteoporosis	Thiazide diuretic	
Pregnancy (current or potential)	Beta-blocker (considerable experience with labetalol; atenolol associated with low birth weight), calcium channel blocker, methyldopa, hydralazine	ACE inhibitor
Demographic factors		
Older patients	Diuretic (especially for isolated systolic hypertension)	ACE inhibitor
Blacks	Calcium channel blocker, diuretic	ACE inhibitor, beta-blocker
Young whites	Beta-blocker, ACE inhibitor	

*Growing evidence supports a role for beta-blockers in some patients with CHF, but these drugs may cause acute deterioration and require careful consideration of the other comorbid conditions.

High blood pressure that is due to an **identifiable** organic cause. **Surgically correctable** causes of hypertension, which account for < 5% of cases of hypertension, include renal artery stenosis (most common), coarctation of the aorta, pheochromocytoma, Conn's syndrome (primary hyperaldosteronism), Cushing's syndrome, unilateral renal parenchymal disease, hyperthyroidism, and hyperparathyroidism.

- **Renal disease:** Any primary renal disease can lead to high blood pressure. **ACE inhibitors** will treat the hypertension and slow the progression of renal disease.
- **Renal artery stenosis:** Especially common in patients < 25 years old as well as in patients > 50 years old with recent-onset hypertension. Etiologies include **fibromuscular dysplasia** (usually seen in **younger** patients) and **atherosclerosis** (more common in older patients). Diagnosis can be made by arteriography as well as by renal vein renin ratio (RVRR). Screening is performed with the captopril provocation test or nuclear perfusion scan. Treat with **angioplasty** and **stenting** if possible; also consider ACE inhibitors as adjunctive or temporary therapy in unilateral disease **(in bilateral disease, ACE inhibitors can accelerate kidney failure by preferential vasodilation of the efferent arteriole).** Surgery is a secondary option if angioplasty is not effective or feasible. *IM2.34*
- **Oral contraceptive use:** Common in women > 35 years old, obese women, and those with long-standing OCP use. Discontinue the OCP (it can take time to see an effect).
- **Pheochromocytoma:** Classically associated with **episodic hypertension, diaphoresis, and headache.** Patients are often misdiagnosed with anxiety disorder. Look for this in patients who are **young,** have severe and/or **paroxysmal symptoms,** or have a history of endocrine tumors (MEN IIA and IIB syndromes). Pheochromocytoma is diagnosed by **elevated** 24-hour **urinary catecholamines** and/or **VMA** (vanillylmandelic acid) or by the clonidine suppression test. Imaging studies (CT, MRI) or scintigraphy (MIBG scan) can also be used for diagnosis. Treatment consists of **surgical resection** (pretreat with alpha- and beta-blockers). *[handwritten: primary tumor of adrenal gland] [handwritten: suprarenal mass]*
- **Primary hyperaldostonerism:** Due to excess aldosterone (Conn's syndrome) or glucocorticoid production (Cushing's syndrome). Primary hyperaldosteronism usually stems from an **adrenal adenoma,** although the lesion can be malignant. Screen for hyperaldosteronism by looking for **hypokalemia,** elevated urinary potassium, and **elevated plasma/urine aldosterone.** Screen for Cushing's syndrome by physical exam (e.g., **central obesity,** hirsutism, "buffalo hump," **striae**) and by testing for **glucose intolerance;** think of iatrogenesis if the patient is on chronic steroid therapy. *[handwritten: Conn's syndrome]*

Hypertensive urgency consists of an asymptomatic or moderately symptomatic (headache, chest pain, syncope) BP > 200/120. Hypertensive emergency includes **symptoms** and **signs of** impending **end-organ damage.** Signs can include acute renal failure or **hematuria, altered mental status** or other evidence of neurologic disease, intracranial hemorrhage (see Clinical Images, p. 6), ophthalmologic findings suggesting retinal damage (**papilledema,** vascular changes), unstable angina/MI, or pulmonary edema. "Malig-

> **Causes of secondary hypertension—**
>
> **CHAPS**
> **C**ushing's syndrome
> **H**yperaldosteronism
> **A**ortic coarctation
> **P**heochromocytoma
> **S**tenosis of renal arteries

nant hypertension" is defined as progressive **renal failure** and/or **encephalopathy** with papilledema.

Evaluation

Cardiovascular, neurologic, ophthalmologic, and abdominal exams. Obtain head and/or abdominal CT, UA, BUN/creatinine, CBC, and electrolytes to assess the extent of end-organ damage.

Treatment

- **Hypertensive urgency:** To prevent cerebral hypoperfusion or coronary insufficiency, BP should be brought down slowly (over a few hours) with **oral agents** such as beta-blockers, clonidine, and ACE inhibitors. Avoid short-acting calcium channel blockers. If oral therapy is not sufficient, try IV agents (see below).
- **Hypertensive emergency:** Use **IV agents** to reduce BP by approximately 25% **within one hour.** Treat with **nitroprusside** (very potent; use carefully), nitroglycerin, labetalol, nicardipine, and hydralazine. Add a **diuretic** if there is evidence of pulmonary edema/fluid overload.

UCV EM.5

CARDIAC STRESS TESTING

Exercise or pharmacologic testing aimed at **increasing cardiac workload** to assess myocardial perfusion, cardiac ischemia, and the risk of subsequent MI. Cardiac stress testing should be performed on patients with suspected or known CAD, patients who present with chest pain for the first time, and those with progressively worsening symptoms. If patients can achieve a peak heart rate that is 85% of predicted for age/sex and have an interpretable EKG (e.g., no LBBB), an exercise stress test is preferred (with **nuclear imaging** to look for myocardial **perfusion defects**). If a patient cannot achieve sufficient physical activity (e.g., disabled or older patients), a **pharmacologic** stress test such as adenosine, Persantine thallium scan, or dobutamine echocardiogram is commonly performed.

Signs of active ischemia during stress testing include angina, ST-segment changes on EKG, or decreased BP. A premature rise in heart rate to > 90% of the patient's predicted heart rate (predicted maximum heart rate = 220 – age) is indicative of **cardiac deconditioning** secondary to a sedentary lifestyle. Patients whose stress tests reveal reversible myocardial ischemia should have **cardiac catheterization** if they are appropriate candidates for PTCA or CABG. Exercise stress testing is fairly sensitive but not perfect, so a negative test does not rule out disease, especially if the patient has classic symptoms of CAD.

HYPERCHOLESTEROLEMIA

Elevated blood cholesterol increases the incidence of coronary heart disease.

History/PE

Most patients with hypercholesterolemia have **no specific signs or symptoms.** Only in patients with extremely elevated triglycerides or LDL levels are there clinical manifestations. Xanthomas (eruptive and/or tendinous), xanthelasmas, and lipemia retinalis (creamy appearance of retinal vessels) can be seen in association with such high levels and are usually related to a familial hypercholesterolemia.

Etiologies

Obesity, diabetes mellitus, alcoholism, hypothyroidism, nephrotic syndrome, hepatic disease, Cushing's disease, OCP use, diuretic use, and familial hypercholesterolemia.

Evaluation

All men > 35 and womem > 45 should be screened, unless there is a strong family history. If normal blood levels are found, patients should be reevaluated every five years. **Risk factors for CAD include a family history of premature CAD, hypertension, male gender, smoking, HDL < 35, and diabetes.** Males > age 45 and women > age 55 are at greater risk. Guidelines are as follows:

- **Total cholesterol < 200 (mg/dL):** Retest in five years.
- **Total cholesterol > 200:** Test lipid fractions; treat on the basis of LDL.
- **LDL 130–159:** Borderline risk. Treat with dietary modification and exercise.
- **LDL > 130 + CAD, LDL > 160 with two risk factors, or LDL > 190:** High risk. Begin medical therapy.
- **Triglycerides < 200 mg/dL:** Normal.

Treatment

- **Diet:** A modest (10–15%) reduction in cholesterol results in a 15–30% reduction in cardiovascular events.
- **HMG-CoA reductase inhibitors ("statins"):** The most effective cholesterol-lowering drugs. May cause LFT abnormalities, warfarin potentiation, and/or myositis.
- **Bile acid sequestrants (cholestyramine):** May interfere with the absorption of other drugs (digoxin, warfarin, thiazides). Constipation and gas are common.
- **Niacin:** Cheap and effective. Compliance is a problem because of facial flushing and pruritic side effects. Aspirin can be used to ameliorate the flushing.

AORTIC ANEURYSM

Most commonly secondary to **atherosclerosis** (versus aortic dissection, which is most commonly due to hypertension). Most aortic aneurysms are abdominal, and > 90% originate below the renal arteries. Risk factors include **hypertension,** other vascular disease (atherosclerosis), family history, and tobacco use; **males** are affected more frequently than females, and risk increases with age.

History

Usually **asymptomatic** and discovered coincidentally on physical exam or on a radiologic study. However, a ruptured aneurysm can cause hypotension as well as severe, tearing abdominal pain radiating to the back. Many individuals with rupture die before they arrive at the hospital.

PE

Pulsatile abdominal mass, abdominal bruits, hypotension (if ruptured).

Differential

Pancreatitis/pseudocyst, neoplasms (pancreatic, colonic, other), orthopedic causes of back pain, appendicitis, gallbladder disease.

Evaluation

Abdominal ultrasound for diagnosis or to follow an aneurysm over time, although CT determines the precise anatomy and may be helpful as an adjunct.

Treatment

- In asymptomatic patients, **monitoring** is appropriate for lesions < 5 cm. If the lesion is **> 5 cm (abdominal) or > 6 cm (thoracic) or is enlarging rapidly, surgical repair** is indicated.
- Emergent surgery is indicated for symptomatic or ruptured aneurysms.

UCV *EM.15*

AORTIC DISSECTION

Occurs when an intimal tear allows blood to enter the aortic media, splitting the medial lamellae and causing a **second "false" lumen** to form. Stanford *proximal* **type A** dissections involve the ascending aorta; **type B** are distal to the left subclavian artery. Risk factors include **hypertension,** trauma, coarctation of the aorta, syphilis, Ehlers–Danlos syndrome, and **Marfan's syndrome.**

History/PE *Interscapular back pain*

Patients present with acute-onset, severe **"tearing"** or **"ripping" chest pain** or back pain. Occlusion of aortic branch vessels may lead to asymmetric or decreased peripheral pulses, syncope, stroke, MI, or paraplegia. Aortic regurgitation with diastolic murmur may occur in type A dissection. Shock may develop as the condition worsens.

Patients classically present with sudden onset of tearing chest pain radiating to the back and with asymmetric upper extremity blood pressures.

Differential

MI, pulmonary embolus, angina, thoracic aortic aneurysm, esophageal rupture.

Evaluation

CXR often demonstrates a **widened superior mediastinum.** Diagnosis can be made via **CT with IV contrast,** transesophageal echocardiography, MRI/MRA, or **angiography (the gold standard).** An intimal flap or pseudolumen may be seen. Workup should also include EKG (look for LVH and ischemic changes).

Treatment

- Stabilize the patient by treating high or low blood pressure. Treat high blood pressure with **IV nitrates and beta-blockers.** Pressure may bottom out with nitrates (e.g., sublingual nitroglycerin), so exercise caution.
- Type A dissections require **emergent surgery.** Consider medical management in patients with type B dissections.

UCV EM.1

embolization in an extremity

PERIPHERAL VASCULAR DISEASE (PVD)

Defined as occlusion of blood supply to the extremities by atherosclerotic plaques. Clinical manifestations depend on the vessel involved, the extent and rapidity of obstruction, and the presence of collateral blood flow. The lower extremities are most commonly affected.

History/PE

Patients initially present with **intermittent claudication** (reproducible leg pain that occurs with walking and is always relieved with rest). In worsening disease, there is progression to rest pain and to ischemia that affects the distal aspects of the extremities. A painful, cold, and numb foot is characteristic of severe ischemia. Dorsal foot ulcerations may also develop.

- In aortoiliac disease, claudication is present and femoral pulses are absent. **Impotence is** common in males.
- In femoropopliteal disease, claudication is present in the calves and pulses below the femoral are absent.
- In patients with small vessel disease, foot pulses are absent.
- Acute ischemia is most often caused by **embolization from the heart.** Acute occlusions commonly occur at bifurcations distal to the last palpable pulse.
- With severe chronic ischemia, lack of blood perfusion results in muscle atrophy, pallor, cyanotic discoloration, hair loss, and gangrene/necrosis.

Differential

stroke / heart attack
pul. embolism

Thromboangiitis obliterans, Raynaud's phenomenon, arterial embolism, acrocyanosis, erythromelalgia.

Evaluation

Careful **palpation of pulses and auscultation for bruits** are necessary. Measurement of the ankle and brachial systolic BP **(ankle–brachial index [ABI])** can provide objective evidence of atherosclerotic changes (rest pain occurs with ABIs < 0.4). **Doppler ultrasound** can help identify stenosis and occlusion; doppler readings of ankle systolic pressure that are > 90% of brachial readings are normal. Arteriography and digital subtraction angiography are necessary for surgical evaluation.

Treatment

Exercise (as tolerated) is important to help develop collateral circulation. Tobacco use must be eliminated. Hygiene and foot care must be carefully followed. Control of underlying causes (diabetes) is also crucial. **Pentoxifylline,** calcium antagonists, and thromboxane inhibitors may improve symptoms. PTCA has a variable success rate that is dependent on the area of occlusion. Surgery (arterial bypass) or amputation can be employed when conservative treatment fails.

EKG shows Wenckebach pattern of heart block: possible offending drugs?	Beta-blockers, digoxin, Ca²⁺ channel blockers
Patient develops complete heart block following MI treatment.	Atropine (inferior MI)
Eight surgically correctable causes of hypertension.	Renal artery stenosis, coarctation of the aorta, pheochromocytoma, Conn's syndrome, Cushing's syndrome, unilateral venous parenchymal disease, hyperthyroidism, hyperparathyroidism
Patient treated for hypercholesterolemia experiences flushing and pruritus; which drug was used?	Niacin
Treatments for atrial fibrillation.	Anticoagulation, rate control, cardioversion
Treatment for ventricular fibrillation.	Immediate cardioversion
Autoimmune complication occurring 2–4 weeks post-MI.	Dressler's syndrome: fever, pericarditis, increased ESR
Pharmacologic causes of dilated cardiomyopathy.	Cocaine, doxorubicin
IV drug user with JVD, holosystolic murmur in left sternal border. Treatment?	Treat any existing left-sided heart failure; replace tricuspid valve
Diagnostic test for hypertrophic cardiomyopathy.	Echocardiogram showing thickened LV wall and outflow obstruction
Fall in systolic BP > 10 mmHg with inspiration.	Pulsus paradoxus, seen in cardiac tamponade
Classic EKG findings in pericarditis.	Low-voltage, diffuse ST-segment elevation
Major criteria for rheumatic fever.	Polyarthritis, carditis, subcutaneous nodules, erythema marginatum, Sydenham's chorea
Pulsatile abdominal mass and bruit; evaluation?	Abdominal ultrasound
Indications for surgical repair of abdominal aneurysm.	> 5 cm, rapidly enlarging, symptomatic, or ruptured
Beck's triad for cardiac tamponade.	Hypotension, distant heart sounds, and JVD

HIGH-YIELD FACTS

Cardiovascular

77

Questions 1, 2, and 5: Reproduced, with permission, from Berk SL, *PreTest: Medicine*, 9th ed., New York: McGraw-Hill, 2001.
Questions 3 and 4: Reproduced, with permission, from Reteguiz J, *PreTest: Physical Diagnosis*, 4th ed., New York: McGraw-Hill, 2001.

Questions

1. A 36-year-old white female nurse comes to the ER due to a sensation of fast heart rate, slight dizziness, and vague chest fullness. The following rhythm strip is obtained which shows

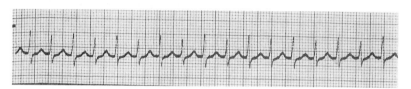

   a. Atrial fibrillation
   b. Atrial flutter
   c. Supraventricular tachycardia ‒ *Atrial Tachycardia*
   d. Ventricular tachycardia

2. The initial therapy of choice in this stable patient is
   a. Adenosine 6 mg rapid IV bolus
   b. Verapamil 2.5 to 5 mg IV over 1 to 2 minutes
   c. Diltiazem 0.25 mg/kg IV over 2 minutes
   d. Digoxin 0.5 mg IV slowly
   e. Lidocaine 1.5 mg/kg IV bolus
   f. Electrical cardioversion at 50 joules

3. A 71-year-old man complains of occasional lower back pain. His blood pressure is 150/85 mm Hg and his pulse is 80/min. Cardiac examination reveals an S4 gallop. Abdominal examination reveals a pulsatile mass approximately 5.0 cm in diameter palpable in the epigastric area. Peripheral pulses are normal. Which of the following is the most likely diagnosis?
   a. Abdominal aortic aneurysm
   b. Cancer of the proximal colon
   c. Peptic ulcer disease
   d. Chronic pancreatitis
   e. Lipoma of the abdominal wall

4. A 47-year-old man has been at home recovering from an anterior myocardial infarction that occurred 10 days ago. He presents to your office complaining of persistent chest pain that is worse on inspiration and that is different from his "heart attack" pain. The pain radiates to both clavicles. The pain is worse when the patient is lying down and improves with sitting up and leaning forward. The patient has a temperature of 101.2°F and a normal blood pressure. Heart auscultation reveals a pericardial rub. Lung examination is positive for dullness and diminished breath sounds at the right base. Chest radiograph reveals a small right-sided pleural effusion. Laboratory data reveal that the patient has a mild leukocytosis and an increased erythrocyte sedimentation rate (ESR). Which of the following is the most likely diagnosis?

Dressler's Syndrome

fever pericarditis

a. Extension of the myocardial infarction
b. Unstable angina
c. Prinzmetal's angina
d. Pulmonary embolus
e. Postmyocardial infarction syndrome *Dressler*

5. A 55-year-old obese woman develops pressure-like substernal chest pain of one-hour duration. Her EKG is shown below. The most likely diagnosis is

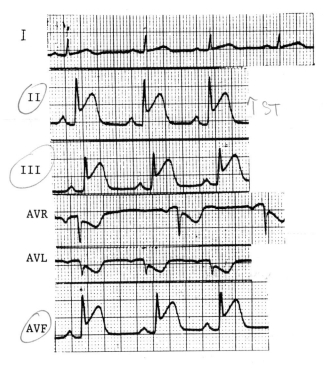

a. Costochondritis
b. Acute anterior myocardial infarction
c. Acute inferior myocardial infarction   *lead II, III and AVF*
d. Pericarditis
e. Esophageal reflux
f. Cholecystitis

Answers

1. **The answer is c.** Paroxysmal supraventricular tachycardia typically displays a narrow QRS complex without clearly discernible P waves, with rate in the 160 to 190 range. The rate is faster in atrial flutter. Atrial fibrillation would show an irregularly irregular rate. Wide QRS complexes would be expected in ventricular tachycardia.

2. **The answer is a.** Adenosine is the drug of choice for supraventricular tachycardia, with verapamil the next alternative. Adenosine has an excellent safety profile, making it the preferred drug for supraventricular tachycardia.

3. **The answer is a. Abdominal aortic aneurysms (AAAs)** are usually due to atherosclerosis and > 90% originate below the renal arteries. The aneurysms are typically asymptomatic until they rupture, but patients may complain of lower back or hypogastric pain. The aneurysms may be associated with emboli to the feet and kidneys. Normal diameter of the aorta is < 2 cm. **When the diameter of the AAA is > 4.5 cm, repair is generally suggested.** Risk of rupture is 1–2% over 5 years when the AAA is < 5 cm, but 20–40% when the AAA reaches 6 cm in diameter. The best method of evaluating the AAA is by **ultrasound or CT scan.**

4. **The answer is e.** Postmyocardial infarction syndrome or **Dressler syndrome** is an autoimmune complication of myocardial infarction. It occurs from three days to six weeks after the infarction and usually responds quickly to salicylates. The fever, pericarditis, leukocytosis, elevated ESR, and pleural effusion are all part of the autoimmune process.

5. **The answer is c.** The EKG shows ST-segment elevation in inferior leads II, III, and aVF with reciprocal ST-depression in aVL, consistent with an acute inferior MI. An anterior MI would give ST-segment elevation in the precordial leads. Pericarditis classically gives pleuritic chest pain and diffuse ST-segment elevation (except aVR) on EKG. Costochondritis, esophageal reflux, cholecystitis, and duodenal ulcer disease can all cause the symptoms of substernal chest pain, but not these EKG findings.

HIGH-YIELD FACTS

Cardiovascular

Dermatology

A delayed (type IV—cell-mediated) hypersensitivity reaction in the form of a skin rash that develops from contact with a substance to which the patient has **previously been sensitized.** Common offending agents include **poison ivy, poison oak, nickel,** perfumes, **soaps** and detergents, and **cosmetics.**

History

Patients most commonly complain of **pruritus and rash.** Rarely they may present with edema, fever, lymphadenopathy, and generalized malaise.

PE

Erythematous, weepy, crusted patches, plaques, or **papulovesicles** grouped in **linear arrays** or **geometric shapes** with sharp angles and straight borders (Figure 2.2–1). Characteristic locations are where makeup, clothing, perfume, jewelry, and plants come into contact with the skin.

Differential

Impetigo, herpes simplex, herpes zoster, seborrheic dermatitis, eczema.

Evaluation

Diagnosis is based on **clinical impression** and, if necessary, on skin patch testing.

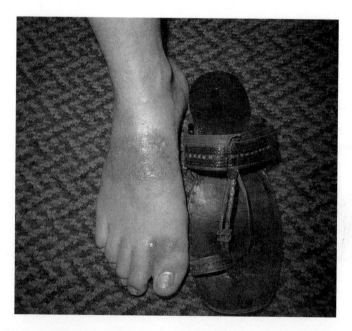

FIGURE 2.2–1. Contact dermatitis. Erythematous papules, vesicles, and serous weeping localized to areas of contact with the offending agent are characteristic. (Reproduced, with permission, from Hurwitz RM, *Pathology of the Skin: Atlas of Clinical–Pathological Correlation,* 2nd ed., Stamford, CT: Appleton & Lange, 1998: p. 3, Fig. 1–5.)

Treatment

- **Mild cases:** **Cool compresses** or oatmeal preparation; apply topical steroids 3–4 times a day to reduce pruritus.
- **Severe cases:** **Systemic corticosteroids** may be required; use antihistamines for relief of itching.

SEBORRHEIC DERMATITIS

Chronic, superficial inflammatory disorder commonly involving the face; thought to be a reaction to *Pityrosporum* yeast. The rash is most common during the **neonatal** and **postpubertal** periods.

History

Patients present with mild to moderate **pruritus.**

PE

Yellowish, greasy, and **erythematous scaling patches and plaques** of the **scalp, ears,** and **face.** In severe cases, the rash may extend to the chest, back, and intertriginous areas. Scaling of the scalp (**"cradle cap"**) may be present.

Differential

Fungal infection, allergic contact dermatitis, psoriasis, immune deficiencies (e.g., histiocytosis X).

Evaluation

Diagnosis is based on **clinical suspicion.** KOH preparation can rule out **fungal infection.** A biopsy is rarely necessary except in atypical presentations.

Treatment

- **Therapy for the face, body, and intertriginous areas:** 1% hydrocortisone or stronger BID depending on the thickness of the affected skin. In some cases a 2% ketoconazole cream can be used as a substitute for, or in conjunction with, topical steroids. Mild tar cream can be used as an adjunct to topical steroids. *Topical steroid*
- **Therapy for the scalp:** Medicated shampoos with selenium sulfide, tar, or zinc pyrithione (Selsun or Head and Shoulders) 2–3 times a week. In more severe cases, topical steroids may be used.

An idiopathic inflammatory disorder that results in **epidermal hyperproliferation.**

History

Pruritus may be present. Pain, tenderness, and joint stiffness may occur with **psoriatic arthritis** (characterized by involvement of the DIP joints). **Generalized toxicity,** fever, and malaise may occur with the generalized pustular form.

PE

Dark **red plaques with silvery-white scales** and **sharp margins** (Figure 2.2–2). Lesions are classically found over **areas of extension.** Characteristic nail findings include **nail pitting,** "oil spots," and **onycholysis** (lifting of the nail plate).

Differential

SLE (possibly without systemic symptoms), syphilis, allergic contact dermatitis, fungal infections, seborrheic dermatitis, cutaneous T-cell lymphoma, eczema.

Evaluation

Diagnosis is based on the **gross appearance** and pattern of distribution of the lesions. **Skin biopsy** shows a thickened epidermis with an absent granular cell layer and preservation of the nuclei within the hyperkeratotic stratum corneum. Neutrophils in the stratum corneum are classic. Blood tests may show elevated uric acid levels, increased ESR, and mild anemia.

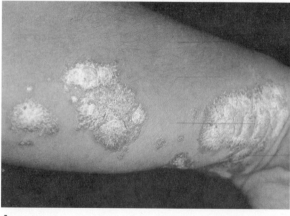
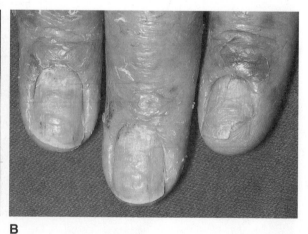

A   B

FIGURE 2.2–2. Psoriasis. (A) Skin changes. The classic sharply demarcated plaques with silvery scales are commonly located on extensor surfaces (e.g., elbows, knees). These plaques are fully developed. (B) Nail changes. Note the pitting, onycholysis, and "oil spots." (Reproduced, with permission, from Hurwitz RM, *Pathology of the Skin: Atlas of Clinical–Pathological Correlation*, 2nd ed., Stamford, CT: Appleton & Lange, 1998: p. 18, Fig. 1–64, p. 15, Fig. 1–55.)

Treatment

- **Mild to moderate disease: Topical steroids,** intralesional corticosteroid therapy, tars, anthralin, salicylic acid, tretinoin, 5-FU, topical antifungal agents, systemic antibiotics.
- **Severe or generalized psoriasis: Phototherapy,** PUVA, methotrexate, etretinate.

UCV *IM2.6*

PITYRIASIS ROSEA

A mild, idiopathic, self-limited cutaneous eruption seen primarily in children.

History

Patients present with mild to moderate pruritus.

PE

A diffuse eruption of round to **oval erythematous papules** and plaques covered with a fine "cigarette paper" white scale, with the distribution of the rash on the trunk following skin lines in a <u>**Christmas-tree pattern**</u> (Figure 2.2–3). A **herald patch**—a solitary patch 2–6 cm in diameter that precedes the rest of the rash—is pathognomonic.

A herald patch is pathognomonic for pityriasis rosea.

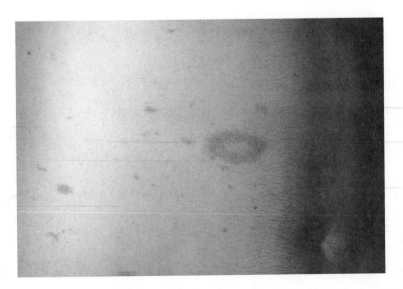

FIGURE 2.2–3. Pityriasis rosea. The round to oval erythematous plaques are often covered with a fine white scale ("cigarette paper") and are often found on the trunk and proximal extremities. The plaques are often preceded by a larger herald patch (arrow). (Reproduced, with permission, from Hurwitz RM, *Pathology of the Skin: Atlas of Clinical–Pathological Correlation,* 2nd ed., Stamford, CT: Appleton & Lange, 1998: p. 13, Fig. 1–42.)

Differential

Secondary syphilis, psoriasis, cutaneous T-cell lymphoma (parapsoriasis).

Evaluation

A **skin biopsy** is required if the lesions do not resolve in two months. A serologic test is indicated to rule out secondary syphilis.

Treatment

The lesions are **self-limited.** A mild topical steroid or talc may be used for relief of pruritus. Natural sunlight or daily UVB treatments may hasten healing.

ACTINIC KERATOSIS

A **premalignant lesion** resulting from **sun exposure** which can lead to squamous cell carcinoma. Actinic keratosis is also known as solar keratosis.

History

Lesions are usually **asymptomatic** unless they are irritated or inflamed.

PE

Physical exam reveals **discrete, rough, scaling patches** and papules 1–5 mm in diameter. Lesions usually have a poorly demarcated erythematous base with an area of rough, **white superficial scaling** and are generally found in sun-exposed areas of the body (Figure 2.2–4).

Differential

Squamous cell carcinoma, eczema.

Evaluation

Skin biopsy shows areas of **dysplastic squamous epithelium** (hyperkeratosis, with cells of the lower epidermis showing loss of polarity, pleomorphism, and hyperchromatic nuclei) **without invasion.**

Treatment

Treat with **topical 5-FU,** cryosurgery, curettage, and chemical peel. **Prevent with UVA/UVB sunscreens** and by avoiding prolonged and unnecessary sun exposure.

UCV *IM2.1*

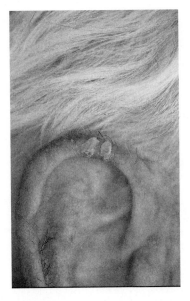

FIGURE 2.2–4. Actinic keratosis. The discrete patch has an erythematous base and rough white scale. Actinic keratosis is a premalignant lesion that may progress to squamous cell carcinoma. It is most commonly found in sun-exposed areas. (Reproduced, with permission, from Hurwitz RM, *Pathology of the Skin: Atlas of Clinical–Pathological Correlation,* 2nd ed., Stamford, CT: Appleton & Lange, 1998: p. 359, Fig. 31–3.)

SQUAMOUS CELL CARCINOMA

Risk factors include **exposure** to sun and ionizing radiation, actinic keratosis, immunosuppression, arsenic, and industrial carcinogens.

History

Lesions are usually slowly evolving and **asymptomatic;** occasionally, bleeding or pain may develop.

PE

Physical examination reveals small, red, **exophytic nodules** with varying degrees of scaling or crusting (Figure 2.2–5). Lesions are commonly found in **sun-exposed areas.** Lesions are usually found on the ears, cheeks, lower lip, and dorsum of the hands.

Differential

Basal cell carcinoma, warts, actinic keratosis.

Evaluation

Biopsy shows irregular masses of anaplastic epidermal cells proliferating down to the dermis.

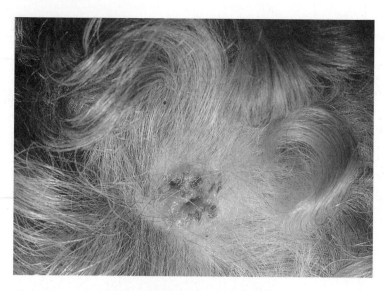

FIGURE 2.2–5. Squamous cell carcinoma. Note the crusting and ulceration of this erythematous plaque. Most lesions are exophytic nodules with erosion or ulceration. (Reproduced, with permission, from Hurwitz RM, *Pathology of the Skin: Atlas of Clinical–Pathological Correlation*, 2nd ed., Stamford, CT: Appleton & Lange, 1998: p. 360, Fig. 31–20.)

Treatment

Surgical excision is necessary for larger lesions and for those involving the periorbital, periauricular, perilabial, genital, and perigenital areas. **Mohs' micrographic surgery** (serial excisions with fresh-tissue microscopic examination to maximize cosmesis) may be performed for recurrent lesions and on areas of the face that are difficult to reconstruct, as well as for poorly differentiated tumors and those with ill-defined margins. **Radiation** may be necessary in cases where surgery is not a viable option. **Prevent with UVA/UVB sunscreens** and by avoiding prolonged and unnecessary sun exposure.

UCV *IM2.8*

BASAL CELL CARCINOMA

The **most common type of skin cancer.** Basal cell carcinoma is associated with excessive sun exposure and may take many different forms, including nodular, ulcerative, pigmented, and superficial.

History

Lesions are usually asymptomatic unless secondarily infected or inflamed or in advanced disease.

PE

Pearly-colored papule of variable size. The external surface is frequently covered with fine **telangiectasias** and appears **translucent** (Figure 2.2–6). Lesions may be found anywhere on the body but are most commonly found in sun-exposed areas.

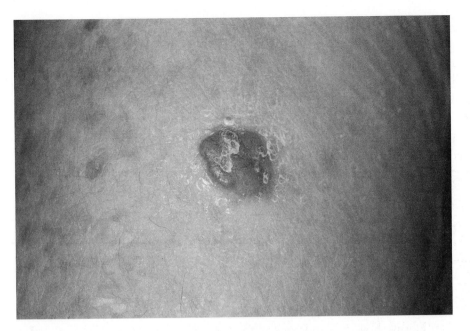

FIGURE 2.2–6. Basal cell carcinoma. Erythematous, fleshy, telangiectasic nodule with translucent surface. (Reproduced, with permission, from Hurwitz RM, *Pathology of the Skin: Atlas of Clinical–Pathological Correlation,* 2nd ed., Stamford, CT: Appleton & Lange, 1998: p. 362, Fig. 31–24.)

Differential

Squamous cell carcinoma, actinic keratosis, seborrheic keratosis.

Evaluation

Skin biopsy shows characteristic basophilic **palisading cells.**

Treatment

Therapy depends on the size and location of the tumor, the histologic type, the history of prior treatment, the underlying health of the patient, and cosmetic considerations. Options include curettage, surgical excision, Mohs' micrographic surgery, cryosurgery, and radiation. **Prevent with UVA/UVB sunscreens** and by avoiding prolonged and unnecessary sun exposure.

MELANOMA

An **aggressive** skin malignancy of melanocytic origin. Risk factors include sun exposure, fair skin, a positive family history (e.g., dysplastic nevus syndrome), xeroderma pigmentosum, a large number of nevi, and the presence of dysplastic nevi. Melanoma is the leading cause of death from skin disease.

History

Melanoma is usually **asymptomatic** until late in the disease process. Patients may present with pruritus and mild discomfort. **A pigmented skin lesion that has recently changed in size or appearance should raise concern.** Lesions may be seen on sun-exposed areas as well as on the plantar aspect of the feet.

PE

Lesions are characterized by the **ABCD**s of melanoma (see sidebar) and may occur anywhere on the body (Figure 2.2–7).

Differential

Nevi, seborrheic keratosis, freckles, pigmented basal cell carcinoma.

Evaluation

Skin biopsy shows **melanocytes with marked cellular atypia** (vacuolated cytoplasm, hyperchromatic nuclei with prominent nucleoli, and pleomorphism) and melanocytic invasion into the dermis.

Treatment

Surgical excision is the treatment of choice. In cases of metastases, lymph node dissection and **chemotherapy** are necessary. Advanced disease may not respond to therapy. The thickness of the melanoma **(depth of invasion)** is the most important prognostic factor.

UCV *Surg.4*

> **ABCDs of melanoma:**
>
> **A**symmetry
> **B**order irregularity
> **C**olor variation
> **D**iameter (large)

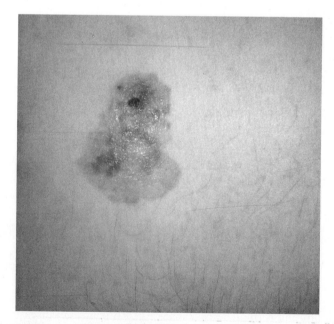

FIGURE 2.2–7. Melanoma. Note the **a**symmetry, **b**order irregularity, **c**olor variation, and large **d**iameter of this plaque. (Reproduced, with permission, from Hurwitz RM, *Pathology of the Skin: Atlas of Clinical–Pathological Correlation*, 2nd ed., Stamford, CT: Appleton & Lange, 1998: p. 432, Fig. 36–8.)

An acute, usually self-limited reaction of the skin and mucous membranes characterized by macules, papules, vesicles, and bullae. Erythema multiforme is an immune-mediated disorder that is due to drugs (e.g., penicillin, sulfonamides, phenytoin), infection (especially herpes simplex and *Mycoplasma*), vaccination, or malignancy.

Erythema multiforme is due to drugs, infection, vaccination, or malignancy.

History

The appearance of skin lesions may be preceded by a mild **prodrome** consisting of malaise and myalgias. Lesions may be associated with pain and fever. Mucosal involvement may result in dysphagia and dysuria.

Stevens–Johnson syndrome can be fatal and is commonly treated in a burn unit.

PE

Pink-red to red-blue **macules, papules, gyrate erythematous plaques, target lesions,** and **bullae** are found on physical examination (Figure 2.2–8). Lesions can be found anywhere but are most common on the **extremities, palms, and soles.** Erythema multiforme major (Stevens–Johnson syndrome) may present with systemic toxicity, involvement of the oral mucosa and conjunctiva, and skin denudation.

Differential

Urticaria, viral exanthem, staphylococcal scalded skin syndrome, bullous pemphigoid, pemphigus vulgaris.

Evaluation

Diagnosis is based on a clinical history of **exposure** to agents known to cause erythema multiforme. An elevated eosinophil count or positive serologic tests for

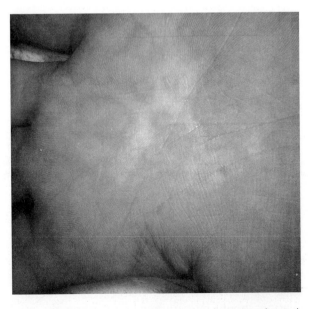

FIGURE 2.2–8. Erythema multiforme. Evolving erythematous plaques and papules with a target appearance: dull red center, pale zone, and darker outer ring. This acute self-limited reaction may occur with infection, antibiotic use, exposure to radiation or chemicals, or malignancy. (Reproduced, with permission, from Hurwitz RM, *Pathology of the Skin: Atlas of Clinical–Pathological Correlation*, 2nd ed., Stamford, CT: Appleton & Lange, 1998: p. 24, Fig. 2–2.)

HIGH-YIELD FACTS

Dermatology

hepatitis, infectious mononucleosis, histoplasmosis, or mycoplasma may be seen. Skin biopsy may show perivascular lymphocytes and necrotic keratinocytes.

Treatment

Mild cases resolve on their own. If the condition is drug-induced, **discontinue the inciting agent** immediately. If due to herpes simplex, acyclovir should be given. Severe forms require **corticosteroids** and analgesia for painful eruptions and may also necessitate hospitalization for dehydration due to poor PO intake and/or skin loss in Stevens–Johnson syndrome.

UCV *EM.7*

ERYTHEMA NODOSUM

An inflammation of the subcutaneous fat that produces tender erythematous nodules, usually on the **anterior tibial areas,** most commonly in young women. Lesions result from hypersensitivity reactions to drugs or infections (including beta-hemolytic strep, coccidioidomycosis, histoplasmosis, TB, and syphilis), sarcoid, rheumatic fever, or inflammatory bowel disease (IBD).

History

Lesions are usually **painful** and located on the anterior aspects of both legs. Malaise, arthralgias, and fever may precede the rash.

PE

Tender, erythematous pretibial nodules without ulceration (Figure 2.2–9). Lesions rarely occur on the face, arms, or trunk.

Differential

Polyarteritis nodosa, other types of panniculitis.

Evaluation

Skin biopsy provides a definitive diagnosis. Other helpful laboratory findings include an elevated ESR, mild leukocytosis, a high ASO titer, and a false-positive VDRL. CXR, cultures, and a Gram stain of the lesion may also be performed. (Gram stain should be negative, since erythema nodosum is a reactive lesion.)

Treatment

Therapy is supportive and includes elevation of the leg, bed rest, and **NSAIDs. Potassium iodide** may be given as well. Systemic corticosteroids may be necessary for persistent cases. Before steroid therapy is initiated, a thorough evaluation should be performed to confirm the etiology of the lesion.

UCV *IM2.4*

Erythema nodosum results from hypersensitivity reactions to drugs, infections, sarcoid, or IBD.

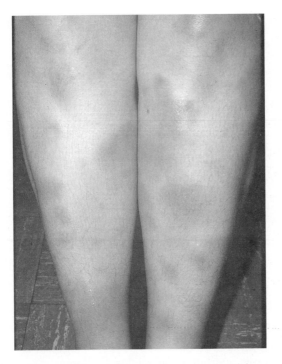

FIGURE 2.2–9. Erythema nodosum. The erythematous plaques and nodules are commonly located on pretibial areas. Lesions are painful and indurated and heal spontaneously without ulceration. (Reproduced, with permission, from Hurwitz RM, *Pathology of the Skin: Atlas of Clinical–Pathological Correlation,* 2nd ed., Stamford, CT: Appleton & Lange, 1998: p. 132, Fig. 10–1A.)

IMPETIGO

A contagious and autoinoculable infection of the skin caused by **staphylococcal or streptococcal organisms,** impetigo is more common in **children** than in adults. Bullous impetigo is due to coagulase-positive staphylococci that produce exfoliatin, a toxin that leads to vesicle or bulla formation. Nonbullous impetigo is caused by group A streptococci, which produce superficial pustular lesions.

History

Patients often present with **pruritic facial lesions** that develop over a few days.

PE

Classically, **honey-colored crusts** are seen on the lesions, which often involve the face. **Bullous impetigo** begins as small, erythematous macules that develop into thin-walled vesicles or bullae on an erythematous base. **Nonbullous impetigo** is characterized by superficial pustules with surrounding erythema. Common sites of distribution are the **face, neck,** and **extremities** (Figure 2.2–10).

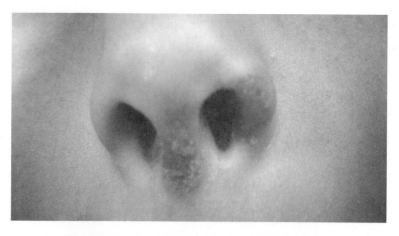

FIGURE 2.2–10. Impetigo. Dried pustules with superficial golden-brown crust are most commonly found around the nose and mouth. (Reproduced, with permission, from Hurwitz RM, *Pathology of the Skin: Atlas of Clinical–Pathological Correlation,* 2nd ed., Stamford, CT: Appleton & Lange, 1998: p. 165, Fig. 12–12.)

Differential

Ecthyma (thick crust overlying a deep ulcer), allergic contact dermatitis.

Evaluation

A bacterial culture may help assess sensitivity to the chosen antibiotic therapy.

Treatment

Affected areas should be gently washed with a mild soap. **Systemic antibiotics** should have activity against both staphylococcus and streptococcus, since the distinction may at times be difficult to make. Because of contagion, the patient's towels and washcloths should be segregated from other household members.

UCV *Ped.4*

CELLULITIS

A primary skin infection commonly caused by **group A streptococci** or **staphylococci.** Risk factors include diabetes, IV drug use, venous stasis, and immune-compromised states.

History

The area of involvement is **red, swollen,** and either **painful** or burning. Fever and chills may be present.

PE

Red, hot, swollen, tender skin lesions. Tinea pedis with resultant skin fissures is a common portal of bacterial entry (often not apparent on physical exam). Look for signs of compartment syndrome.

Differential

Necrotizing fasciitis, osteomyelitis, abscess, urticaria, allergic contact dermatitis, phlebitis.

Evaluation

A culture of material obtained from the wound may aid in diagnosis. Blood cultures should be obtained when bacteremia is suspected. Otherwise, the diagnosis is based on clinical signs and symptoms.

Treatment

For mild to moderate cases, prescribe **oral antibiotics** (usually cephalexin or dicloxacillin for penicillinase-producing organisms) for 7–10 days. Hospitalization and IV antibiotics (e.g., oxacillin) are necessary if there are any signs of systemic toxicity, comorbid conditions, extremes of age, hand or orbital involvement, or other concerns.

HERPES SIMPLEX

A painful, **recurrent** vesicular eruption of the mucocutaneous surfaces due to herpes simplex virus infection. The **oral-labial** form of HSV is usually due to herpes simplex type 1. The **genital** form is usually due to herpes simplex type 2.

History

Primary eruptions are more severe and longer-lasting than recurrent eruptions. **Primary** outbreaks may be accompanied by **lymphadenopathy, fever,** discomfort, **malaise,** and edema of the involved tissue. **Recurrent** infections are limited to the mucocutaneous area innervated by the **involved nerve.** Onset is preceded by **tingling,** burning, or frank pain.

PE

Physical exam reveals **grouped vesicles on an erythematous base** (Figure 2.2–11A).

Differential

Aphthous stomatitis, pemphigus vulgaris, Behçet's disease, syphilis, chancroid, trauma.

Evaluation

Multinucleated giant cells and acantholytic cells on **Tzanck smear** yield a **presumptive** diagnosis (Figure 2.2–11B). However, herpes zoster has the same appearance on the Tzanck, so definitive diagnosis requires culture or direct fluorescent antibody testing.

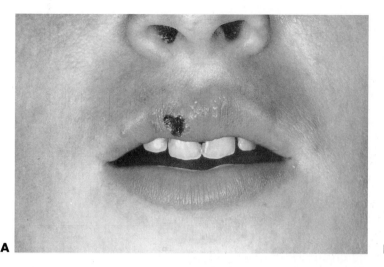
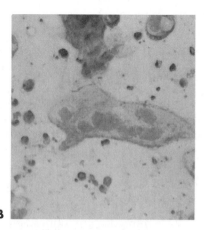

A   B

FIGURE 2.2–11. Herpes simplex. (A) Primary infection. Grouped vesicles on an erythematous base on the patient's lips and oral mucosa may progress to pustules before resolving. (B) Tzanck smear. The multinucleated giant cells from vesicular fluid provide a presumptive diagnosis of HSV infection. The Tzanck smear cannot distinguish between HSV and VZV infection. (Reproduced, with permission, from Hurwitz RM, *Pathology of the Skin: Atlas of Clinical–Pathological Correlation,* 2nd ed., Stamford, CT: Appleton & Lange, 1998: p. 145, Fig. 11–9.)

Treatment

Acyclovir ointment is somewhat effective in reducing the duration of viral shedding but not in preventing recurrence. The mainstay of therapy is oral or IV acyclovir (use IV acyclovir for severe cases or immune-compromised patients), which reduces both the frequency and the severity of recurrences. Daily acyclovir suppressive therapy may be used in patients with > 6 outbreaks per year.

UCV *IM2.3*

VARICELLA

Infection by the varicella-zoster virus (a member of the herpesvirus family), also known as **chickenpox**. Transmission is via **respiratory droplet contamination** or contact with **skin lesions.** Varicella has an incubation period of 10–20 days. Contagion begins **24 hours** before the eruption appears and continues until crusting has occurred.

History

A **prodrome** of malaise, fever, headache, and myalgia commonly occurs 24 hours before the onset of the rash. **Pruritic lesions appear in crops** over a period of 3–4 days.

PE

Lesions start as pink to red macules and then progress to grouped central vesicles, giving the classic appearance of a **"dewdrop on a rose petal,"** finally crusting over. Lesions are commonly found on the **trunk, face,** and **scalp.**

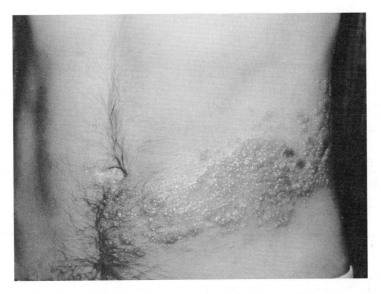

FIGURE 2.2–12. Herpes zoster. The unilateral dermatomal distribution of the grouped vesicles on an erythematous base is characteristic. (Reproduced courtesy of the Yale Department of Dermatology.)

Differential

Disseminated herpes zoster, exanthem due to coxsackievirus.

Evaluation

Diagnosis is based on **clinical examination** and history and, if necessary, can be confirmed by culture or direct fluorescent antibody testing.

Treatment

The disease is **self-limited** in healthy children. For healthy adults with uncomplicated primary varicella, **oral acyclovir** is the appropriate therapy. For adults with severe disease, immune-compromised patients, and those with primary varicella pneumonia, **IV acyclovir** may be required. A **vaccine** is now available for infants, children, and adults (immune-compromised patients and adults without previous infection). Recurrent infection can present as **shingles (herpes zoster,** Figure 2.2–12), which can be quite painful and serious. *IM2.20*

UCV *Ped.35*

MOLLUSCUM CONTAGIOSUM

A poxvirus infection that is most common in **young children** and is also among the most common cutaneous findings in **AIDS patients.**

History

Lesions are **asymptomatic** unless inflamed or irritated.

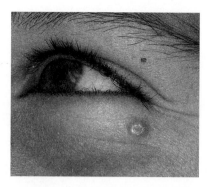

FIGURE 2.2–13. Molluscum contagiosum. The dome-shaped, fleshy, umbilicated papule on the child's eyelid is characteristic. (Reproduced, with permission, from Hurwitz RM, *Pathology of the Skin: Atlas of Clinical–Pathological Correlation,* 2nd ed., Stamford, CT: Appleton & Lange, 1998: p. 149, Fig. 11–19.)

PE

Physical exam reveals discrete, **dome-shaped, shiny papules,** frequently with central **umbilication** (Figure 2.2–13). Lesions are usually 2–5 mm in diameter. In children, the lesions are commonly found on the trunk, extremities, and face. In adults they are more frequently found in the perianal and perigenital areas.

Differential

Warts, acne, milia. See "Genital Lesions," p. 229.

Evaluation

Expressing and staining the contents confirms the diagnosis. Giemsa or Wright's stain allows for the identification of large inclusion or molluscum bodies. Ask adults about HIV risk factors.

Treatment

Treatment consists of curretting the lesion, liquid nitrogen cryotherapy, or application of **trichloroacetic acid.** Lesions resolve spontaneously over periods of months or years and are often left untreated in children.

TINEA VERSICOLOR (PITYRIASIS VERSICOLOR)

A common superficial skin infection caused by the fungus *Malassezia furfur.*

History

Lesions are usually asymptomatic but may cause mild itching.

PE

Physical exam reveals **small, scaling macules** that tend to enlarge and sometimes coalesce. They can be pinkish, lightly pigmented, or **hypopigmented.** The usual sites are the chest and back, but lesions can be found anywhere (Figure 2.2–14).

Differential

Vitiligo, eczema, psoriasis, seborrheic dermatitis.

Evaluation

KOH examination reveals **short, blunt hyphae and small spores** ("spaghetti and meatballs"). Wood's light examination distinguishes pigmented from hypopigmented areas and is helpful in evaluating the extent of the disease.

Treatment

Initial treatment is with a **topical antifungal agent,** with resolution occurring in approximately 2–3 weeks. Selenium sulfide shampoo may be used 1–3 times a week for three weeks; the lotion is applied to the skin for 10 minutes and is then scrubbed off. In light of their serious side effects, systemic antifungals should be used only in the most resistant cases. Oral ketoconazole therapy is used in some cases. Eighty percent of cases recur within two years, since the organism colonizes the skin.

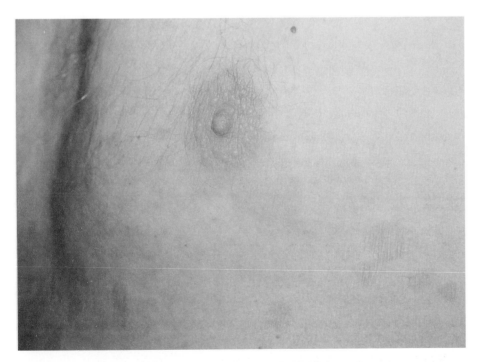

FIGURE 2.2–14. Tinea versicolor. Hypo- and hyperpigmented, scaly patches commonly appear on the back, chest, and shoulders. (Reproduced, with permission, from Hurwitz RM, *Pathology of the Skin: Atlas of Clinical–Pathological Correlation,* 2nd ed., Stamford, CT: Appleton & Lange, 1998: p. 202, Fig. 17–19.)

Tinea corporis, or ringworm, is a fungal infection on the body.

History

Patients complain primarily of pruritic scaly plaques.

PE

Ring-shaped, erythematous, and **scaling plaques** are seen, often with central clearing and **elevated borders.** The lesions are usually few in number (Figure 2.2–15).

Differential

Pityriasis rosea, psoriasis, SLE, secondary syphilis, nummular eczema.

Evaluation

Diagnosis is based on physical findings and on **hyphae** seen on **KOH preparation.** Culture is confirmatory.

Treatment

Topical antifungal cream should be applied twice a day for four weeks. Griseofulvin may be necessary if the lesions do not respond to topical therapy.

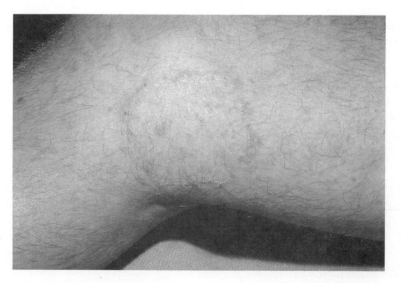

FIGURE 2.2–15. Tinea corporis. A ring-shaped, erythematous, scaling patch with central clearing seen here on the leg is characteristic. (Reproduced, with permission, from Hurwitz RM, *Pathology of the Skin: Atlas of Clinical–Pathological Correlation,* 2nd ed., Stamford, CT: Appleton & Lange, 1998: p. 200, Fig. 17–1.)

An infection of the skin caused by *Candida albicans*. Predisposing factors include **obesity, diabetes, recent antibiotic therapy,** and a **warm, moist environment.**

History

Pruritus and **pain** are the most common presenting symptoms.

PE

Well-demarcated, beefy-red **erythematous patches** surrounded by satellite pustules. The infection is usually restricted to **intertriginous areas** (see Clinical Image, plate 1). In infants, it often presents as a rash in the **diaper area.**

Differential

Tinea cruris, irritant intertrigo, psoriasis, eczema, seborrheic dermatitis, erythrasma.

Evaluation

Diagnosis can be confirmed by scraping a satellite lesion, placing it in **KOH,** and observing **pseudohyphae** under a microscope.

Treatment

Reduce moisture and friction through **weight loss** and **body powder.** A **topical antifungal agent** should be used and may be combined with a low-potency topical steroid to alleviate the pruritus associated with the lesions.

An extremely common pruritic rash that develops when *Sarcoptes scabiei,* the human itch mite, burrows into the skin to lay its eggs. Symptoms occur as a result of a hypersensitivity reaction against the mite feces. Mites are passed from person to person. Infection is associated with crowded and dirty living conditions.

History/PE

Presents with intense itching that worsens at night and after a hot shower. Excoriations, small papules and vesicles, and sometimes mite burrows are seen on the wrists and between the fingers, elbows, and intertriginous areas. The face, scalp, and neck are generally spared except in infants. Others in the household may be affected.

Evaluation

Diagnosis is made clinically; scrapings of burrows may be examined under a microscope for the mite or its eggs.

Treatment

First-line treatment consists of 5% permethrin cream. Treat close contacts. Antihistamines for symptomatic relief. Wash bedding and clothing in hot water to prevent reinfestation.

Lesion characteristically occurring in a linear pattern in areas where skin comes into contact with clothing or jewelry.	Contact dermatitis
Treatment for "cradle cap."	Medicated shampoos (e.g., selenium sulfide) +/− topical steroids
Presents with herald-patch, Christmas-tree pattern.	Pityriasis rosea
Prophylactic treatment for recurrences of herpes simplex.	Oral or IV acyclovir
Treatment for varicella in healthy children.	None; disease is self-limited
"Dew drop on a rose petal."	Lesions of primary varicella
Premalignant lesions found in sun-exposed areas of skin.	Actinic keratosis, or "solar" keratosis
Necessary evaluation for actinic keratosis.	Skin biopsy
Risk factors for squamous cell carcinoma.	Exposure to sun or radiation, actinic keratosis, immunosuppression, arsenic, industrial carcinogens
The most common type of skin cancer; lesion is a pearly-colored papule with a translucent surface.	Basal cell carcinoma
Leading cause of death from skin disease; pigmented skin lesion with irregularity or recent change in appearance.	Melanoma
Four characteristics of a nevus suggestive of melanoma.	Asymmetry, border irregularity, color variation, large diameter
"Target" lesions with a red center, pale zone, and dark outer ring appearing on the palms and soles. Preceded by a prodrome of malaise and myalgias.	Erythema multiforme
Drugs associated with erythema multiforme.	Penicillin, sulfonamides, phenytoin s/e.
A young woman presents with erythematous plaques and nodules on the anterior tibial area bilaterally. Gram stain of lesion is negative.	Erythema nodosum
Treatment for erythema nodosum.	A hypersensitivity reaction; supportive therapy and NSAIDs
Pinkish, scaling flat lesions on the chest and back. KOH prep has "spaghetti and meatballs" appearance. Treatment?	Use topical antifungal agent for tinea versicolor
Child with flesh-colored, umbilicated lesions on face. When occurring in adults, where do the lesions appear?	Molluscum contagiosum appears in the perigenital and perianal area in adults
Beefy-red patches and satellite pustules appearing in intertriginous areas. How to diagnose?	KOH prep of satellite lesion scraping; pseudohyphae indicate candidal intertrigo

handwritten annotation: m/c bullous Dz. · Iris lesion graycenter w red rim.

The following clinical questions and accompanying answers are reproduced, with permission, from Reteguiz J, *PreTest: Physical Diagnosis*, 4th ed., New York: McGraw-Hill, 2001.

Questions

1. A 16-year-old student with a history of herpetic gingivostomatitis develops a generalized and symmetric rash. The lesions are 1–2 cm in diameter and look like round patches. They consist of two concentric rings surrounding a central disk. The rash is burning and pruritic. A few erosive lesions are visible in the oral mucosa. Which of the following is the most likely diagnosis?
    a. Erythema multiforme
    b. Secondary syphilis
    c. Systemic lupus erythematosus
    d. Pemphigus vulgaris
    e. Urticaria

2. A 17-year-old patient presents with severe pruritus that is worse at night. Upon examination of the skin, areas of excoriated papules are observed in the interdigital area. Family members report similar symptoms. Which of the following is the most likely diagnosis?
    a. Scabies
    b. Cutaneous larva migrans
    c. Contact dermatitis
    d. Dermatitis herpetiformis
    e. Impetigo

3. A 6-year-old child presents complaining of patchy hair loss on the back of the scalp. Examination reveals well-demarcated areas of erythema and scaling, and although there are still some hairs in the area, they are extremely short and broken in appearance. Which of the following is the most likely diagnosis?
    a. Androgenic hair loss
    b. Psoriasis of the scalp
    c. Seborrheic dermatitis
    d. Tinea capitis
    e. Carbuncle

4. Five days after going on a nature walk, a 13-year-old boy develops well-demarcated, erythematous plaques and vesicles over his arms and face. The plaques are arranged in a linear fashion and are crusting. The boy has some facial edema. He has no history of fever or chills but complains of pruritus. Which of the following is the most likely diagnosis?
    a. Rubeola
    b. Atopic dermatitis
    c. Acute contact dermatitis
    d. Impetigo
    e. Erythema infectiosum

5. A 6-year-old child presents with flesh-colored papules on the hand that are not pruritic. Examination reveals lesions that are approximately 4 mm in diameter with central umbilication. A halo is seen around those lesions undergoing regression. Which of the following is the most likely diagnosis?
    a. Verruca vulgaris
    b. Molluscum contagiosum
    c. Keratoacanthoma
    d. Herpetic whitlow
    e. Hemangioma

Answers

1. **The answer is a. Erythema multiforme** (EM) **minor** due to the herpes infection is the most likely diagnosis in this patient. The lesions of EM are classically target lesions; they are burning and pruritic. They are generalized and often involve the oral mucosa. Etiologies of **EM major** include drugs such as phenytoin, sulfonamides, barbiturates, and allopurinol. Finger pressure in the vicinity of a lesion in EM major leads to a sheetlike removal of the epidermis **(Nikolsky sign)**. Pemphigus vulgaris is a chronic, bullous, autoimmune disease usually seen in middle-aged adults. The Nikolsky sign is positive in pemphigus vulgaris. **Secondary syphilis** appears 2–6 months after a primary infection and consists of round to oval, maculopapular lesions 0.5–1.0 cm in diameter. The eruptions typically involve the palms and soles. Secondary syphilis lesions that are flat and soft with a predilection for the mouth, perineum, and perianal areas are called **condylomata lata.** The skin lesions of SLE range from the classic butterfly malar rash to the discoid plaques of chronic cutaneous lupus erythematosus (CCLE). Urticaria is characterized by pruritic wheals typically lasting several hours.

2. **The answer is a.** The history is classic for scabies. Scabies is an infestation by the mite *Sarcoptes scabiei* that is spread by skin-to-skin contact. Although there are few skin findings on physical examination, patients usually complain of intense pruritus. Contact dermatitis is unlikely in this location, and cutaneous larva migrans (most commonly from *Ancylostoma braziliense* due to the dog and cat hookworm) typically has large, erythematous, serpiginous tracks. **Dermatitis herpetiformis** is associated with a gluten-sensitive enteropathy and is characterized by tiny papules, vesicles, and urticarial wheals. **Impetigo** is an infectious skin disease due to either *Staphylococcus aureus* or *Streptococcus pyogenes* seen typically on the face and characterized by discrete vesicles that rupture to form a yellowish crust.

3. **The answer is d.** The history is most consistent with tinea capitis due to either *Trichophyton tonsurans* or *Microsporum canis*. It is usually seen in school-age children and may be transmitted from person to person. **Psoriasis** is a hereditary disorder characterized by scaling patches and plaques appearing in specific areas of the body, such as the scalp, elbows, lumbosacral region, and knees. The lesions are "salmon pink" with a silver-colored scale that on removal produces blood **(Auspitz sign)**. The **Koebner phenomenon** (with trauma, the lesion jumps to a new location) is also elicited in patients with psoriasis. **Seborrheic dermatitis** is a common chronic dermatosis occurring in areas with active sebaceous glands (face, scalp, and body folds) and may occur either in infancy or in people over the age of 20. The eczematous plaques of seborrheic dermatitis are yellowish red and are often greasy with a sticky crust. Androgenic hair loss is a progressive hereditary bitemporal, frontal, or vertex balding that may begin any time after puberty. A **carbuncle** is a deep infectious collection of interconnecting abscesses **(furuncles)** arising from several hair follicles.

4. **The answer is c.** Contact dermatitis can be due to an allergen causing a type IV, cell-mediated, delayed hypersensitivity reaction. It may also be due to a nonallergen such as a chemical irritant. This patient presents with typical symptoms of acute contact dermatitis due to **poison ivy** resin. This results in sensitization within a week of exposure. Contact dermatitis due to poison ivy is usually pruritic, localized to one region, and often linear. **Impetigo** is an epidermal bacterial infection seen on the face characterized

by vesicles that rupture and crust. Erythema infectiosum or **fifth disease** is a childhood disease due to parvovirus B19 and is characterized by edematous, erythematous plaques on the cheeks (**"slapped cheek" disease).** Atopic dermatitis or eczema is an autosomal dominant pruritic inflammation with a predilection for the neck, face, flexor areas, feet, wrists, and hands. Usually there is a personal or family history of asthma, allergic rhinitis, or hay fever. **Rubeola (measles)** is a viral infection characterized by conjunctivitis and cough and a confluent erythematous maculopapular rash that spreads centrifugally. **Koplik spots** (bright red spots with blue-white specks in the center), which appear on the buccal mucosa opposite the premolar teeth, are pathognomonic for rubeola.

5. **The answer is b.** The description of the skin lesions is most consistent with **molluscum contagiosum.** This is a self-limited viral infection due to a pox virus (molluscum contagiosum virus) seen in children, sexually active adults, and HIV-infected patients. These lesions characteristically have a central keratotic plug that gives them the appearance of being dimpled (umbilication). The lesions resolve spontaneously. Common **warts or verrucae vulgaris** are due to human papillomavirus (HPV). Warts are firm, hyperkeratotic, round papules that are 1–10 mm in diameter. They have no umbilication but have a predilection for sites of trauma, including hands, fingers, and knees. A **keratoacanthoma** is a skin-colored, isolated, dome-shaped nodule with a central hyperkeratotic core usually found on the face. A **herpetic whitlow,** due to herpes simplex virus, consists of a painful group of vesicles on the volar finger. Capillary **hemangiomas** are bright red or purple nodules or plaques that develop at birth and spontaneously disappear by the fifth year.

Endocrinology

Type I vs. type II diabetes mellitus

	Type I—juvenile onset (IDDM)	Type II—adult onset (NIDDM)
Incidence	15%	85%
Insulin necessary in treatment	Always	Sometimes
Age (exceptions commonly occur)	Under 30	Over 40
Association with obesity	No	Yes
Genetic predisposition	Weak, polygenic	Strong, polygenic
Association with HLA system	Yes (HLA-DR3 and 4)	No
Glucose intolerance	Severe	Mild to moderate
Ketoacidosis	Common	Rare
Beta cell numbers in the islets	Reduced	Variable
Serum insulin level	Reduced	Variable
Classic symptoms of polyuria, polydipsia, thirst, weight loss	Common	Sometimes
Basic cause	?Viral or immune destruction of beta cells	?Increased resistance to insulin

Diabetic ketoacidosis

One of the most important complications of type I diabetes. Usually due to an increase in insulin requirements from an increase in stress (e.g., infection). Excess fat breakdown and increased ketogenesis from the increase in free fatty acids, which are then made into ketone bodies.

Signs/symptoms

Kussmaul hyperpnea (rapid/deep breathing), hyperthermia, nausea/vomiting, abdominal pain, psychosis/dementia, dehydration. Fruity breath odor.

Labs

Hyperglycemia, increased H^+, decreased HCO_3^- (anion gap metabolic acidosis), increased blood ketone levels, leukocytosis.

Complications

Life-threatening mucormycosis, *Rhizopus* infection, cerebral edema, cardiac arrhythmias, heart failure.

Treatment

Fluids, insulin, and potassium; glucose if necessary to prevent hypoglycemia.

Diabetes mellitus

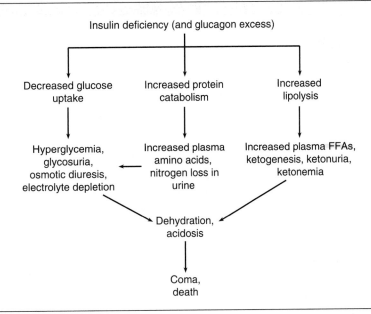

Insulin deficiency (and glucagon excess)

Decreased glucose uptake → Hyperglycemia, glycosuria, osmotic diuresis, electrolyte depletion

Increased protein catabolism → Increased plasma amino acids, nitrogen loss in urine

Increased lipolysis → Increased plasma FFAs, ketogenesis, ketonuria, ketonemia

Dehydration, acidosis

Coma, death

Adrenal cortex and medulla

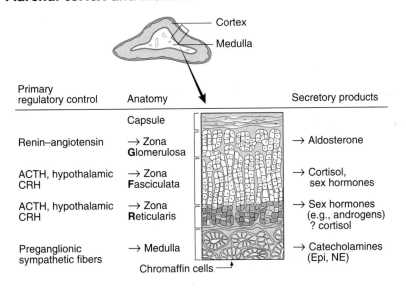

Cortex
Medulla

Primary regulatory control	Anatomy	Secretory products
	Capsule	
Renin–angiotensin	→ Zona **G**lomerulosa	→ Aldosterone
ACTH, hypothalamic CRH	→ Zona **F**asciculata	→ Cortisol, sex hormones
ACTH, hypothalamic CRH	→ Zona **R**eticularis	→ Sex hormones (e.g., androgens) ? cortisol
Preganglionic sympathetic fibers	→ Medulla	→ Catecholamines (Epi, NE)

Chromaffin cells

GFR corresponds with salt (Na⁺), sugar (glucocorticoids), and sex (androgens). "The deeper you go, the sweeter it gets."

PTH parathyroid Hormone

Source — Chief cells of parathyroid.

Function
1. Increases bone resorption of calcium
2. Increases kidney reabsorption of calcium in DCT
3. Decreases kidney reabsorption of phosphate
4. Increases 1,25 (OH)$_2$ vit. D (cholecalciferol) production by stimulating kidney 1α-hydroxylase

Regulation — Decrease in free serum Ca^{2+} increases PTH secretion.

PTH: increases serum Ca^{2+}, decreases serum PO$_4^{3-}$, phosphate increases urine PO$_4^{3-}$.
PTH stimulates both osteoclasts and osteoblasts.

PTH = **P**hosphate **T**rashing **H**ormone

Thyroid hormones (T_3/T_4)

Iodine-containing hormones that control the body's metabolic rate.

Source	Follicles of thyroid.	T_4 functions: **4B's**
Function	1. Bone growth (synergism with GH)	**B**rain maturation
	2. CNS maturation	**B**one growth
	3. Beta-adrenergic effects	**B**eta-adrenergic effects
	4. Increased basal metabolic rate via increased Na^+/K^+ ATPase activity = increased O_2 consumption, increased body temp	**B**MR increased
	5. Increased glycogenolysis, gluconeogenesis, lipolysis	
	6. CV: Increased CO, HR, SV, contractility, RR	
Regulation	TRH (hypothalamus) stimulates TSH (pituitary), which stimulates follicular cells. Negative feedback by T_3 to anterior pituitary decreases sensitivity to TRH. TSI, like TSH, stimulates follicular cells (Graves' disease).	

Cushing's syndrome

Increased cortisol due to a variety of causes.

Etiologies include:

1. Cushing's disease (1° pituitary adenoma); increased ACTH
2. Primary adrenal (hyperplasia/neoplasia); decreased ACTH
3. Ectopic ACTH production (e.g., carcinoid); increased ACTH
4. Iatrogenic; decreased ACTH

The clinical picture includes hypertension, weight gain, moon facies, truncal obesity, buffalo hump, hyperglycemia (insulin resistance), skin changes (thinning, striae), osteoporosis, and immune suppression.

Propylthiouracil

Mechanism	Inhibits organification and coupling of thyroid hormone synthesis. Also decreases peripheral conversion of T_4 to T_3.
Clinical use to treat:	Hyperthyroidism.
Toxicity	Skin rash, agranulocytosis (rare), aplastic anemia.

TYPE I

Also known as juvenile-onset insulin-dependent diabetes mellitus (IDDM), type I DM is thought to be due to autoimmune destruction of the beta cells of the pancreas. It manifests as hyperglycemia secondary to insulin deficiency, ultimately requiring exogenous insulin therapy. It is usually diagnosed in children or adolescents. Type I DM is associated with HLA-DR3 and -DR4.

History/PE

Patients commonly present with **polyuria** (including nocturia), **polydipsia, polyphagia,** and rapid or unexplained weight loss.

Differential

Pancreatic disease (e.g., chronic pancreatitis), glucagonoma, Cushing's disease, iatrogenic factors (e.g., corticosteroids, thiazide diuretics, phenytoin), gestational diabetes, diabetes insipidus.

Evaluation

At least one of the following is required to make the diagnosis:

- Random plasma glucose concentration > 200 mg/dL with classic symptoms of diabetes.
- Fasting plasma glucose ≥ 126 mg/dL on two separate occasions.
- Two-hour postprandial glucose > 200 on 75-g oral glucose tolerance test (on two separate occasions).

The presence of urine glucose and urine ketones supports the diagnosis. **Hemoglobin A$_{1c}$** is used to monitor the efficacy of and compliance with treatment, since it reflects glucose levels over the three months prior to measurement. The goal is to maintain HbA$_{1c}$ < 8, as near-normalization of blood glucose has been shown to slow the development and progression of retinopathy, nephropathy, and neuropathy.

Treatment

Treat with a regular regimen of insulin injections (see Table 2.3–1). Patients must be taught to monitor their glucose levels by fingerstick at home. Patients should be carefully monitored for diabetes-related complications (see Table 2.3–2).

TABLE 2.3–1. Insulin Formulations		
Type	**Time of Onset of Action**	**Peak Effect**
Lispro	10–15 minutes	1–2 hours
Regular	45 minutes	2–5 hours
NPH	2–4 hours	6–10 hours
Lente	3–4 hours	6–12 hours
Ultralente	6–8 hours	none 18–24 hrs

TYPE II

Also known as adult-onset non-insulin-dependent diabetes mellitus (NIDDM). In contrast to type I, hyperglycemia is secondary to end-organ insulin resistance. It is most commonly diagnosed in obese patients over the age of 40 years. Type II DM often has a strong family history, although there is no known HLA linkage.

History/PE

Patients may present with symptoms similar to those of type I DM, including polyuria, polydipsia, and polyphagia. However, onset is typically insidious, so patients may initially present with symptoms of diabetic complications such as blurry vision or recurrent infections. Patients with type II DM rarely develop diabetic ketoacidosis, but with very poor glycemic control, hyperosmolar nonketotic coma may occur.

Differential

Same as for type I DM. Additionally, blurry vision may be due to primary visual disorders such as glaucoma, cataracts, or macular degeneration.

Evaluation

Same as for type I DM.

Treatment

Consider in stages:

- Diet, weight loss, and exercise
- Oral-agent monotherapy
- Combination oral therapies (see below)
- Insulin (alone or in conjunction with oral agents)

Educate and monitor the patient with the goal of gaining glucose control at the lowest possible stage. Oral agents include the following:

- **Metformin:** Unknown mechanism. May cause lactic acidosis.
- **Thiazolidinediones** (the "glitazones"): Increase peripheral response to insulin.
- **Troglitazone** has recently been linked to life-threatening hepatotoxicity.
- **Sulfonylureas** (tolbutamide, glyburide, glipizide): Increase pancreatic secretion of insulin. The main toxicity is hypoglycemia.
- **Alpha-glucosidase inhibitors:** Decrease intestinal absorption of carbohydrate. A side effect is GI upset.
- **Strict control of blood pressure** in type II patients with hypertension has been shown to reduce the development of diabetes-related complications.

Complications

See Table 2.3–2.

TABLE 2.3–2. Complications of Diabetes

Complications of Treatment	Description
Somogyi effect	Nocturnal hypoglycemia causing elevated morning glucose due to release of counterregulatory hormones (reduce insulin to treat). at ?m
Dawn phenomenon	Early-morning hyperglycemia caused by reduced effectiveness of insulin at that time.

Acute Complications	Description
Diabetic ketoacidosis (DKA)	Hyperglycemia-induced crisis that occurs most commonly in **type I diabetics**. It is often precipitated by stress, including infections, MI, alcohol, drugs (e.g., corticosteroids, thiazide diuretics), or pancreatitis, or by noncompliance with insulin therapy. Patients often present with **abdominal pain, vomiting, Kussmaul respirations** (slow, deep breaths), and a **fruity, acetone odor.** Patients are severely dehydrated with many electrolyte abnormalities (e.g., hypokalemia, hypophosphatemia, **increased anion gap metabolic acidosis**) and may also develop mental status changes. Treatment includes fluids, potassium, and insulin to correct electrolyte abnormalities and treatment of initiating event.
Hyperosmolar hyperglycemic nonketotic coma (HHNK)	Presents as **profound dehydration,** mental status changes, and an extremely high plasma glucose (> 600 mg/dL) without acidosis; occurs most commonly in **type II diabetics,** is precipitated by acute stress, and is often fatal. Treatment includes aggressive rehydration, **insulin,** and **aggressive fluid and electrolyte replacement.**

Chronic Complications	Description
Retinopathy	Appears when diabetes has been present for at least **3–5 years.** Preventive measures include control of hyperglycemia and hypertension and **laser therapy for neovascularization.**
Diabetic nephropathy	Characterized by glomerular hyperfiltration followed by **microalbuminuria.** Begin therapy with an **ACE inhibitor;** control hyperglycemia; control hypertension.
Neuropathy	Peripheral, symmetric, sensorimotor neuropathy leading to foot trauma and diabetic ulcers. Treat with preventive **foot care, analgesics,** and tricyclic antidepressants.
Macrovascular complications	Cardiovascular, cerebrovascular, peripheral vascular disease. **Cardiovascular disease is the most common cause of death in diabetic patients.** Goal BP is 135/85; lower LDL to < 130. In the presence of known CAD, lower LDL to < 100 and triglycerides to < 200 mg/dL.

UCV *IM1.18, 19, 26*

HIGH-YIELD FACTS

Endocrinology

Graves' disease is the most common etiology of hyperthyroidism. It is most often seen in **women 20–40** years of age. Other etiologies include toxic nodular goiter, toxic adenomas, and subacute thyroiditis (initial phase). Less common etiologies include pituitary TSH hypersecretion, exogenous iodide (Jod–Basedow disease), struma ovarii, and Hashimoto's thyroiditis.

History

Weight loss and increased appetite as well as **heat intolerance, nervousness,** weakness, **increased bowel frequency,** and menstrual abnormalities.

diarrhea

PE

Warm, moist skin, goiter, sinus **tachycardia** or **atrial fibrillation,** thyroid bruit, fine **tremor,** and hyperactive reflexes. **Exophthalmos** and pretibial myxedema are seen only in Graves' disease (Figure 2.3–1).

Differential

Anxiety, neurosis, mania, pheochromocytoma, malignancy, chronic alcoholism, primary myopathy.

Evaluation

TSH receptor antibodies are seen in patients with Graves' disease.

Suppressed TSH is the most sensitive test for primary hyperthyroidism; also look for elevated T_4, increased free T_4, and elevated free T_4 index. ESR will be elevated in thyroiditis.

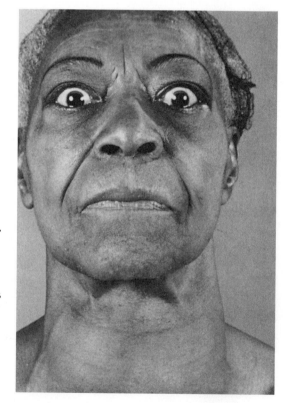

FIGURE 2.3–1. Graves' ophthalmopathy. Proptosis with lid retraction that results from lymphocytic infiltration and edema of the extraocular muscles. May progress to fibrosis with limited eye movement and blindness from optic nerve compression. Patient also demonstrates impressive goiter. (Reproduced, with permission, from Stobo JD, *The Principles and Practice of Medicine*, 23rd ed., Stamford, CT: Appleton & Lange, 1996: p. 295, Fig. 4.4–1.)

Treatment

Administer **propranolol** for catecholamine symptoms followed by **radioablation.** Give **antithyroid drugs** (methimazole, carbimazole, propylthiouracil) for patients with mild thyrotoxicosis or goiter. **Thyroidectomy** is indicated for large goiters with postoperative levothyroxine to prevent hypothyroidism.

s/e Rash/ aplastic anemia

Complications

Thyroid storm—extreme hyperthyroidism often precipitated by surgery or infection. Symptoms include high fever, dehydration, tachycardia with **high-output cardiac failure,** and coma. Carries a **25% mortality.**

UCV EM.8

HYPOTHYROIDISM

A condition characterized by low levels of thyroid hormone. Hypothyroidism is most commonly caused by **Hashimoto's thyroiditis;** other causes include subacute or postpartum thyroiditis, drugs (e.g., iodide, amiodarone, sulfonamides, lithium), iatrogenic factors (radioablation or excision with inadequate supplementation), and pituitary dysfunction (with low TSH). Myxedema refers to severe hypothyroidism with deposition of mucopolysaccharides in the dermis. Cretinism refers to untreated congenital hypothyroidism leading to cognitive defects and physical abnormalities.

History

Patients present with weakness, fatigue, **cold intolerance, constipation,** weight gain, **depression,** menstrual irregularities, and **hoarseness.**

PE

Dry, cold, puffy skin, edema, thin eyebrows, **bradycardia,** and delayed relaxation of deep tendon reflexes.

Differential

Chronic fatigue, malnutrition, CHF, primary amyloidosis, depression.

Antimicrosomal and antithyroglobulin antibodies are seen in patients with Hashimoto's thyroiditis.

Evaluation

Elevated **TSH** is the most sensitive measure for primary hypothyroidism. Also look for decreased serum T_4, decreased free T_4, and radioiodine uptake < 10% in 24 hours.

Treatment

- **Uncomplicated hypothyroidism** (e.g., Hashimoto's disease): Administer levothyroxine.
- **Subacute thyroiditis:** Usually self-limited; treat with ASA and add cortisol in severe cases.
- **Myxedema coma:** IV levothyroxine +/– hydrocortisone.

UCV IM1.21, 24, Ped.5

Thyroid nodules are found in 1% of individuals between the ages of 20 and 30 and in 5% of individuals > 60 years. The vast majority of thyroid nodules are benign. There is a higher risk of malignancy in patients with a **history of neck irradiation,** "cold" **nodules** (on radionuclide scan), firm and fixed solitary nodules, and **rapidly growing nodules** with **hoarseness** or **dysphagia.**

History

Malignant thyroid nodules are usually cold and solid.

Usually **asymptomatic** on initial presentation. Note the presence of systemic symptoms (e.g., hypo/hyperthyroidism), local symptoms (dysphagia, dyspnea/respiratory difficulties, odynophagia, hoarse voice), family history (especially **medullary thyroid cancer**), and history of neck irradiation (for thyroid cancer, hyperthyroidism, or salivary gland tumors).

PE

Carcinoma will likely be palpable, **firm, fixed,** and **nontender.** Check for anterior cervical lymphadenopathy.

Differential

Lymphocytic thyroiditis, multinodular goiter, colloid nodule, benign follicular adenoma, papillary or follicular carcinoma.

Evaluation/Treatment

- TSH and **thyroid function tests.**
- **Ultrasound** can determine if the nodule is cystic; a radioactive scan can determine if it is cold or hot (cancers are usually cold and solid).
- The best method of assessing a nodule for malignancy is **fine needle aspiration** (high sensitivity and moderate specificity).
- If the FNA is benign, treat with **thyroxine** (suppresses TSH and shrinks nodule) and follow with ultrasound.
- If malignant, perform **surgical resection.**
- If the distinction between benign and malignant is not clear (this is often a difficult diagnosis), perform a lobectomy and wait for final pathology.
- Medullary thyroid cancer/anaplastic carcinomas are aggressive variants with a worse prognosis. Medullary thyroid carcinoma is associated with MEN IIA and IIB cancer syndromes.
- Look for metastases with radioactive iodine scans.

UCV *Surg.8*

Occurs in 0.1% of the population. Ninety percent of cases result from a single **adenoma;** 10% result from parathyroid hyperplasia. Parathyroid carcinoma accounts for < 1% of all cases.

History

Seventy percent of cases are **asymptomatic.**

PE

The following mnemonic describes common presenting symptoms and signs: **stones** (nephrolithiasis or nephrocalcinosis), **bones** (bone pain, muscle aches, arthralgias, fractures [osteitis fibrosa]), **groans** (PUD, pancreatitis), and **psychic overtones** (fatigue, depression, anxiety, irritability, sleep/concentration disturbances).

Differential

Consider all major causes of hypercalcemia (see "Hypercalcemia," p. 427 in Renal).

Evaluation

Hypercalcemia, hypophosphatemia, and **hypercalciuria** are the classic hallmarks. PTH will be elevated relative to ionized calcium.

Treatment

Treat with **parathyroidectomy** if symptomatic; administer bisphosphonates preoperatively. For acute hypercalcemia, give **IV fluids** and **loop diuretics** (once adequately hydrated).

UCV *IM1.22*

ADRENAL INSUFFICIENCY

Can be either primary (Addison's disease) or secondary (due to decreased ACTH production by the pituitary). Addison's disease is caused by destruction of the adrenal cortices, leading to deficiencies of both mineralocorticoids and glucocorticoids. **Autoimmune destruction** is the most common etiology and accounts for 80% of spontaneous cases. Addison's disease may be isolated or may occur as part of a polyglandular autoimmune syndrome (hypothyroidism, type I diabetes, vitiligo, premature ovarian failure, testicular failure, and pernicious anemia). Other causes include congenital enzyme deficiencies, adrenal hemorrhage (often as part of DIC, as in Waterhouse–Friderichsen syndrome), TB, and other infections.

> **AdD**ison's disease is due to **Ad**renocortical **D**eficiency.

Secondary adrenal insufficiency is most often due to abrupt cessation of chronic glucocorticoid treatment.

History

Presenting symptoms include **weakness, weight loss, nausea,** and **vomiting.**

PE

- Addison's disease: Increased skin pigmentation, hypotension, and anorexia.
- Secondary adrenal insufficiency: No hyperpigmentation.

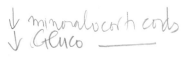

Differential

Anorexia nervosa, malabsorption states, occult malignancy, hypoparathyroidism, thyrotoxicosis, panhypopituitarism, hemochromatosis.

Evaluation

- **Addison's disease:** Elevated plasma **ACTH** and low cortisol levels in response to ACTH challenge.
- **Secondary adrenal insufficiency:** Decreased plasma ACTH and increased cortisol levels in response to ACTH.

Additional lab findings include **hyponatremia, hyperkalemia,** and **eosinophilia.**

Treatment

Treat with replacement **glucocorticoids** and **mineralocorticoids.** Administer **stress-dose** steroids during periods of stress (e.g., major surgery, trauma, infection). Avoid secondary adrenal insufficiency by tapering off glucocorticoids, allowing endogenous production of ACTH to return to normal.

UCV *IMI.16*

CUSHING'S SYNDROME

A term that refers to the manifestations of **hypercortisolism.** Cushing's syndrome is most commonly caused by **excessive** administration of corticosteroids. Noniatrogenic causes include ACTH hypersecretion by the pituitary (70%) (i.e., Cushing's disease) or by nonpituitary neoplasms (15%) such as small cell lung cancer, or cortisol secretion by an adrenal tumor or bilateral adrenal hyperplasia (15%).

History

Depression, oligomenorrhea, growth retardation, weakness, acne, and **excessive hair growth.** Symptoms of **diabetes** (e.g., polydipsia, polyuria, dysuria) may also be present secondary to decreased glucose tolerance.

PE

High ACTH: ectopic or pituitary source. Low ACTH: adrenal or exogenous source.

Hypertension, **central obesity,** muscle wasting, thin skin with easy **bruisability** and purple **striae,** psychological changes, **hirsutism, moon facies,** and "buffalo hump."

Differential

Chronic alcoholism, depression, diabetes mellitus, exogenous steroid administration, adrenogenital syndrome.

Evaluation

- Screen for elevated **free urinary cortisol.**
- Administer a **low-dose dexamethasone suppression test** (an abnormal result consists of persistently elevated cortisol levels after suppression the previous night).
- Localize the lesion; ACTH is high with an ectopic or pituitary source and is low or undetectable in the presence of an adrenal source. If high, a **high-dose dexamethasone suppression test** will suppress cortisol secretion in pituitary disease.
- CT (adrenal) or MRI (sphenoid) can further localize lesions.
- Other lab values suggestive of the diagnosis include **hyperglycemia,** glycosuria, and **hypokalemia.**

Treatment

Treat with **resection** of the hypersecretory source (pituitary, adrenal). Irradiation may be a consideration in pituitary disease. **Ketoconazole, metyrapone,** or **octreotide** may be used in adrenal carcinoma or small cell lung cancer (inhibits cortisol secretion).

Complications

Increased susceptibility to infection; vertebral compression fractures, avascular necrosis of the femoral head.

UCV *IM1.17*

PRIMARY HYPERALDOSTERONISM

A condition that most commonly results from a unilateral adrenal tumor **(Conn's syndrome).** The remaining cases (30%) result from bilateral adrenocortical hyperplasia.

History

Patients present with **hypertension, headache, polyuria** (secondary to hypokalemic nephropathy), and **muscle weakness** (secondary to hypokalemia).

PE

Hypertension, tetany (secondary to hypokalemia), paresthesias, and, in severe cases, peripheral edema.

Differential

Essential hypertension, diuretic toxicity, nephrogenic diabetes insipidus, secondary hyperaldosteronism (renal artery stenosis, CHF, cirrhosis, renal failure associated with high plasma renin).

Evaluation

Hypokalemia, hypernatremia, metabolic alkalosis, **low plasma renin,** and elevated 24-hour urine <u>aldosterone</u>; CT or MRI may reveal an adrenal mass.

Treatment

Treat with laparoscopic or open **adrenalectomy** for Conn's syndrome and with **spironolactone** (an aldosterone receptor antagonist) for bilateral hyperplasia.

UCV *EM.7, Ped.5, Surg.6*

PHEOCHROMOCYTOMA

> **Rule of 10's:**
>
> **10%** malignant
> **10%** extra-adrenal
> **10%** calcify
> **10%** occur in kids
> **10%** familial

The most common primary tumor of the adrenal gland in adults. Pheochromocytomas secrete epinephrine and norepinephrine, thus stimulating the sympathetic nervous system.

History/PE

Symptoms include intermittent rapid heart rate, palpitations, chest pain, diaphoresis, hypertension, headaches, and anxiety.

> **The 5 P's:**
>
> **P**ressure (↑ BP)
> **P**ain (headache)
> **P**erspiration
> **P**alpitations
> **P**allor/diaphoresis

Evaluation

CT or MRI shows a <u>suprarenal mass.</u> Elevated urinary catecholamines (e.g., vanillylmandelic acid, homovanillic acid) are also found.

Treatment

Symptoms may be alleviated with alpha-antagonists (phenoxybenzamine). Definitive treatment is removal of the tumor.

UCV *Surg.7*

ACROMEGALY

A condition of adults in which a usually benign pituitary tumor secretes high levels of growth hormone.

History/PE

Patients present with enlargement of jaw, hands, feet and have a characteristic coarsening of facial features (see Figure 2.3–2). These symptoms may be accompanied by visual disturbances, including loss of peripheral vision due to compression of the optic chiasm by a <u>pituitary adenoma.</u> Excess growth hormone may also lead to glucose intolerance. Children with excess growth hormone production present with gigantism.

Evaluation

MRI or CT shows <u>sellar lesion.</u> Elevated serum growth hormone levels are also found.

Treatment

Transsphenoidal surgical resection or irradiative ablation of the tumor. Octreotide can be used for symptomatic management of refractory cases.

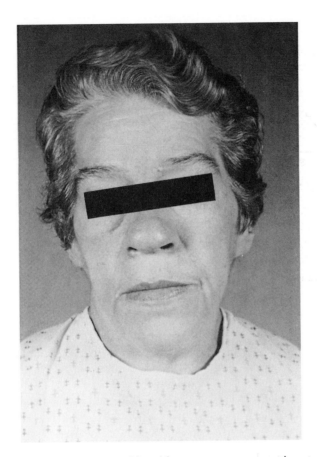

FIGURE 2.3–2. Acromegaly. Coarsening of facial features in a woman with active disease. (Reproduced, with permission, from Stobo JD, *The Principles and Practice of Medicine*, 23rd ed., Stamford, CT: Appleton & Lange, 1996: p. 276, Fig. 4.2–1.)

Symptoms of pallor, high pressure, palpitations, headache pain, and perspiration.	Pheochromocytoma
Exophthalmos, pretibial myxedema, and decreased TSH.	Hyperthyroidism with these symptoms is due to Graves' disease
First-line treatment for growth-hormone-secreting pituitary adenoma.	Transsphenoidal surgical resection
Source of lesion in Cushing's syndrome with high ACTH levels.	Either ectopic or pituitary
Patient complains of headache, weakness, and polyuria; exam reveals hypertension and tetany. Labs include hypernatremia, hypokalemia, and metabolic alkalosis.	Primary hyperaldosteronism due to Conn's syndrome or bilateral adrenal hyperplasia
Oral diabetic agent associated with fulminant hepatic failure.	Troglitazone
Antidiabetic agent associated with lactic acidosis.	Metformin
Morning hyperglycemia that is a rebound response to nighttime hypoglycemia, not a need for more insulin.	Somogyi effect
Patient presents with weakness, nausea and vomiting, weight loss, and new skin pigmentation. Labs show hyponatremia and hyperkalemia.	Addison's disease ‡ (Cushing hypokalemia)
"Stones, bones, groans, psychic overtones."	Signs and symptoms of hyperparathyroidism

Questions reproduced, with permission, from Berk SL, *PreTest: Medicine*, 9th ed., New York: McGraw-Hill, 2001, and from Reteguiz J, *PreTest: Physical Diagnosis*, 4th ed., New York: McGraw-Hill, 2001.

Questions

1. A 50-year-old obese female is taking oral hypoglycemic agents. While being treated for an upper respiratory infection, she develops lethargy and is brought to the emergency room. On physical exam, there is no focal neurologic finding or neck rigidity. Laboratory results are as follows:

Na^+	134 mEq/L
K^+	4.0 mEq/L
HCO_3	25 mEq/L
glucose	900 mg/dL
BUN	84 mg/dL
creatinine	3.0 mg/dL
BP	120/80 sitting
BP	105/65 lying

   The most likely cause of this patient's coma is
   a. Diabetic ketoacidosis
   b. Hyperosmolar coma
   c. Inappropriate ADH
   d. Bacterial meningitis

2. The most important treatment in this patient is
   a. Large volumes of fluid, insulin; seek concurrent illnesses
   b. Bicarbonate infusion 100 mEq/L
   c. Rapid glucose lowering with intravenous insulin
   d. 30 mEq/hr of KCl.

3. This 30-year-old female complains of palpitations, fatigue, and insomnia. On physical exam, her extremities are warm and she is tachycardic. There is diffuse thyroid gland enlargement and proptosis. There is an orange thickening of the skin in the pretibial area. Which of the following lab values would you expect in this patient?
   a. Increased TSH, total thyroxine, total T_3
   b. Decreased TSH, increased total thyroxine   *hyper T.*
   c. Increased T_3 uptake, decreased T_3
   d. Normal T_4, decreased TSH

4. The cause of this patient's thyrotoxicosis is   *Grave's Dz*
   a. Autoimmune disease
   b. Benign tumor
   c. Malignancy
   d. Viral infection of the thyroid

Answers

1. **The answer is b.** This obese patient on oral hypoglycemics has developed hyperglycemia and lethargy during an upper respiratory infection. The patient's serum osmolality is as follows:

$$\frac{900}{18} \text{ (glucose)} + 2 \text{ (Na}^+ + \text{K}^+\text{)} + \frac{84}{2.8} = 50 + 276 + 30 = 356$$

Hence the serum osmolality is greater than 350 mOsm/kg. The serum bicarbonate is too high to be consistent with diabetic ketoacidosis. The hyponatremia is related to hyperglycemia. SIADH could not be diagnosed in this clinical setting. The patient's diabetes likely went out of control due to infection. There is no clinical evidence for meningitis.

2. **The answer is a.** The primary treatment for hyperosmolar nonketotic states is fluid replacement, usually normal saline. Hypotonic saline may be given for severe hypernatremia or congestive heart failure. Hyperglycemia can be corrected slowly. The patient is not acidotic and would not require bicarbonate treatment (used in severe DKA when pH is less than 7.0). The patient's serum potassium is in the normal range and would not be expected to fall rapidly.

3. **The answer is b.** This patient has clinical symptoms of thyrotoxicosis. Most patients with thyrotoxicosis have increases in total and free concentrations of T_3 and T_4. (Some may have isolated T_3 or T_4 increases.) Most thyrotoxicosis results in suppression of pituitary TSH secretion, so low TSH levels can also confirm the diagnosis.

4. **The answer is a.** This patient has, in addition to thyrotoxicosis, orbitopathy as well as the characteristic dermopathy of Graves' disease, called *pretibial myxedema*. Graves' disease is an autoimmune phenomena. Biopsy of the thyroid shows lymphocytic infiltration. Toxic multinodular goiter produces thyrotoxicosis caused by benign, functionally autonomous tumors. It would not produce the protopsis or dermopathy of Graves' disease. Subacute thyroiditis (de Quervain's) is probably caused by a viral infection. It produces a transient hyperthyroidism followed by hypothyroidism.

Epidemiology and Preventive Medicine

Length Bias

The tendency of a screening test to detect a disproportionate number of slowly progressive diseases or cases and to miss rapidly progressive ones (which have a small window of detection, since afflicted individuals are present in the population only briefly). Length bias may lead to **overestimation of the effectiveness of screening.**

Lead-Time Bias

Lead-time bias occurs when screening advances the time of diagnosis, thereby prolonging the period of time between diagnosis and death without actually prolonging true survival. Since a disease is identified earlier but its natural course is not altered, survival will only **appear** to be greater.

Enrollment Bias

Enrollment bias occurs when subjects are assigned to a study group in a non-random fashion. One example of an enrollment bias is the assignment of sicker patients to the intervention group compared to the placebo group.

Self-Selection

Patients who choose to enroll in a study or respond to a survey may introduce **confounding variables** to that study; for example, patients with a disease that has been resistant to conventional therapy may be more likely to enroll in some studies.

Observational Bias

Participants' responses to subjective questions may be affected by their awareness of the particular leg of the study in which they are enrolled. An observer's evaluation of a participant's clinical status may also be affected by such information. This is an important **reason for blinding a study.**

Recall Bias

Confounders may be introduced (e.g., in case-control studies) through **errors of memory** on the part of participants, since they may be asked to recall past events and exposures. People who have had a negative experience, such as a disease, may be more likely to reflect upon the circumstances that led to that experience and thus more likely to remember risk factors than those who did not have the disease.

	Disease Present	No Disease	
Positive test	a	b	*PPV* = *a* / (*a* + *b*)
Negative test	c	d	*NPV* = *d* / (*c* + *d*)
	Sensitivity = a / (a + c)	Specificity = d / (b + d)	

FIGURE 2.4–1. Sensitivity, specificity, PPV, and NPV.

SENSITIVITY

***PID** = **P**ositive **I**n **D**isease (note that PID is a sensitive topic).*

Sensitivity is the probability that a diseased patient will have a positive test result (number of true positives divided by the number of all people with the disease; Figure 2.4–1). False negative ratio is 1 – sensitivity. High sensitivity is desirable for a **screening test.**

SPECIFICITY

***NIH** = **N**egative **I**n **H**ealth.*

Specificity is the probability that a healthy patient will have a negative test result (number of true negatives divided by the number of all people without the disease; see Figure 2.4–1). False positive ratio is 1 – specificity. High specificity is desirable for a **confirmatory test.**

POSITIVE PREDICTIVE VALUE (PPV)

Positive predictive value is the probability that a patient with a positive test result has the disease (true positives divided by the total number who tested positive). A test will have higher positive predictive value for diseases with a higher prevalence. **Both positive and negative predictive value are affected by the prevalence of the disease.**

NEGATIVE PREDICTIVE VALUE (NPV)

Negative predictive value is the probability that a patient with a negative test result is disease-free. A test will have a higher negative predictive value for diseases with a low prevalence.

RELATIVE RISK (RR)

Used in **prospective studies,** relative risk compares the risk of disease in a group exposed to a particular factor with the risk in the unexposed group (Figure 2.4–2).

	Disease Develops	No Disease	
Exposure	a	b	$RR = \dfrac{a\,/\,(a+b)}{c\,/\,(c+d)}$
No exposure	c	d	$OR = ad/bc$

FIGURE 2.4–2. Odds ratio and relative risk.

ODDS RATIO (OR)

The odds ratio is used in **retrospective studies** (e.g., case-control studies) and describes the odds of exposure in diseased individuals compared with those without the disease (see Figure 2.4–2). For rare diseases, the odds ratio approximates the relative risk.

CASE-CONTROL STUDY

An observational study, usually **retrospective,** in which cases (with disease) and controls (without disease) are identified. Information collected about past exposure to possible etiologic factors is used to calculate an OR.

- **Advantages:** Studies can use smaller study groups, are less costly, focus on **rare diseases,** and examine multiple potential etiologic factors.
- **Limitations:** Data may be inaccurate due to **recall bias** (exposures happened in the past) and **survivorship bias** (many of those with disease have already died) and cannot be used to calculate RR.

COHORT STUDY

An observational study that is usually **prospective.** A sample group (cohort) with matched controls (selected based on the presence or absence of exposure to a factor of interest) is **followed to see if disease develops.** A **relative risk** is calculated from these data.

- **Advantages:** Data are often more accurate, since they can be collected as the exposures occur (not based on recall of past events). Studies can examine the effects of **rare exposures** and multiple outcomes for the same exposure.
- **Limitations:** Studies take a long time to complete and may be costly. Confounders may be introduced (since exposure is not randomly distributed), rare diseases cannot be studied, and cases may be lost to follow-up.

CLINICAL TRIAL

An experimental, **prospective** study in which subjects are assigned to a treatment group or a control group. Studies are usually **randomized** to eliminate selection bias and to balance prognostic factors, as well as **double-blinded** to prevent observer bias on the part of those performing the study (since they often have a vested interest in the outcome). A new therapy should be compared to the established standard of care if this standard of care has been shown to be preferable to placebo.

- **Advantages:** Highest-quality study; can control for many potential confounders with careful inclusion/exclusion criteria; can potentially prove causality.
- **Limitations:** Very costly; can take a long time to complete.

CROSS–SECTIONAL SURVEYS

A survey of the population at a single point in time.

- **Advantages:** Can be used to estimate disease prevalence and for hypothesis formation.
- **Limitations:** Risk factors and presence of disease are collected simultaneously; thus, a cause-and-effect relationship cannot be established.

META-ANALYSIS

Pooling together data from several studies (often via literature search).

- **Advantages:** Can achieve greater statistical power. Can be used to resolve controversial issues in the clinical literature (conflicting studies).
- **Limitations:** Cannot overcome limitations of different studies. There are methodologic and statistical issues in combining means and variances in different studies.

CONFOUNDING VARIABLES

Confounding variables are variables in a study that are associated with both the exposure of interest and the disease and may thus disrupt the relationship between these two variables, leading to erroneous conclusions. Confounders such as socioeconomic status, gender, or age can be controlled for by design (matching for case control; stratification) or by analysis (multivariate analysis; adjustment).

Epidemiology and
Preventive Medicine

LEADING CAUSES OF DEATH

Table 2.4–3 presents the leading causes of death in different age groups.

TABLE 2.4–3. Leading Causes of Death by Age*

Age	Most Common Causes of Death
Birth to 18 months	Perinatal conditions, congenital abnormalities, injuries, pneumonia
2–6	Injuries, motor vehicle accidents (MVAs), congenital abnormalities, homicide, heart disease
7–12	MVAs, injuries, congenital abnormalities, leukemia, homicide, heart disease
13–39	MVAs, homicide, suicide, injuries, heart disease
40–60	Heart disease, lung cancer, CVA, breast cancer, COPD
Over age 60	Heart disease, cerebrovascular disease, COPD, pneumonia, lung cancer, colorectal cancer

*From U.S. Preventative Services Task Force, 1996.

HEALTH CARE SCREENING

Table 2.4–4 summarizes recommended screening measures by age.

TABLE 2.4–4. Health Care Screening

Age	Screening Measure
Birth to 10 years	Height and weight, BP, vision screen, hemoglobinopathy screen (in high-risk populations*), phenylalanine level (at birth), TSH and/or T_4 (at birth).
11–24	Height and weight, BP, Pap smear (beginning when sexually active or at 18 years), chlamydia screen (sexually active), rubella serology or vaccination (women only), screen for alcohol abuse.
25–64	BP (< 140/90), height and weight, cholesterol, Pap smear, fecal occult blood test (FOBT) and/or sigmoidoscopy (> 50 years), mammography/clinical breast exam (50–69 years), screen for alcohol abuse, rubella serology or vaccination (women).
65 and older	BP, height and weight, FOBT and/or sigmoidoscopy, mammography/breast exam, Pap smear (sexually active), vision screening, hearing screening, screen for alcohol abuse.

* Individuals of African, Caribbean, Latin American, Mediterranean, Middle Eastern, or Southeast Asian descent.

Table 2.4–5 summarizes recommended screening measures.

CXR is not effective in lung cancer screening.

TABLE 2.4–4. Recommended Cancer Screening Measures*

Screening Measure	Ages and Intervals
Flexible sigmoidoscopy**	Q 3–5 years after 50
Fecal occult blood test	Q year after 50
Digital rectal examination**	Q year after 40
Prostate examination**	Q year after 50
Pap smear	Sexually active or 18, Q 1 year; after three normal smears, Q 3 years
Pelvic exam	20–40, Q 1–3 years; after 40, Q year
Endometrial tissue sample**	At menopause
Breast self-exam**	Q month after 20
Breast exam by clinician	20–40, Q 3 years; after 40, Q year
Mammography	Q year after 40–50 (exact timing controversial)
CXR	Not recommended as a screening test

*From U.S. Preventative Services Task Force, 1996.
**Additional recommendations from the American Cancer Society.

COLORECTAL CANCER SCREENING

- Patients with **large/multiple adenomas** on sigmoidoscopy or colonoscopy should have a follow-up colonoscopy within three years.
- Patients with one or more **first-degree relatives** (parent, child, sibling) with a history of colorectal cancer should be screened with sig-moi-doscopy beginning at age 40.
- Patients with **IBD of eight years' duration** should consider surveillance colonoscopy.
- Patients with **FAP** should be screened by genetic analysis and followed with serial colonoscopy/sigmoidoscopy starting at age 10.
- Patients with **FAP** or with long-standing **ulcerative colitis (10+ years)** should consider prophylactic colectomy to eliminate the risk of colon cancer.
- Patients with a first-degree relative with adenomatous polyps before age 60 should consider early screening.

HEPATITIS B VACCINE

Give the hepatitis B vaccine to Alaskan natives, Pacific Islanders, Native Americans, homosexual men, IV drug users, military personnel, and health care/lab workers.

PNEUMOCOCCAL VACCINE

Give the pneumococcal vaccine to patients with cardiopulmonary disease, diabetes, nephrotic syndrome, cirrhosis, or asplenia (including patients with sickle cell disease), to Native American/Alaskan native populations, and to all people > 65. The standard pneumococcal vaccine (PPV23) is not effective in children < 2 years of age. A new conjugate vaccine (PPV7) has been approved for children of this age.

INFLUENZA A VACCINE

Give the influenza A vaccine to patients with cardiopulmonary disease, diabetics, elderly patients (especially in **chronic care facilities**), patients with hemoglobinopathies, immune-compromised individuals, patients with renal dysfunction, health care workers (to reduce nosocomial transmission), and all people > 65.

CHOLESTEROL

**Cardiovascular
risk factors—**

CAD HDL
Cigarettes
Age and sex
Diabetes mellitus

Hypertension
Death from MI in
family
LDL high and **L**ow
HDL

Target LDL in patients with

CAD < 100.

Elevated cholesterol levels are a strong risk factor for cardiovascular disease. Screening should be done for men at age 35 and then every five years; for women, screening should be conducted once at age 45 and then every five years. Additional risk factors for CAD include a family history of premature CAD, hypertension, smoking, HDL < 35, and diabetes. Males > 45 years of age and women > 55 are at greatest risk. Guidelines are as follows:

- **Total cholesterol < 200** (mg/dL): Retest in five years.
- **Total cholesterol > 200:** Test lipid fractions; treat on basis of LDL.
- **LDL 130–159:** Borderline risk. Treat with dietary modification and exercise.
- **LDL > 130 + CAD, LDL > 160 with two risk factors, or LDL > 190:** High risk. Begin drug therapy.
- **Triglycerides < 200 mg/dL:** Considered normal.

Management is as follows:

- **Diet:** Modest (10–15%) reduction in cholesterol results in 15–30% reduction in cardiovascular events.
- **HMG-CoA reductase inhibitors:** Most effective cholesterol-lowering drugs. Can cause LFT abnormalities, warfarin potentiation, and/or myositis.
- **Bile acid sequestrants:** May interfere with the absorption of other drugs (digoxin, Coumadin, thiazides). Constipation and gas are common.

- **Niacin:** Cheap and effective, but facial flushing limits patient compliance.

Lifetime risks for a 50-year-old Caucasian woman:

- CAD 46%, hip fracture 15%, breast cancer 10%, endometrial cancer 3%.
- Leading causes of death in women 50–75: CAD > cancer > stroke.

Benefits of HRT:

- Reduction of CAD risk.
- Reduction of osteoporosis and fracture risk (all fractures) by 50%.
- Possibly decreases colon cancer risk and stroke risk; delays onset of Alzheimer's.
- Minimizes vasomotor and genitourinary symptoms.

Risks of HRT:

- Endometrial cancer risk increased (reduced by giving progesterone).
- Increase in incidence of thromboembolic disease.

Management:

- HRT is currently recommended for postmenopausal women.
- Family or personal history of breast cancer is a relative contraindication.

HIGH-YIELD FACTS

Epidemiology and Preventive Medicine

Bias introduced when a clinician is aware that his patient belongs to a particular study group.	Observational bias
Bias introduced when screening detects a disease earlier and thus lengthens the time from diagnosis to death.	Lead-time bias
In a study of 100 subjects, 50 receive a new medication and 50 receive placebo. Of the 50 receiving the medication, 30 develop a purple rash; 20 do not. Of the 50 receiving placebo, 5 report a purple rash, while 45 do not. What is the relative risk of developing a purple rash on the medication?	Relative risk is 1.5
Type of study useful for examining the etiology of a relatively rare disease.	Retrospective case-control study
Standard annual screening measures in patients > 50 years.	FOBT, pelvic exam, mammography/breast exam
Age to begin mammography in a patient without family history of breast cancer.	40–50
In which patients do you initiate colorectal cancer screening early?	Patients with IBD, FAP, first-degree relatives with adenomatous polyps (< 60 years) or colorectal cancer
Indications for beginning cholesterol-lowering medication.	Total cholesterol > 200 with LDL > 190. Begin with LDL > 130 if there is coexisting coronary artery disease; LDL > 160 with two risk factors (family history, hypertension, smoking, low HDL, diabetes)
When do you give a pneumococcal vaccine?	Indications include patients > 65, cardiopulmonary disease, diabetes, cirrhosis, asplenia, sickle cell disease
Name three benefits of hormone replacement therapy in menopausal women.	1. Reduced risk of cardiovascular disease 2. Reduced risk of osteoporosis 3. Decreased symptoms, including flushing, vaginal dryness, and loss of urinary control

The following clinical questions and accompanying answers are reproduced, with permission, from Ratelle S, *PreTest: USMLE Step 2: Preventive Medicine and Public Health*, 9th ed., New York: McGraw-Hill, 2001.

Questions

Lou Stewells, a pioneer in the study of diarrheal disease, has developed a new diagnostic test for cholera. When his agent is added to the stool, the organisms develop a characteristic ring around them. (He calls it the "Ring-Around-the-Cholera" [RAC] test.) He performs the test on 100 patients known to have cholera and 100 patients known not to have cholera with the following results:

	Cholera	No Cholera
RAC test +	91	12
RAC test −	9	88
Totals	100	100

1. Which of the following statements is INCORRECT about the RAC test?
   a. The sensitivity of the test was about 91%
   b. The specificity of the test was about 12%
   c. The false negative rate was about 9%
   d. The predictive value of a positive result cannot be determined from the preceding information
   e. The predictive value of a negative result cannot be determined from the preceding information

2. In a study of the cause of lung cancer, patients who had the disease were matched with controls by age, sex, place of residence, and social class. The frequency of cigarette smoking was then compared in the two groups. What type of study was this?
   a. Prospective cohort
   b. Retrospective cohort
   c. Clinical trial
   d. Case-control
   e. Correlation

3. For which patient is pneumococcal vaccine PPV23 not beneficial?
   a. A 15-month-old HIV-infected infant
   b. A 20-year-old about to undergo a splenectomy for ITP
   c. A 70-year-old healthy female
   d. A 5-year-old with sickle cell disease
   e. A 10-year-old with nephrotic syndrome who received the vaccine five years ago

A 53-year-old woman presents to your office with questions about hormonal replacement therapy (HRT). She has been experiencing hot flashes and night sweats. She has not menstruated for one year. She has no risk factors for cardiovascular disease. She is 5'6" and weighs 120 lbs. Her gynecological examination is normal as well as her Pap smear. Her breast examination and mammography are also normal. She wonders about the risks and benefits of HRT given her health status.

4. HRT most increases her risk of developing which of the following conditions?
   a. Hypertension
   b. Thrombosis
   c. Alzheimer's disease
   d. Gallbladder disease
   e. Endometrial cancer

Answers

1. **The answer is b.** Sensitivity and specificity are measures of how often a diagnostic test gives the correct answer. Sensitivity reflects the test's performance in people who have the disease, and specificity measures the test's performance in people who do not have the disease. These definitions can be illustrated as follows:

	Disease Present	**Disease Absent**
Test positive	True positive (TP)	False positive (FP)
Test negative	False negative (FN)	True negative (TN)
Sensitivity = TP/(TP + FN)	Specificity = TN/(TN + FP)	

Among people who have the disease, there are two possibilities: either the test correctly identifies them (TP), or it falsely classifies them as negative (FN). Thus, among those with disease, sensitivity measures how often the test gives the right answer. (A good way to remember sensitivity is by the initials PID: positive in disease.) Similarly, among people who do not have the disease, there are also two possibilities: either the test will correctly identify them as not having disease (TN), or it will falsely classify them as diseased (FP). Thus, specificity measures how often the test gives the right answer among those who do not have the disease. (A good way to remember specificity is by the initials NIH: negative in health.)

As opposed to sensitivity and specificity, which measure the test's performance in groups of patients who do and do not have the disease, predictive value measures how often the test is right in patients grouped another way: by whether the test result is positive or negative. Thus, predictive value of a positive test is the proportion of positive tests that are true positives [TP/(TP + FP)], and predictive value of a negative result is the proportion of negative test results that are true negatives [TN/(TN + FN)].

But predictive value is a little tricky because it also depends on the prevalence of the disease in the population tested. In this case, Dr. Stewells assembled groups of 100 patients with and without cholera, and the prevalence is not given. Therefore, predictive value cannot be calculated in this question, and the correct answer is B, since specificity is 88%, not 12%.

2. **The answer is d.** The study described was a case-control study. In this type of study, people who have a disease (cases) are compared with people whom they closely resemble except for the presence of the disease under study (controls). Cases and controls are then studied for the frequency of exposure to a suspected risk factor. In case-control studies, the validity of inferences about the causal relationship between the exposure (cigarette smoking) and the disease (lung cancer) depends on how comparable the cases and controls are for all variables that may be related to both the risk factor and disease under study (e.g., age, sex, race, place of residence, and occupation). Matching is a method to control for confounding in case-control studies to eliminate the effect of any extraneous variable that is not under study but may have an effect on the results. In clinical trials, or experimental/intervention studies, the investigators allocate the exposure. Correlation studies are used to compare disease frequencies between entire populations (as opposed to individuals). For example, a correlation study could examine the consumption of animal fat and the rates of colon cancer among 20 different countries.

3. **The answer is a.** Pneumococcal vaccine PPV23 is not effective in children < 2 years of age. A heptavalent pneumococcal conjugate vaccine (PCV7) has been approved for use in children 23 months and younger. PCV7 is now recommended for universal use for all children under 23 months, including those at high risk (which includes HIV infection). Other indications for pneumococcal vaccine include persons over the age of 65 and those with anatomical or functional asplenia, nephrotic syndrome, sickle cell disease, chronic heart and lung disease, cirrhosis of the liver, and diabetes. As this is a rapidly evolving field and includes more complicated regimens for children, consultation with local health departments should be made for the latest recommendations for immunization series and boosters.

4. **The answer is e.** Menopause is associated with substantial rises in total and LDL cholesterol. Some studies have suggested that HRT appears to decrease the incidence of Alzheimer's disease. HRT has no effect on gallbladder disease and hypertension. Unopposed estrogen therapy particularly increases the risk of endometrial cancer. Adding progesterone to the regimen significantly reduces this risk, but does not eliminate it. Thin, white women are particularly at risk of osteoporosis. Although there is definitely a benefit from reduction of CVD, this patient has little risk factors for developing the disease and may benefit more from the reduction of fractures. HRT may increase the risk of developing breast cancer and may slightly increase the risk of deep venous thrombosis (DVT). On a population basis, the benefits of HRT (reduction in cardiovascular diseases and osteoporosis) are of greater magnitude than the risks (DVT, endometrial, and breast cancer). On an individual basis, risks and benefits should be assessed based on risk profile.

HIGH-YIELD FACTS

Epidemiology and Preventive Medicine

Ethics

Incompetent patients cannot refuse treatment.

All competent patients have the right to refuse care. For example, **Jehovah's Witnesses can refuse blood products.** However, a patient who has been deemed incompetent, such as an acutely intoxicated patient with altered mental status, cannot refuse treatment.

UCV *Psych.32*

DISCLOSURE

Physicians must be honest and open with patients. Patients have a right to know about their medical status, their prognosis, and all potential treatment options **(full disclosure). Physicians are obligated to inform patients of mistakes made in their medical treatment.** A patient's family cannot make a physician withhold information from the patient. In the rare situation where disclosure would harm the patient or potentially undermine his or her decision-making capacity, it may be ethically acceptable to withhold information **(therapeutic privilege).**

UCV *Psych.34*

INFORMED CONSENT

Before any procedure or medical therapy, a patient must be told the **indications** for that intervention, its **risks and benefits,** the potential **alternatives** (including the likely outcome of undergoing no treatment), and a **description** of the intervention. This information must be provided in a manner that the patient can understand. Patients cannot be coerced into giving **informed consent** and may change their minds at any time. Exceptions are as follows:

- In cases where treatment is needed emergently and the individual is unable to give consent, **consent to treatment is implied.** Likewise, it is not necessary to wait for parental consent (unless parents are present) before initiating emergent treatment on minors (implied consent).
- For patients lacking decision-making capacity, consent should be obtained from the **designated surrogate** decision maker or closest relative.
- Patients who have signed a waiver to the right of informed consent.

CONFIDENTIALITY

When in doubt, always maintain patient confidentiality.

Any information disclosed by a patient to his or her physician, as well as any information about a patient's medical condition, is considered to be **confidential** and should not be divulged without the expressed consent of the patient. When in doubt, always maintain patient confidentiality. However, it is ethically and legally **necessary to override confidentiality in order to prevent harm to a third party** (e.g., in cases involving child/elder/spousal abuse or threats against an individual that you feel the patient has the potential to carry out) as well as in specific legally defined situations (e.g., mandatory reporting of gunshot and knife wounds, intoxicated automobile drivers, and reportable diseases).

UCV *Psych.33*

HIGH-YIELD FACTS

Ethics

MINORS

Parental consent is not necessary in emergent life-threatening situations, since consent to treat is implied. For minors needing medical care **during pregnancy** or those requesting **treatment for STDs or substance abuse,** parental consent is not necessary, and confidentiality with the patient should be maintained. Confidentiality in such situations can be broken only with the patient's expressed permission, even if a parent requests information. Also remember that **confidentiality can be broken if a minor is a danger to himself or to others** (e.g., in instances where a minor expresses suicidal or homicidal intent).

UCV *Psych.30*

Parental consent is not necessary for pregnant minors or those requesting treatment for STDs or substance abuse.

DURABLE POWER OF ATTORNEY (DPOA)

Durable power of attorney (DPOA) is a written advance directive that legally designates an individual as the surrogate health care decision maker if a patient loses decision-making capability. This is **more flexible** than a living will. The designated individual should make decisions consistent with the patient's stated wishes whenever possible.

UCV *Psych.29*

LIVING WILL

A living will is a written advance directive addressing the patient's wishes in limited, specific medical situations. Examples include **DNR** ("do not resuscitate") and **DNI** ("do not intubate") directives. Note: DNR/DNI orders do not imply "do not treat"; patients with such orders should still receive the maximal medical intervention available short of resuscitation and/or intubation.

UCV *Psych.29*

DNR/DNI orders do not imply "do not treat."

SURROGATE

When patients are unable to make decisions regarding their health care and no living will or DPOA exists, decisions should be made by **close family members, friends,** or **personal physicians,** in that order. In such situations, the individuals in question will make decisions consistent with what they believe to be the patient's wishes.

END-OF-LIFE ISSUES

Patients and their decision makers have the right to forgo life-sustaining treatments even when this requires the withdrawal of care. This includes mechanical ventilation, IV hydration, parenteral/enteral nutrition, and the administration of medications, including antibiotics. It is important to know that from an ethical perspective, **there is no distinction between the withholding and the withdrawal of life-sustaining interventions.** It is also ethical to provide palliative treatment to relieve pain and suffering even though it may hasten a patient's death.

UCV *Psych.35*

It is ethical to provide palliative treatment even though it may hasten the patient's death.

FUTILITY

Physicians are not ethically obligated to provide treatment when:

- There is no pathophysiologic rationale for treatment.
- Maximal intervention is currently failing.
- A given intervention has already failed.
- Treatment will not achieve the goals of care.

In such circumstances, physicians are permitted to **refuse** a family's request for further intervention.

EUTHANASIA

Euthanasia is the administration of a **lethal agent** with the intent of **relieving suffering.** This is a highly controversial issue that is currently the subject of intense debate both in court and in the media. The AMA Code of Medical Ethics currently **opposes** such practices. **Inadequate pain control** or comorbid depression are common causes for requests for euthanasia.

True or false: Once patients sign a statement giving consent, they are bound to continue treatment.	False. Patients may change their minds at any time.
Exceptions to the requirement of informed consent.	In emergency situations, in patients deemed incapable of decision making, and when a waiver to the right of informed consent has been signed.
A 15-year-old pregnant girl requires hospitalization for preeclampsia. Should parents be informed?	No. Parental consent for minors is not necessary for medical treatment during pregnancy.
When confidentiality may be overridden.	Only to prevent harm to a third party or to self (suicide) or with reportable diseases.
True or false: Withdrawing care is a more serious measure than withholding care.	False. Patients have the right to forgo life-sustaining treatments; withdrawing or withholding care are considered the same measures from an ethical standpoint.
When is a physician allowed to refuse to continue to treat a patient on the grounds of futility?	When there is no rationale for treatment, maximal intervention is failing, the requested intervention has already failed, and treatment will not achieve the goals of care.

HIGH-YIELD FACTS

Ethics

Gastrointestinal

Portal-systemic anastomoses

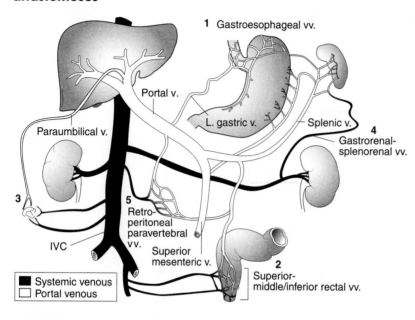

1. Left gastric-azygous → **esophageal varices.**
2. Superior-middle/inferior rectal → **hemorrhoids.**
3. Paraumbilical-inferior epigastric → **caput medusae** (navel).
4. Retroperitoneal → renal.
5. Retroperitoneal → paravertebral.

Gut, butt, and caput, the anastomoses 3. Commonly seen in alcoholic cirrhosis.

GI blood supply

Artery	Gut region	Structures supplied
Celiac	Foregut	Stomach to duodenum; liver, gallbladder, pancreas
SMA	Midgut	Duodenum to proximal $2/3$ of transverse colon
IMA	Hindgut	Distal $1/3$ of transverse colon to upper portion of rectum

Cirrhosis/ portal hypertension

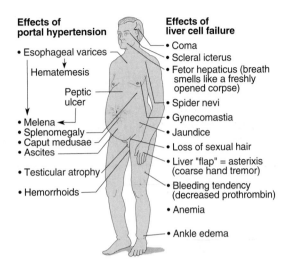

Effects of portal hypertension
- Esophageal varices
  ↓ Hematemesis
  Peptic ulcer
  ↓
- Melena ◄
- Splenomegaly
- Caput medusae
- Ascites
- Testicular atrophy
- Hemorrhoids

Effects of liver cell failure
- Coma
- Scleral icterus
- Fetor hepaticus (breath smells like a freshly opened corpse)
- Spider nevi
- Gynecomastia
- Jaundice
- Loss of sexual hair
- Liver "flap" = asterixis (coarse hand tremor)
- Bleeding tendency (decreased prothrombin)
- Anemia
- Ankle edema

(Adapted, with permission, from Chandrasoma P, Taylor CE, *Concise Pathology*, 3rd ed., Stamford, CT: Appleton and Lange, 1998: p. 654.)

Cirrho (Greek) = tawny yellow. Diffuse fibrosis of liver, destroys normal architecture.
Nodular regeneration.
Micronodular: nodules < 3 mm, uniform size. Due to metabolic insult (e.g., alcohol).
Macronodular: nodules > 3 mm, varied size. Usually due to significant liver injury leading to hepatic necrosis (e.g., postinfectious or drug-induced hepatitis).
Increased risk of hepatocellular carcinoma.

Hepatocellular carcinoma

Also called hepatoma. Most common primary malignant tumor of the liver in adults. Increased incidence of hepatocellular carcinoma is associated with hepatitis B and C, Wilson's disease, hemochromatosis, α_1-antitrypsin deficiency, alcoholic cirrhosis, and carcinogens (e.g., aflatoxin B1).

Hepatocellular carcinoma, like renal cell carcinoma, is commonly spread by hematogenous dissemination.

Gallstones

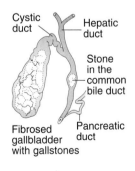

Cystic duct
Hepatic duct
Stone in the common bile duct
Fibrosed gallbladder with gallstones
Pancreatic duct

Form when solubilizing bile acids and lecithin are overwhelmed by increased cholesterol and/or bilirubin.
Three types of stones:
1. Cholesterol stones: associated with obesity, Crohn's disease, cystic fibrosis, advanced age, clofibrate, estrogens, multiparity, rapid weight loss, and Native American origin.
2. Mixed stones: have both cholesterol and pigment components. Most common type.
3. Pigment stones: seen in patients with chronic RBC hemolysis, alcoholic cirrhosis, advanced age, and biliary infection.
Diagnose with ultrasound. Treat with cholecystectomy.

Risk factors (**4 F's**):
1. **F**emale
2. **F**at
3. **F**ertile
4. **F**orty
May present with "Charcot's triad" of epigastric/RUQ pain, fever, jaundice.

Pancreatic adenocarcinoma

Prognosis averages six months or less; very aggressive; usually already metastasized at presentation; tumors more common in pancreatic head (obstructive jaundice).

Often presents with:

1. Abdominal pain radiating to back
2. Weight loss
3. Anorexia
4. Migratory thrombophlebitis (Trousseau's syndrome)
5. Pancreatic duct obstruction (malabsorption with palpable gallbladder)

H₂ blockers

Cimetidine, ranitidine, famotidine, nizatidine

Mechanism   Reversible block of histamine H₂ receptors.

Clinical use   Peptic ulcer, gastritis, esophageal reflux, Zollinger–Ellison syndrome.

Toxicity   Cimetidine is a potent inhibitor of P450; it also has an antiandrogenic effect and decreases renal excretion of creatinine. Other H₂ blockers are relatively free of these effects.

Omeprazole, lansoprazole

Mechanism   Irreversibly inhibits H⁺/K⁺ ATPase in stomach parietal cells.

Clinical use   Peptic ulcer, gastritis, esophageal reflux, Zollinger–Ellison syndrome.

Regulation of gastric acid secretion

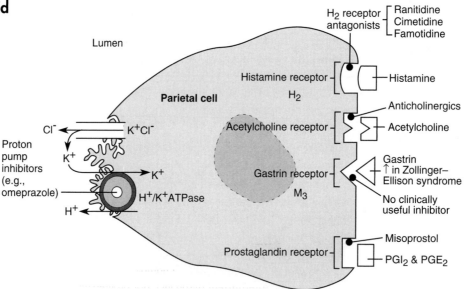

Difficulty swallowing due to difficulty getting food through the oropharynx (**oropharyngeal dysphagia**), difficulty getting it through the esophagus (**esophageal dysphagia**), or pain with swallowing (**odynophagia**).

History

Oropharyngeal dysphagia usually involves **liquids** more than solids and may be accompanied by dysarthria or dysphonia. Esophageal dysphagia usually involves **both** liquids and solids and is generally progressive.

PE

Examine for masses (goiter, tumor) and anatomic defects.

Differential

- **Oropharyngeal dysphagia:** Neurologic disorders (e.g., cranial nerve disease or bulbar injury), muscular disease, thyroid disease, sphincter dysfunction, Zenker's diverticulum, neoplasm, postsurgery/radiation.
- **Esophageal dysphagia:** Schatzki's ring (lower esophageal webs; usually due to reflux), neoplasm (Surg.15), achalasia (Surg.9), spasm, peptic stricture, scleroderma (Table 2.6–1).
- **Odynophagia:** Infectious agents (in HIV+ patients, consider *Candida*, CMV, and herpesvirus), chemical agents (lye ingestion or pill-induced).

Evaluation

- **Oropharyngeal dysphagia:** Videoesophagography.
- **Esophageal dysphagia:** Barium swallow followed by endoscopy, manometry, or pH monitoring. If an obstructive lesion is suspected, proceed straight to endoscopy.
- **Odynophagia:** Barium study or endoscopy.

Diagnostic hints:
Patient who smokes and drinks: esophageal cancer.
Patient with iron deficiency anemia: esophageal webs.
Patient with AIDS: Candida esophagitis.

HIGH-YIELD FACTS

Gastrointestinal

TABLE 2.6–1. Causes of Esophageal Dysphagia

Cause	Clues
Mechanical obstruction	Solid foods more than liquids
Schatzki's ring	Intermittent dysphagia; not progressive
Peptic stricture	Chronic heartburn; progressive dysphagia
Esophageal cancer	Progressive dysphagia; age > 50
Motility disorder	Solid and liquid foods
Achalasia	Progressive dysphagia
Diffuse esophageal spasm	Intermittent; not progressive; may have chest pain
Scleroderma	Chronic heartburn; Raynaud's phenomenon

ESOPHAGEAL CANCER

Squamous cell carcinoma is the most common (90%) cancer of the esophagus. Risk factors include alcohol, smoking, male gender, and age > 50. Approximately 10% of esophageal cancers are adenocarcinomas. These cancers are associated with Barrett's esophagus (columnar metaplasia of the distal esophagus secondary to chronic GERD).

History/PE

Progressive dysphagia, initially to solids and later to liquids as well. Weight loss, odynophagia (painful swallowing), reflux, GI bleeding, and vomiting are also common.

Evaluation

Barium study shows narrowing of the esophagus with an irregular mass protruding into the lumen. Esophagogastroduodenoscopy (EGD) and biopsy confirm the diagnosis. MRI or CT is used to evaluate for metastases.

Treatment

Chemotherapy and radiation therapy are used, but the prognosis is poor. Surgical or endoscopic debulking of the tumor may alleviate the symptoms.

UCV *Surg.22*

GASTROESOPHAGEAL REFLUX DISEASE (GERD)

Risk factors for GERD include hiatal hernia, obesity, and pregnancy.

Symptomatic reflux of gastric contents into the esophagus. **Transient lower esophageal sphincter (LES) relaxation** is the most common etiology of GERD. GERD can be due in part to an incompetent LES, abnormally acidic gastric contents, and hiatal hernia. Risk factors include obesity, pregnancy, and scleroderma/Raynaud's disease. Alcohol, caffeine, nicotine, chocolate, and fatty foods can reduce LES tone.

History

GERD may mimic asthma.

Patients present with **"heartburn"** (substernal burning) that commonly occurs 30–90 minutes **after a meal,** frequently **worsens with reclining,** and often improves with antacids, standing, or sitting. Other symptoms include sour taste ("water brash"), regurgitation, dysphagia, and cough/wheezing/dyspnea (symptoms may mimic or exacerbate asthma).

PE

Usually **normal** unless there is evidence of associated systemic disease (e.g., Raynaud's disease/scleroderma).

Differential

PUD, CAD, infectious (CMV, candidal) or chemical esophagitis, gallbladder disease, achalasia, esophageal spasm, pericarditis.

Evaluation

Diagnosis is based primarily on history. **Upper endoscopy** should be performed if the patient has long-standing symptoms (to look for Barrett's esophagus and adenocarcinoma). Evaluation may include abdominal x-ray (AXR), CXR, barium swallow (of limited usefulness, but can diagnose associated hiatal hernia), and esophageal manometry/pH monitoring.

Treatment

- **Lifestyle:** Lifestyle modifications include weight loss, elevation of the head of the bed, and avoidance of nocturnal meals and substances reducing LES tone.
- **Pharmacologic:** Start with **antacids** in patients with mild to moderate disease; use H_2 **receptor antagonists** (cimetidine, ranitidine) or **proton pump inhibitors** (omeprazole, lansoprazole) in patients with severe or refractory disease. For patients who have problems with LES function, a **pro-motility agent** (cisapride) may be beneficial.
- **Surgical:** For refractory or severe disease, **Nissen fundoplication** or hiatal hernia repair may offer significant relief.
- **Health maintenance:** Monitor for Barrett's esophagus and esophageal adenocarcinoma with **serial endoscopy/biopsy.**

Complications

Esophageal ulceration, esophageal stricture, aspiration of gastric contents, upper GI bleeding, and **Barrett's esophagus** (columnar metaplasia of the distal esophagus secondary to chronic acid irritation; associated with an increased risk of esophageal **adenocarcinoma**).

UCV IM1.32

BARReff's—

Becomes
Adenocarcinoma,
Results from **R**eflux.

GASTRITIS

Inflammation of the stomach lining.

- **Acute (stress) gastritis** occurs as rapidly developing, superficial lesions. It is often due to NSAIDs, alcohol, and stress from severe illness (e.g., burns).
- **Chronic gastritis** has two types. **Type A** (< 10%) occurs in the fundus and is due to autoantibodies to parietal cells. It is associated with other autoimmune disorders, including pernicious anemia and thyroiditis. **Type B** (> 90%) occurs in the antrum and may be caused by NSAID use or *H. pylori* infection. It is often asymptomatic but is associated with an increased risk for peptic ulcer disease and gastric cancer.

History/PE

The patient may be asymptomatic or may complain of indigestion, nausea, vomiting, hematemesis, or melena.

Evaluation

Upper endoscopy to visualize gastric lining. *H. pylori* infection can be detected by urease breath test, serum IgG antibody (indicating exposure, not current infection), or endoscopic biopsy.

Treatment

Treatment depends on the underlying cause. Decrease intake of offending agents (e.g., NSAIDs, alcohol), and give antacids, sucralfate, H_2 blockers, and/or proton pump inhibitors. *H. pylori* infection should be treated with triple therapy (metronidazole, clarithromycin, bismuth salicylate/amoxicillin) +/− a proton pump inhibitor. Patients at risk for stress ulcers (e.g., ICU patients) should be given an H_2 blocker for prophylaxis.

PEPTIC ULCER DISEASE (PUD)

Damage to the gastric or duodenal mucosa caused by a combination of impaired mucosal defense and increased acidic gastric contents. **H. pylori** plays a causative role in > 90% of duodenal ulcers as well as in 70% of gastric ulcers. Other risk factors include **corticosteroid, NSAID, alcohol,** and **tobacco** use. Males are affected more often than females.

History

Patients present with chronic/periodic, **dull/burning/aching epigastric pain** (dyspepsia) that **improves with meals** (especially duodenal ulcers), worsens 2–3 hours after eating, and can radiate to the back. Patients may also complain of nausea, hematemesis ("coffee-ground" emesis), and blood in the stool (melena or hematochezia).

PE

Varying degrees of **epigastric tenderness** and **positive stool guaiac** if there is active bleeding. An acute perforation will commonly present with a rigid abdomen, rebound tenderness, guarding, or other signs of peritoneal irritation.

Differential

GERD, CAD, gastritis, pancreatitis (acute or chronic), cholecystitis, Zollinger–Ellison syndrome, aortic aneurysm, and other causes of acute abdomen, depending on the severity of the pain and on physical findings (severe pain suggests perforation).

Evaluation

AXR to **rule out perforation** (free air under the diaphragm) and CBC to assess for GI bleeding (low or falling hematocrit). **Upper endoscopy** with biopsy to confirm the diagnosis and to rule out active bleeding or gastric adenocarcinoma (10% of gastric ulcers). *H. pylori* testing involves urease breath test, serum IgG (less expensive but less sensitive and indicates exposure, not active infection), or endoscopic biopsy. PUD can also be diagnosed with a barium swallow if endoscopy is not available. Elevated amylase suggests pancreatic involvement. In recurrent or refractory cases, serum gastrin should be measured to screen for Zollinger–Ellison syndrome.

Rule out Zollinger–Ellison syndrome with serum gastrin levels in cases of GERD and PUD that are refractory to medical management.

Treatment

- **Acute:** Rule out active bleeding with nasogastric lavage, stool guaiac, and serial hematocrits. If perforation is likely (based on exam and AXR), **surgery** is usually indicated. For GI bleeding, carefully monitor the patient's hematocrit and BP and initiate IV hydration, transfusion, endoscopy, and surgery as needed.
- **Pharmacologic:** Therapy consists of three arms: (1) mucosal protection, (2) decreasing acid production, and (3) eradicating *H. pylori* infection. Mild disease may be treated with antacids, which neutralize gastric acid. Sucralfate, bismuth, and misoprostol (a prostaglandin analog) can be used for mucosal protection. Either proton pump inhibitors (e.g., omeprazole) or H_2 receptor antagonists (e.g., ranitidine, cimetidine) may be used to reduce acid secretion. In patients without *H. pylori* infection, this may suffice. Patients with confirmed *H. pylori* infection should receive a course of **antibiotic treatment** (e.g., metronidazole + clarithromycin or + amoxicillin) plus treatment with a proton pump inhibitor or H_2 receptor antagonist therapy. Discontinue use of exacerbating agents (NSAIDs, alcohol, cigarettes). Patients with recurrent or severe disease may require chronic symptomatic therapy.
- **Surgery/endoscopy:** All patients with symptomatic gastric ulcers who have been symptomatic for **> 2 months** despite standard medical therapy must undergo endoscopy with biopsy to rule out gastric adenocarcinoma. Truly refractory cases may require a surgical procedure such as **parietal cell vagotomy** (most selective; preferred) or antrectomy/vagotomy.

Misoprostol can help patients with PUD who require NSAID therapy (e.g., patients with arthritis).

Complications

Hemorrhage (especially with posterior ulcers that erode into the gastroduodenal artery), gastric outlet obstruction, perforation (usually anterior ulcers; look for a perforated viscus on x-rays), and intractable disease.

UCV *IM1.38, Surg.14*

Complications of PUD—

HOPI
Hemorrhage
Obstruction
Perforation
Intractability (pain)

HIATAL HERNIA

A condition in which a portion of the stomach protrudes upward into the chest through the diaphragmatic opening. There are two common types: 95% are **sliding hiatal hernias** in which the gastroesophageal (GE) junction and a portion of the stomach protrude; 5% are **paraesophageal hiatal hernias** in which the GE junction remains below the diaphragm while a neighboring portion of the fundus herniates into the mediastinum.

History/PE

Patients may be asymptomatic but often present with reflux due to the compromised location of the GE junction.

Evaluation

Barium study. Sometimes an incidental finding on CXR.

Treatment

- **Sliding hernias:** Medical therapy and lifestyle modifications to reduce symptoms of reflux (see GERD entry).
- **Paraesophageal hernias:** Surgery (gastropexy: attachment of the stomach to the rectus sheath and closure of the hiatus) is often recommended to prevent torsion and ensuing complications.

CHOLELITHIASIS AND BILIARY COLIC

Symptoms of gallstones are due to transient cystic duct blockage from impacted stones. Risk factors include the **"5 F's"**: female, fat, fertile, forty, and flatulent—although the disorder is common and can occur in any patient. Other risk factors include oral contraceptive use, rapid weight loss, chronic hemolysis (pigment stones), small bowel resection, and total parenteral nutrition.

History

Patients present with **postprandial abdominal pain** (usually in the **RUQ**) radiating to the right subscapular area or epigastrium. Pain is of abrupt onset followed by gradual relief and is often associated with **nausea and vomiting.** Presenting symptoms may also include fatty food intolerance, dyspepsia, and flatulence. Gallstones may be asymptomatic in up to 80% of patients.

PE

RUQ tenderness and palpable gallbladder.

Differential

Acute cholecystitis, PUD, MI, acute pancreatitis, GERD, hepatitis, appendicitis.

Evaluation

RUQ ultrasound may show gallstones (95% sensitive). Consider upper GI series to rule out hiatal hernia or ulcer.

> **Patients with gallstones—**
>
> **The 5 F's**
> **F**emale
> **F**at
> **F**ertile
> **F**orty
> **F**latulent

Only 15–20% of gallstones are radiopaque.

Treatment

Cholecystectomy is both definitive and curative and can be performed on an elective basis. For patients who are not surgical candidates, treat with **dietary modification** (avoid triggering substances like fatty foods) and **pharmacologic dissolution** (with bile salts) with or without **lithotripsy** (associated with a high recurrence rate).

Complications

Recurrent biliary colic, acute cholecystitis, choledocholithiasis, gallstone ileus, and gallstone pancreatitis.

ACUTE CHOLECYSTITIS

Prolonged blockage of the cystic duct, usually by an impacted stone, resulting in postobstructive distention, inflammation, superinfection, and, in extreme cases, gangrene of the gallbladder. In chronically debilitated patients, those on TPN, and trauma or burn victims, acute cholecystitis may occur in the absence of cholelithiasis (**acalculous cholecystitis**).

History

Patients present with **RUQ pain, nausea, and vomiting** similar to that seen in biliary colic, but typically more severe and of longer duration.

PE

RUQ tenderness, inspiratory arrest during deep palpation of the RUQ (**Murphy's sign**), low-grade fever, mild icterus, and possibly guarding or rebound tenderness.

Differential

Biliary colic, cholangitis, GERD, hepatitis, acute pancreatitis, MI, acute appendicitis, renal colic, Fitz-Hugh–Curtis syndrome (acute gonococcal perihepatitis), PUD, pneumonia.

Evaluation

CBC (**leukocytosis**), amylase, and LFTs (normal or elevated). **Ultrasound** may demonstrate stones, bile sludge, pericholecystic fluid, a thickened gallbladder wall, and gas in the gallbladder (Figure 2.6–1). Obtain a **HIDA scan** when ultrasound is equivocal (Figure 2.6–2); absence of the gallbladder on HIDA scan suggests acute cholecystitis. Diagnosis is made on the basis of clinical suspicion and imaging modalities.

Treatment

Hospitalize patients, administer **IV antibiotics** and **IV fluids,** and replete electrolytes. Perform **early cholecystectomy** (within 72 hours of onset of

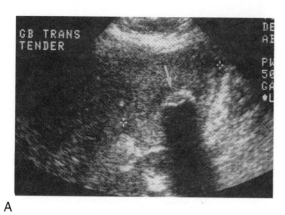
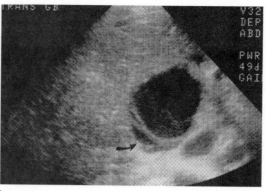

A   B

FIGURE 2.6–1. Acute cholecystitis, ultrasound. (A) Note the sludge-filled, thick-walled gallbladder with a hyperechoic stone and acoustic shadow (arrow). (B) This patient exhibits sludge and pericholecystic fluid (arrow) but no gallstones. (Reproduced, with permission, from Grendell J, *Current Diagnosis and Treatment in Gastroenterology*, 1st ed., Stamford, CT: Appleton & Lange, 1996: p. 212, Fig. 15–14A and B.)

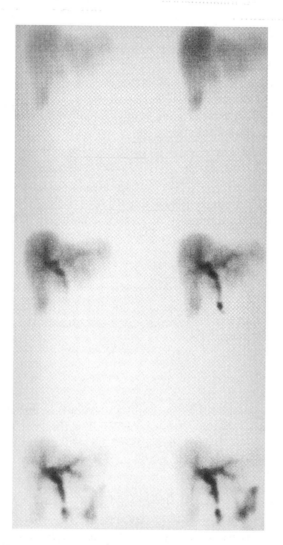

FIGURE 2.6–2. Acute cholecystitis, HIDA scan. Intravenous dye is taken up by hepatocytes, conjugated, and excreted into the common bile duct. The gallbladder is not visualized, although activity is present in the liver, common duct, and small bowel, suggesting cystic duct obstruction due to acute cholecystitis. (Reproduced, with permission, from Grendell J, *Current Diagnosis and Treatment in Gastroenterology*, 1st ed., Stamford, CT: Appleton & Lange, 1996: p. 217, Fig. 15–18.)

symptoms) in patients without significant operative risk factors along with an **intraoperative cholangiogram** to rule out common bile duct stones. An expectant approach should be taken toward patients with significant medical problems (especially diabetes). Since 50% of cases resolve spontaneously, such patients can be treated medically as long as there is no deterioration in their condition, with a four- to six-week delay in surgical treatment.

Complications

Gangrene, empyema, perforation, gallstone ileus, fistulization, sepsis, or abscess formation.

UCV *Surg.17*

CHOLANGITIS

An infection/inflammation of the biliary tree that commonly occurs secondary to **obstruction,** usually from **gallstones or malignancy.** Sclerosing cholangitis is due to progressive inflammation of the biliary tree and occurs most commonly in patients with choledocholithiasis or IBD. Other risk factors include bile duct stricture, ampullary carcinoma, and pancreatic pseudocyst. The organisms most commonly associated with cholangitis are gramnegative enterics (e.g., *E. coli, Enterobacter, Pseudomonas*).

History

Patients present with **Charcot's triad: RUQ pain, jaundice,** and **fever/chills. Reynold's pentad** (Charcot's triad plus **shock** and **altered mental status**) may be present in acute suppurative cholangitis.

PE

RUQ tenderness, jaundice, and **fever/chills.**

Differential

Pancreatic cancer, cholangiocarcinoma, carcinoma of the bile ducts, metastatic carcinoma, hepatitis, primary biliary cirrhosis *(IM1.41)*, cholecystitis, pancreatitis, sepsis, liver abscess.

Workup

Look for **leukocytosis, increased bilirubin,** and **increased alkaline phosphatase.** Obtain blood cultures. **Ultrasound** or CT may be a useful adjunct, but diagnosis is often clinical. **ERCP is the diagnostic gold standard.**

Treatment

This is a serious, life-threatening disease. Patients often require **ICU admission** for monitoring and hydration/pressor support along with aggressive **IV antibiotic treatment.** Patients with acute toxic cholangitis require **emergent bile duct decompression** via endoscopic sphincterotomy, percutaneous transhepatic drainage, or operative decompression. After the acute episode has been managed, percutaneous transhepatic cholangiography or ERCP should be performed to locate the cause of the obstruction, followed by stone extraction, stent placement, or sphincterotomy.

UCV *EM.13*

PANCREATITIS (ACUTE AND CHRONIC)

Table 2.6–2 lists the important features of acute and chronic pancreatitis.

TABLE 2.6–2. Acute and Chronic Pancreatitis

	Acute Pancreatitis	Chronic Pancreatitis
Pathophysiology	Leakage of pancreatic enzymes into pancreatic and peripancreatic tissue, often secondary to gallstone disease or alcoholism.	Irreversible parenchymal destruction leading to pancreatic dysfunction.
Time course	Abrupt onset, severe.	Persistent, recurrent.
Risk factors	**Gallstones, alcoholism,** hypercalcemia, hypertriglyceridemia, trauma, drug side effects (including thiazide diuretics), viral infections, and post-ERCP.	**Alcoholism (90%),** pancreatolithiasis, hyperparathyroidism, congenital malformation (pancreas divisum). May also be idiopathic.
Symptoms/ signs	**Severe epigastric pain** (radiating to the back), nausea, vomiting, weakness, fever, shock. Flank discoloration **(Grey–Turner sign).**	**Persistent epigastric pain,** anorexia, nausea, constipation, flatulence, steatorrhea.
Workup	↑ amylase, ↑ lipase, ↓ Ca^{++} if severe; "sentinel loop" or "colon cutoff" sign on x-ray. Ultrasound or CT may show enlarged pancreas, abscess, or pseudocyst (see Figure 2.6–3).	↑ amylase, ↑ lipase, **glycosuria, pancreatic calcifications** and mild ileus on x-ray and CT.
Management	Removal of offending agent if possible (drugs, stone, etc.). Standard supportive measures: 1. IV fluids/electrolyte replacement. 2. Analgesia. 3. Bowel rest, NG suction, nutritional support. 4. Possible respiratory support. May also require surgical debridement.	1. Pain control. 2. Treat exocrine insufficiency: exogenous lipase/trypsin and low-fat diet. 3. Discontinue alcohol use. 4. Surgery for intractable pain or structural causes.
Prognosis	85–90% mild, self-limited; 10–15% severe, requiring ICU; mortality may approach 50%.	Patients may have chronic pain and pancreatic exocrine/endocrine dysfunction.
Complications	Pancreatic **pseudocyst** (see Figure 2.6–3), fistula formation, hypocalcemia, renal failure, pleural effusion, chronic pancreatitis, sepsis.	**Chronic pain,** malnutrition, PUD.

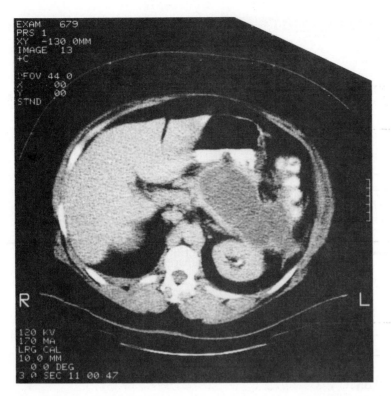

FIGURE 2.6–3. Pancreatic pseudocyst. The large pseudocyst impinges on the posterior wall of the stomach (filled with contrast) on CT scan. (Reproduced, with permission, from Way L, *Current Surgical Diagnosis & Treatment*, 10th ed., Stamford, CT: Appleton & Lange, 1994: p. 578, Fig. 27–3.)

UCV *IM1.29, Surg.13*

PANCREATIC CANCER

Carcinoma of the exocrine pancreas is most often adenocarcinoma occurring in the head of the pancreas. Risk factors are smoking and a high-fat diet. Men in their 60s are most commonly affected.

History/PE

Abdominal pain radiating toward the back, loss of appetite, nausea, vomiting, weight loss, weakness, fatigue, and indigestion. Jaundice develops if the tumor blocks the bile duct. Exam may reveal a palpable, nontender gallbladder **(Courvoisier's sign).** Migratory thrombophlebitis **(Trousseau's sign)** occurs in 10% of patients due to ectopic production of procoagulants.

Evaluation

CT scan is sensitive in detecting a pancreatic mass, dilated pancreatic and bile ducts, and the extent of vascular involvement and metastases. If a mass is not visualized, use ERCP. Transcutaneous pancreatic biopsy is useful in confirming the diagnosis but risks spreading an otherwise resectable tumor.

Treatment

Twenty percent of tumors have no evidence of metastasis and may be resected using the Whipple procedure (pancreaticoduodenectomy). Patients often present after disease is widespread, however, and in this case prognosis is poor, with a mean survival rate of six months.

UCV *Surg.33*

Portal pressure > 5 mmHg above the pressure in the IVC. Causes are divided into presinusoidal (splenic or portal vein thrombosis, schistosomiasis, granulomatous), sinusoidal (cirrhosis, granulomatous disease), and postsinusoidal (right heart failure, constrictive pericarditis, hepatic vein thrombosis). Budd–Chiari syndrome is hepatic or IVC thrombosis secondary to hypercoagulability. It requires clot lysis or hepatic transplantation and has a poor prognosis.

History

Patients can present with ascites, bacterial peritonitis (fever, abdominal pain), hepatic encephalopathy (asterixis, delirium), esophageal varices (hematemesis, GI bleed), and renal dysfunction.

PE

Abdominal fluid wave, shifting dullness, and splenomegaly. Patients with cirrhosis may have easy bruising, spider angiomata, dilated abdominal veins (caput medusae), gynecomastia, and testicular atrophy.

Evaluation

Evaluation should include LFTs, alkaline phosphatase, bilirubin, albumin, PT/PTT to assess hepatic function, and other tests to determine the cause of liver disease (serum ferritin for hemochromatosis, CT scan for Budd–Chiari syndrome). Diagnosis can be made on the basis of clinical findings plus laboratory tests that show evidence of hepatic or other dysfunction. Indirect hepatic vein wedge pressure (a measure of portal pressure) is increased.

Treatment

Treatment is aimed at ameliorating the complications of portal hypertension.

- **Ascites:** **Sodium restriction** and **diuretics** (furosemide and spironolactone); rule out infectious/neoplastic causes (perform paracentesis to obtain serum ascites albumin gradient [SAAG], WBC/cultures); treat underlying liver disease if possible.
- **Spontaneous bacterial peritonitis:** Check peritoneal fluid if there is a question of infection (PMNs > 250 with clinical signs and PMNs > 500 in an asymptomatic patient). Treat with **IV antibiotics** (e.g., third-generation cephalosporin) to cover both gram-positive (*Enterococcus*) and gram-negative (*E. coli, Klebsiella*) organisms until a causative organism is identified.
- **Hepatorenal syndrome:** This is difficult to treat, often requires dialysis, and may be fatal.
- **Hepatic encephalopathy:** Decrease protein consumption; treat with **lactulose** and/or **neomycin.**
- **Esophageal varices:** Monitor for GI bleeding; treat endoscopically or surgically if necessary.
- In some cases a hepatic shunt can be performed surgically or by transjugular intrahepatic portacaval shunt (TIPS), but this is normally a short-term bridge to transplant and may worsen hepatic encephalopathy.

Spontaneous bacterial peritonitis is diagnosed by > 500 PMNs/μL in the ascitic fluid.

UCV *IM1.34, Surg.16*

An **autosomal-recessive** disease that usually occurs in males and is rarely recognized before the fifth decade. Hemochromatosis is caused by hyperabsorption of iron with parenchymal hemosiderin accumulation in the liver, pancreas, heart, adrenals, testes, pituitary, and kidneys. Secondary hemochromatosis may occur with iron overload and is commonly seen in patients receiving **chronic transfusion therapy** and in **alcoholics** (alcohol increases GI absorption of iron).

History

Patients may present with abdominal pain, **diabetic symptoms** (e.g., polydipsia, polyuria), and cirrhosis (e.g., **jaundice**). Patients may also have arthralgias and symptoms of endocrine dysfunction (e.g., **hypogonadism**).

PE

Bronze skin pigmentation, pancreatic dysfunction **(diabetes), cardiac dysfunction** (CHF). Hepatomegaly and testicular atrophy may also be present.

Differential

Other causes of cirrhosis, CHF, or hypopituitarism; diabetes mellitus.

Evaluation

Look for **elevated serum iron,** percentage saturation of iron, and ferritin. Serum transferrin levels are decreased. Other indicators include **glucose intolerance** as well as mildly elevated AST and alkaline phosphatase. Perform a **liver biopsy** (to determine hepatic iron index) or hepatic MRI.

Treatment

Weekly **phlebotomy.** Once serum iron levels decline, patients are placed on maintenance phlebotomy (every 2–4 months). Intramuscular deferoxamine (an iron chelator) may also be used for maintenance therapy.

Complications

Cirrhosis, hepatocellular carcinoma, cardiomegaly leading to CHF and/or conduction defects, diabetes, impotence, arthropathy, hypopituitarism.

UCV *IM1.33*

A rare **autosomal-recessive** disorder characterized by excessive deposition of copper in the liver and brain. Wilson's disease usually occurs in patients < 30 years old. The defect involves a copper-transporting protein and is linked to a defect on chromosome 13.

History

Patients present with **liver abnormalities** (e.g., jaundice secondary to hepatitis/cirrhosis) as well as neurologic and **psychiatric abnormalities.** Neurologic findings include loss of coordination, **tremor,** and dysphagia. Psychiatric abnormalities include psychosis, anxiety, mania, and depression.

PE

Kayser–Fleischer rings in the cornea (green-to-brown deposits of copper in Descemet's membrane), jaundice, hepatomegaly, parkinsonian tremor, and rigidity.

Differential

Other causes of hepatitis, cirrhosis, psychiatric and neurologic disturbances.

Evaluation

Decreased serum ceruloplasmin, elevated urinary copper excretion, and elevated hepatic copper.

Treatment

Begin with **dietary copper restriction** (shellfish, liver, legumes). **Penicillamine** (a copper chelator that increases urinary copper excretion; administer with pyridoxine) and oral zinc (increases fecal excretion) can be used for maintenance therapy.

UCV *Ped.9*

> **Wilson's disease—**
>
> **ABCD**
> **A**sterixis
> **B**asal ganglia deterioration
> **C**eruloplasmin ↓, **C**irrhosis, **C**opper, **C**arcinoma (hepatocellular), **C**horeiform movements
> **D**ementia

APPENDICITIS

Inflammation of the appendix that leads to infection (abscess) and/or perforation if not recognized and treated appropriately. It is the most common abdominal emergency among those < 35 years of age. Appendicitis occurs most frequently in people aged 10–30 years and is more common in the United States than in parts of Africa and Asia (due to the low-fiber diet in the United States). The most common etiologies of appendicitis in the United States are **lymphoid hyperplasia** (60%) and **fecalith obstruction** (35%).

History

Commonly begins as **dull periumbilical pain** that waxes and wanes followed by **nausea,** emesis, and **anorexia.** Classically, **pain then shifts to the RLQ** (secondary to peritoneal irritation) and becomes sharp, continuous, localized, and increasingly severe. With perforation, abdominal pain may worsen and distention may develop (acute abdomen).

PE

Localized tenderness at **McBurney's point** (two-thirds of the way from the umbilicus to the iliac crest), mild to moderate rebound tenderness, pain with cough,

If a patient has pain that moves from the periumbilical area to the RLQ, think appendicitis.

psoas/ obturator signs, Rovsing's sign (RLQ pain on palpation of the LLQ), and low-grade fever. Patients often present before the pain has localized to the RLQ. Perform a **rectal exam** (tenderness suggests an inflamed posterior appendix).

Differential

PID, ovarian torsion, other gynecologic disorders **(always do a gynecologic exam),** volvulus, gastroenteritis, ruptured ectopic pregnancy, pyelonephritis, diverticulitis, colon cancer with perforation, Crohn's disease, perforated peptic ulcer, cholecystitis, mesenteric ischemia, pneumonia, Meckel's diverticulum.

Evaluation

The diagnosis is **clinical** and based on careful observation and serial abdominal examinations. Look for **leukocytosis** with a left shift on CBC; also obtain an AXR. **Appendiceal fecalith** on AXR is suggestive of the diagnosis but not pathognomonic. Look for **free air,** which would suggest perforation. CXR may rule out right middle/lower lobe **pneumonia. Ultrasound/CT** is used in unusual or difficult cases. A β-HCG **test** to rule out ectopic/uterine pregnancy is essential in women of childbearing age.

Always perform a pregnancy test in women of childbearing age with abdominal pain.

Treatment

Appendectomy. With free perforation, emergency surgery is necessary. If the patient has an abscess but is clinically stable, **CT-guided drainage** followed by nonurgent appendectomy may be preferable. A 20% negative appendectomy rate (i.e., removal of a normal appendix) is acceptable to minimize the number of missed cases.

Complications

Abdominal abscess, appendiceal perforation, wound infection, hepatic abscess, and septic pylephlebitis.

UCV *Surg.20*

DIARRHEA

Increased **frequency of bowel movements** or **increased stool liquidity.** Risk factors include viral infection, systemic infection, sick contacts, and recent travel.

History/PE

- **Acute diarrhea:** Acute diarrhea is characterized by acute onset with < 3 weeks of symptoms and is usually **infectious.** Causes include *E. coli, Salmonella, Shigella,* postantibiotic pseudomembranous colitis *(C. difficile),* HIV-related diseases *(Cryptosporidium, Isospora),* bacterial toxins *(S. aureus),* and food poisoning *(Salmonella, Campylobacter,* cholera, giardiasis, amebiasis).
- **Chronic diarrhea:** Chronic diarrhea is characterized by more long-standing symptoms and is due to such factors as **lactose intolerance, malabsorption** (mucosal disease, Whipple's disease, neoplasm, malnutrition), IBD, and **motility disorders.**

Acute diarrhea is usually infectious.

- **Pediatric diarrhea:** Pediatric diarrhea is most commonly due to **rotavirus infection,** bacterial infection (*E. coli, Shigella, Salmonella, Campylobacter*), postantibiotic disease (*C. difficile*), or immunosuppression.

Evaluation

Acute diarrhea usually does not require laboratory investigation unless the patient has a high fever, bloody diarrhea, or diarrhea > 4–5 days. In this case, send stool for fecal leukocytes, bacterial culture, *C. difficile* toxin, and ova and parasites. Consider sigmoidoscopy in patients with severe proctitis, bloody diarrhea, or possible *C. difficile* colitis. See Figure 2.6–4 for the evaluation of chronic diarrhea.

Treatment

- **Acute diarrhea:** Treat with oral or IV **fluids** and electrolyte replacement. **Antidiarrheal agents** such as loperamide or bismuth salicylate

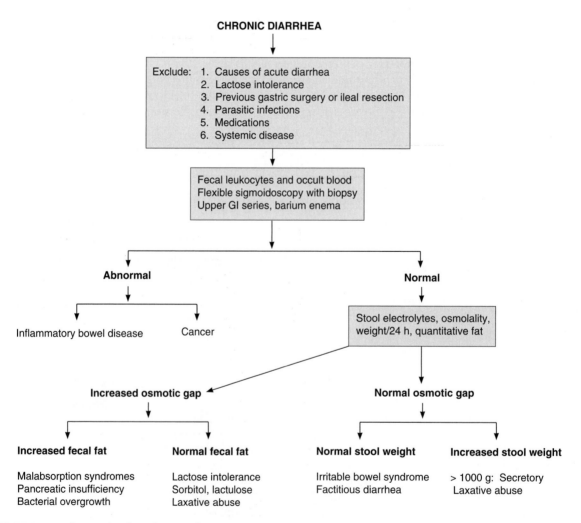

FIGURE 2.6–4. Chronic diarrhea decision diagram. (Reproduced, with permission, from Tierney LM, *Current Medical Diagnosis & Treatment,* 39th ed., New York: McGraw-Hill, 2000: p. 566, Fig. 14–1.)

may improve symptoms. If the patient has evidence of systemic infection (fever, bloody stool, chills, malaise), antibiotics may be started.

- **Chronic diarrhea:** Treatment should be aimed at the underlying cause and can also include loperamide, opioids, clonidine, octreotide, and cholestyramine.
- **Pediatric diarrhea:** For a child who cannot take medication and PO fluids, hospitalize, give IV fluids, and treat the underlying cause.

GASTROINTESTINAL BLEEDING

Bleeding from the GI tract that presents as hematemesis, blood in the stool (hematochezia, melena), or both (see Table 2.6–3).

TABLE 2.6–3. GI Bleeding

	Upper GI Bleeding	Lower GI Bleeding
History/PE	Hematemesis or coffee-ground emesis, melena > hematochezia, depleted volume status (e.g., lightheadedness, hypotension).	Hematochezia > melena, but can be either (upper or lower GI bleed can cause either symptom).
Evaluation	NG tube/lavage, endoscopy if stable.	Colonoscopy if stable. Rule out upper GI bleed with NG tube/lavage.
Common causes	PUD, Mallory–Weiss tear, esophageal varices, vascular abnormalities, neoplasm, esophagitis, gastritis.	Diverticulosis, AVMs, neoplasm, IBD, anorectal disease, mesenteric ischemia.
Initial management	Ensure that the airway is protected. **Two large-bore IV lines ASAP.** Stabilize patient with fluids, blood (hematocrit is not an accurate measure of acute blood loss).	Similar to upper GI bleed.
Management	Endoscopy followed by therapy directed at underlying cause (e.g., H$_2$ blockers or omeprazole if PUD; sclerotherapy for varices).	Rule out upper GI bleed; then anoscopy or sigmoidoscopy; then colonoscopy; then management of cause of bleeding (resect tumor or diverticula, medical therapy for IBD, etc.).

UCV *Surg.26, 27*

Table 2.6–4 describes features that distinguish small and large bowel obstruction.

TABLE 2.6–4. Small and Large Bowel Obstruction

Variable	Small Bowel Obstruction (SBO)	Large Bowel Obstruction (LBO)
History	Moderate to severe abdominal pain; **copious emesis.** Cramping pain with distal SBO. Fever and signs of dehydration/low BP may be seen.	Constipation/obstipation, deep and cramping abdominal pain, abdominal distention, nausea and emesis (less than SBO but more commonly **feculent**).
PE	**Abdominal distention** (distal SBO), abdominal tenderness, visible peristaltic waves, fever, hypovolemia; look for **surgical scars and hernias** and perform rectal exam. **High-pitched "tinkly" bowel sounds,** peristaltic rushes, or absence of bowel sounds.	**Abdominal distention,** tympany, tenderness; look for peritoneal irritation; feel for palpable mass; signs of shock or fever indicate possible perforation/peritonitis vs. ischemia/strangulation. **High-pitched "tinkly" bowel sounds,** peristaltic rushes, or absence of bowel sounds.
Causes	**Adhesions** (postsurgery), hernias, neoplasm, intussusception, volvulus, gallstone ileus, foreign body, Crohn's disease, CF, stricture, hematoma.	**Colon cancer,** diverticulitis, volvulus (Figure 2.6–7B), fecal impaction, benign tumors. **Assume colon cancer until proven otherwise.**
Differential	LBO, paralytic ileus, gastroenteritis, pseudo-obstruction.	SBO (more acute onset, less cramping pain, more emesis, less distention), ileus, pseudo-obstruction (Ogilvie's syndrome), appendicitis, IBD.
Evaluation	Obtain CBC, lactic acid, electrolytes, **abdominal plain films** (Figure 2.6–5A); perform contrast studies (determine if it is partial or complete), CT scan.	Obtain CBC, electrolytes, lactic acid, **abdominal films** (unlike the small bowel, the haustra of the colon do not cross the entire lumen; see Figure 2.6–5), CT scan; obtain barium or water contrast enema (if perforation is suspected); perform sigmoidoscopy/colonoscopy if stable.
Treatment	Hospitalize. Partial SBO can be treated conservatively with **nasogastric decompression,** but complete SBO should be managed aggressively. Make patient NPO, insert NG tube, give IV fluids to rehydrate, and **operate.**	Hospitalize. In some cases, obstruction can be opened colonoscopically or with a **rectal tube,** but **surgery** is usually required. Gangrenous colon requires partial colectomy with a diverting colostomy unless all bowel is well perfused at surgery. Treat underlying cause (e.g., neoplasm).

UCV *EM.20, Surg.23, 30*

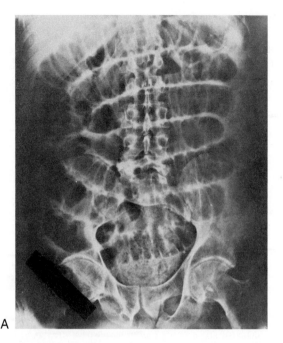
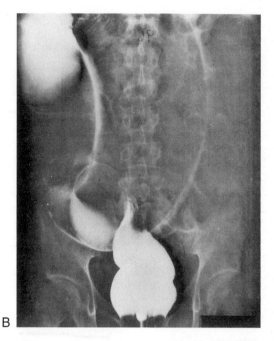

FIGURE 2.6–5. Bowel obstruction. (A) Small bowel obstruction. Supine abdominal x-ray reveals dilated loops of small bowel in a ladder-like pattern. Air–fluid levels may be apparent on an upright x-ray. (B) Sigmoid volvulus. Barium study shows the "bird beak" sign, with juxtaposed adjacent bowel walls in the dilated loop pointing toward the site of torsion. Sigmoid volvulus is a common cause of large bowel obstruction. (Reproduced, with permission, from Way L, *Current Surgical Diagnosis & Treatment,* 10th ed., Stamford, CT: Appleton & Lange, 1994: p. 626, Fig. 30–6; p. 676, Fig. 31–15.)

ILEUS

Loss of peristalsis **without structural obstruction.** Risk factors include recent surgery/GI procedures, severe medical illness, hypothyroidism, diabetes, or medications that slow GI motility (e.g., anticholinergics, opioids). The condition is commonly seen in elderly patients on opioids.

Anticholinergics and opioids slow GI motility.

History

Presenting symptoms include diffuse, constant, moderate abdominal discomfort; **nausea/emesis,** especially with feeding; **abdominal distention;** and an absence of **flatulence or bowel movements.**

PE

Mild, diffuse tenderness and **abdominal distention** with **no peritoneal signs** (no guarding or rebound) along with **reduced or absent bowel sounds.**

Differential

Partial obstruction of the small intestine or colon, appendicitis, gastroenteritis, pancreatitis, neoplasm.

Look for air throughout the small and large bowel on AXR.

Evaluation

Obtain supine and upright plain films of the abdomen to **rule out perforation or obstruction,** as well as CBC/electrolytes. Diagnosis is based on **distended small and large bowel** on AXR and **air–fluid levels;** barium study may be performed to rule out partial obstruction. Obtain CT to rule out obstructing masses. Rule out thyroid disease with TSH.

Treatment

- Decrease use of narcotics and any other drugs that **inhibit bowel motility.**
- Reduce or discontinue oral feeds.
- Initiate **NG suction/parenteral feeds** as necessary.
- Replete electrolytes as needed.

UCV *Surg.24*

IRRITABLE BOWEL SYNDROME

An idiopathic **functional disorder** characterized by abdominal pain and irregular bowel habits. Patients most commonly present in their teens and 20s, but since this syndrome is chronic, patients can present at any age. Half of all patients with this disorder who seek medical care have **comorbid psychiatric disorders** (e.g., depression, anxiety).

Half of all patients with irritable bowel syndrome have psychiatric disorders.

History

Patients present with **abdominal pain,** irregular bowel habits (including **alternating diarrhea and constipation**), and abdominal distention. Irritable bowel syndrome rarely awakens patients from sleep. Vomiting and significant weight loss are also uncommon.

PE

Usually **unremarkable** except for mild abdominal tenderness.

Differential

Crohn's disease/ulcerative colitis, mesenteric ischemia, diverticulitis, gastric/duodenal ulcer, colonic neoplasia, infectious/pseudomembranous colitis, gynecologic disorders.

Evaluation

Irritable bowel syndrome is a diagnosis of exclusion.

A **diagnosis of exclusion** based on clinical history and evaluation, so rule out other causes of GI disease. Tests can include CBC and electrolytes, stool cultures, abdominal films, and barium contrast studies. Some physicians use manometry to assess sphincter function.

Treatment

- **Psychological:** Patients need **assurance** from their physicians. Do not tell patients that their symptoms are "all in their head."

- **Dietary:** A **high-fiber diet** or **fiber supplements** may help.
- **Pharmacologic:** Treat with **antidiarrheal** (loperamide), **antispasmodic** (dicyclomine, anticholinergics), and **psychiatric** medications as indicated.

UCV *IM1.37*

INFLAMMATORY BOWEL DISEASE (IBD)

IBD consists primarily of **Crohn's disease** and **ulcerative colitis** (Figure 2.6–6 A and B). Patients in families with a history of one type of IBD are at risk for both. It is most common in whites and **Ashkenazi Jews** and often presents in patients in their teens or early 20s. Table 2.6–5 presents features of ulcerative colitis and Crohn's disease.

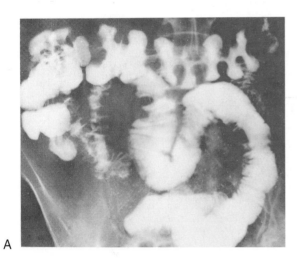

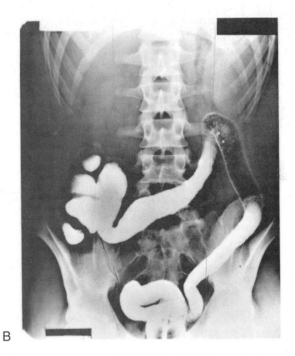

A

B

FIGURE 2.6–6. Inflammatory bowel disease. (A) Crohn's disease. Barium enema x-ray reveals deep transverse fissures, ulcers, and edema of the bowel. (B) Ulcerative colitis. Barium enema x-ray demonstrates shortening of the colon, loss of haustra ("lead pipe" appearance), and fine serrations at the bowel edges from small ulcers. (Reproduced, with permission, from Stobo JD, *The Principles and Practice of Medicine,* 23rd ed., Stamford, CT: Appleton & Lange, 1996: p. 135, Fig. 23–2.)

TABLE 2.6–5. Ulcerative Colitis vs. Crohn's Disease

	Ulcerative Colitis	**Crohn's Disease**
Site of involvement	The **rectum** is always involved. May extend proximally in a **continuous fashion** to involve some or all of the colon. Inflammation and ulceration are limited to the mucosa and submucosa.	May involve **any portion** of the GI tract, particularly the ileocecal region, in a **discontinuous pattern.** The rectum is often spared. Inflammation is transmural.
Symptoms and signs	Bloody diarrhea, lower abdominal cramps, and urgency. Exam may reveal orthostatic hypotension, tachycardia, abdominal tenderness, frank blood on rectal exam, and extraintestinal manifestations (see below).	Abdominal pain, abdominal mass, low-grade fever, weight loss, watery diarrhea. Exam may reveal fever, abdominal tenderness or mass, **perianal fissures, fistulas,** and extraintestinal manifestations (see below).
Extraintestinal manifestations	Aphthous stomatitis, episcleritis/uveitis, arthritis, sclerosing cholangitis, erythema nodosum, and pyoderma gangrenosum.	In addition, nephrolithiasis and fistulas to the skin, biliary tract, urinary tract, or between bowel loops.
Workup	CBC, AXR (see Figure 2.6–6), stool cultures, ova and parasites, stool assay for C. *difficile*, and barium enema/colonoscopy. Colonoscopy shows diffuse and continuous rectal involvement, friability, edema, and pseudopolyps. Definitive diagnosis can be made by biopsy.	Crohn's has the same laboratory workup as colitis (see Figure 2.6–6). Colonoscopy may show aphthoid, linear, or stellate ulcers, strictures, "cobblestoning," and "skip lesions."
Treatment	**Sulfasalazine** or **5-aminosalicylate** (mesalamine). Corticosteroids and immunosuppressants are reserved for refractory disease. **Total colectomy is curative** (done for long-standing or fulminant colitis or toxic megacolon).	**Sulfasalazine;** corticosteroids and immunosuppression are indicated if disease does not improve. If perforation is likely, surgical resection may be necessary, although **Crohn's disease may recur** elsewhere in the GI tract.
Incidence of cancer	Markedly increased risk of **colon cancer** in long-standing cases (monitor with fecal occult blood screening, colonoscopy).	Incidence of secondary malignancy much lower than in ulcerative colitis.

UCV *IM1.30, 40*

DIVERTICULAR DISEASE (DIVERTICULOSIS)

Diverticular disease is the most common cause of acute lower GI bleeding in patients > 40 years old.

Outpouchings of mucosa/submucosa (false diverticula) that herniate through the colonic muscle layers. **Diverticulosis** is asymptomatic unless complicated by diverticulitis or hemorrhage. Diverticular bleeding is due to the erosion of a diverticulum into a colonic blood vessel. Diverticulosis is the most common cause of acute lower GI bleeding in patients > 40 years of age. **Diverticulitis** results from inflammation and resultant perforation of a diverticulum secondary to obstruction, infection, inflammation, or increased luminal pressure.

Intestinal diverticula most commonly occur in the **sigmoid colon** because of increased intraluminal pressure; risk factors include a **low-fiber and high-fat diet,** old age (65% occur in those > 80 years old), and hereditary connective tissue disorders (e.g., Ehlers–Danlos and Marfan syndromes).

History

Diverticular disease is often **asymptomatic** but can manifest as constipation, **lower abdominal pain,** and **abnormal bowel habits.** Diverticulitis presents as acute, mild to severe, steady or cramping lower abdominal pain that is commonly localized to the **LLQ** (but can be suprapubic or in the RLQ) accompanied by fever and nausea/emesis. Diverticular bleeding presents as melena/hematochezia and symptoms of anemia (fatigue, light headedness, dyspnea on exertion).

PE

Diverticular disease without complications usually does not have any physical findings. Findings consistent with diverticulitis include low-grade **fever,** a palpable lower abdominal **mass,** a positive stool guaiac test, and generalized abdominal tenderness with peritoneal signs in the presence of free perforation. Diverticular bleeding presents as a **lower GI bleed.**

Differential

Diverticulitis should be distinguished from **colorectal cancer** with perforation, Crohn's disease, mesenteric ischemia, appendicitis, and gynecologic disease (e.g., ovarian cyst). Diverticular bleeding must be distinguished from **AVMs** and colorectal cancer.

Diverticular disease should be distinguished from colon cancer.

Evaluation

CBC (look for **leukocytosis**) and AXR. Diagnosis is based on AXR, colonoscopy, or barium enema. In patients with severe disease or those who show lack of improvement, CT scans may reveal abscess or free air.

Treatment

- **Diverticular disease without complications:** Patients can be followed and placed on a **high-fiber diet** or fiber supplements.
- **Diverticulitis:** Treat with **bowel rest** (no enteric feeds), NG tube, and **broad-spectrum antibiotics** (metronidazole and second- or third-generation cephalosporin) if the patient is stable. In the presence of free perforation, perform immediate surgical resection of diseased bowel along with anastomosis or temporary colostomy and a Hartmann's pouch/mucous fistula.
- **Diverticular bleeding:** Bleeding usually stops spontaneously; transfuse/hydrate as needed. If bleeding does not stop, angiography with embolization or **surgery** is indicated.

Avoid flexible sigmoidoscopy and barium enemas in the initial stages of diverticulitis because there is a risk of perforation.

Complications

Diverticular bleeding and diverticulitis. Diverticulitis may also lead to abscess formation, intestinal perforation, **fistula formation** (into the bladder, skin, or vagina), hepatic abscess, retroperitoneal fibrosis, and sepsis.

UCV *IM1.34, Surg.11*

Risk factors include a positive **family history,** IBD, colorectal polyps, and a **low-fiber, high-fat** diet. **Familial syndromes** include familial adenomatous polyposis (FAP) and hereditary nonpolyposis colorectal cancer (HNPCC). FAP is characterized by a colon full of polyps (Figure 2.6–7), any of which can progress to cancer, whereas HNPCC is characterized by an increased risk that a single polyp will progress to cancer.

History

Presenting symptoms can include a **change in bowel habits,** pencil-thin stools, **frank or occult blood in the stool,** abdominal obstruction, abdominal pain, symptoms of anemia, and **systemic symptoms** (malaise, fatigue, weight loss).

PE

Physical examination should include a **digital rectal exam,** a **stool guaiac test,** and palpation for an abdominal mass.

Differential

Diverticular disease, IBD, benign polyps of the colon, infectious colitis (amebiasis, *C. difficile* colitis), GI blood loss from the stomach/duodenum (peptic ulcer).

Evaluation

Iron-deficiency anemia in an elderly male patient is colon cancer until proven otherwise.

Colonoscopy or barium enema (Figure 2.6–8) followed by colonoscopy. **Biopsy** suspicious areas. If a diagnosis of cancer is made, stage according to

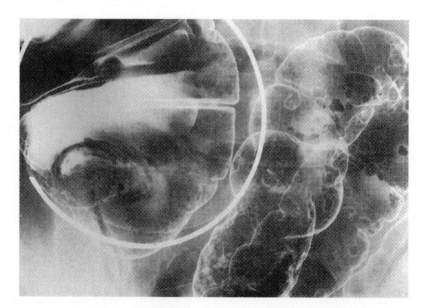

FIGURE 2.6–7. Familial adenomatous polyposis. Double-contrast barium enema x-ray reveals innumerable small polyps. (Reproduced, with permission, from Grendell J, *Current Diagnosis and Treatment in Gastroenterology,* 1st ed., Stamford, CT: Appleton & Lange, 1996: p. 211, Fig. 15–13.)

HIGH-YIELD FACTS

Gastrointestinal

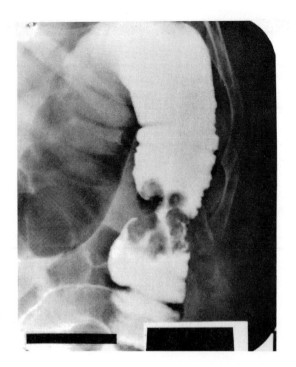

FIGURE 2.6–8. Colon carcinoma. The encircling carcinoma appears as an "apple core" filling defect in the descending colon on barium enema x-ray. (Reproduced, with permission, from Way L, *Current Surgical Diagnosis & Treatment*, 10th ed., Stamford, CT: Appleton & Lange, 1994: p. 658, Fig. 31–8.)

the TNM or the **Dukes system:** Dukes A (tumor within the muscularis propria), Dukes B (tumor invading the muscularis), Dukes C (positive lymph nodes), Dukes D (metastases).

Treatment

- **Surgical resection** following the pattern of lymphatic and vascular drainage is the primary therapy. Rectal cancer is resected by abdominoperineal or low anterior resection.
- Node-negative disease is usually resected and followed.
- **Node-positive** disease is treated with **adjuvant chemotherapy** or radiotherapy following resection.
- Colon cancers are resected even if metastatic. Small to moderate liver mets are resected (with increased five-year survival and the possibility of cure) with subsequent chemotherapy.

Management of colon cancer depends on lymph node status.

Prevention

- **Annual digital rectal examination** beginning at age 40.
- **Annual stool guaiac test** beginning at age 50. If stool guaiac is positive, perform a flexible sigmoidoscopy/colonoscopy.
- A **flexible sigmoidoscopy** should be performed **every 3–5 years** in patients > 50 years of age.
- Conduct earlier screening in patients with a positive family history.
- Consider prophylactic colectomy for patients with FAP or ulcerative colitis.
- CEA levels can help monitor for recurrence.

UCV *Surg.21*

Sign of perforated ulcer on abdominal XR.	Free air under the diaphragm
Most likely cause of acute lower GI bleed in patients > 40 years old.	Diverticulosis
Complications of diverticulitis.	Abscess, perforation, fistulas to bladder, skin, or vagina, sepsis
Does diverticulitis bleed?	No
Diagnostic modality used when ultrasound is equivocal for cholecystitis.	HIDA scan
Sentinel loop on abdominal x-ray.	Acute pancreatitis
Risk factors for cholelithiasis.	Fat, female, fertile, forty, flatulent
Inspiratory arrest during palpation of the RUQ.	Murphy's sign, seen in acute cholecystitis
Intestinal inflammation presenting with watery diarrhea and weight loss; fistulas between bowel and skin, urinary tract, or other parts of bowel may occur.	Crohn's disease
Inflammatory disease of the colon with increased risk of colon cancer.	Ulcerative colitis
Immunosuppressive agent used for both ulcerative colitis and Crohn's.	Sulfasalazine
Charcot's triad.	RUQ pain, jaundice, and fever/chills in the setting of ascending cholangitis
Reynold's pentad.	Charcot's triad plus shock and mental status changes, with ascending cholangitis
Causes of diarrhea with increased fecal fat.	Malabsorption, pancreatic insufficiency, bacterial overgrowth
Dull, waxing/waning periumbilical pain that then shifts to the RLQ and becomes sharp and continuous.	Appendicitis
Clues to distinguish appendicitis from other causes of right lower quadrant abdominal pain.	Appendiceal fecalith or free air on abdominal x-ray, low-grade fever and leukocytosis with left shift, tenderness on rectal exam; negative β-HCG, normal gynecologic exam
Medical treatment for hepatic encephalopathy.	Lactulose, neomycin

The following clinical questions and accompanying answers are reproduced, with permission, from Reteguiz J, *PreTest: Physical Diagnosis*, 4th ed., New York: McGraw-Hill, 2001.

Questions

1. A 40-year-old man presents to the emergency room complaining of severe abdominal pain that radiates to his back accompanied by several episodes of vomiting. He drinks alcohol daily. On physical examination, the patient is found on the stretcher lying in the fetal position. He is febrile and appears ill. The skin of his abdomen has an area of bluish periumbilical discoloration. Abdominal examination reveals decreased bowel sounds. The patient has severe midepigastric tenderness on palpation and complains of exquisite pain when your hands are abruptly withdrawn from his abdomen. Rectal examination is normal. Which of the following is the most likely diagnosis?
   a. Acute cholecystitis
   b. Pyelonephritis
   c. Necrotizing pancreatitis
   d. Chronic pancreatitis
   e. Diverticulitis
   f. Appendicitis

2. A 32-year-old man presents with severe abdominal pain, which he describes as sharp and diffuse. He does not drink alcohol or take any medications. He has a past medical history significant for peptic ulcer disease over five years ago. He has stable vital signs and has no orthostatic changes. You observe the patient to be lying very still on the emergency room stretcher. On physical examination, he has a rigid abdomen and decreased bowel sounds. He has localized left upper quadrant guarding and rebound tenderness. He has referred rebound tenderness on palpation of the right upper quadrant. Rectal examination is fecal occult blood test (FOBT) negative. Which of the following is the best method of confirming the diagnosis in this patient?
   a. Barium swallow
   b. Leukocytosis
   c. Upper endoscopy
   d. Abdominal radiograph
   e. Colonoscopy

3. A 74-year-old man presents with the abrupt onset of pain in the left lower abdomen, which has been progressively worsening over the last two days. He states that the pain is unremitting. He has some diarrhea but no nausea or vomiting. He has no dysuria or hematuria. His temperature is 102°F. Bowel sounds are decreased. The patient has involuntary guarding. There is tenderness and rebound tenderness when the left lower quadrant is palpated. The referred rebound test is positive. A fixed sausage-like mass is palpable in the area of tenderness. There is no costovertebral angle (CVA) tenderness. Rectal examination reveals brown stool, which is FOBT positive. Bloodwork demonstrates a leukocytosis. Which of the following is the most likely diagnosis?
   a. Colon cancer
   b. Diverticulitis
   c. Pancreatitis
   d. Pyelonephritis
   e. Appendicitis

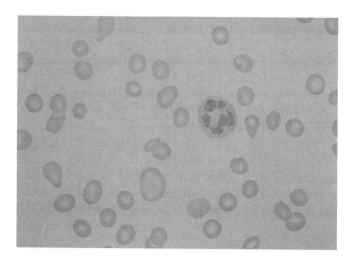

FIGURE 2.7–2. Hypersegmentation. The nucleus of this hypersegmented neutrophil has six lobes (six or more nuclear lobes are required). This is a characteristic finding of megaloblastic anemia.

- **Macrocytic (MCV > 100):**
  - B$_{12}$/folate deficiency (Figure 2.7–2) *(IM1.56)*
  - Hemolytic anemia (increased reticulocyte count, mechanical [e.g., heart valve; Figure 2.7–3] vs. immunologic [positive Coombs' test])
  - Drug exposure (MTX, phenytoin, phenobarbital, etc.)
  - Other: alcohol use, liver disease, hypothyroidism
- **Normocytic (MCV 80–100):**
  - Hemorrhage
  - Intravascular hemolysis (G6PD, microangiopathic hemolysis)
  - Extravascular hemolysis (hereditary spherocytosis [Figure 2.7–4] *(IM1.48)*, cold agglutinins, hypersplenism)
  - Infection (osteomyelitis, HIV, *Mycoplasma*, EBV)

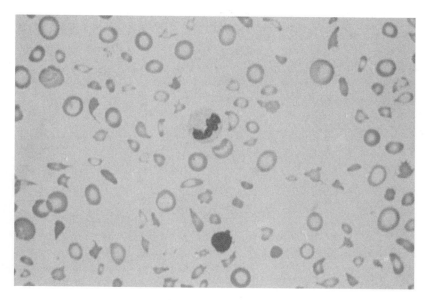

FIGURE 2.7–3. Schistocytes. These fragmented red blood cells may be seen in microangiopathic hemolytic anemia and mechanical hemolysis.

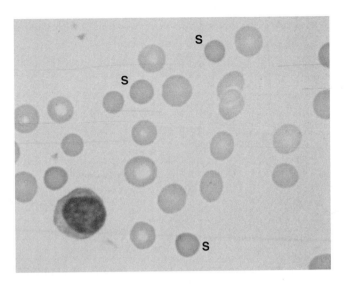

FIGURE 2.7–4. Spherocytes. These RBCs (S) lack areas of central pallor. Spherocytes are seen in autoimmune hemolysis and hereditary spherocytosis.

- Bone marrow disease (leukemia, lymphoma, metastatic cancer, myelodysplasia)
- Renal failure
- Any cause of microcytic/macrocytic anemia

Evaluation

Assess <u>hematocrit</u>, <u>MCV</u> (to distinguish microcytic from normocytic/macrocytic), and <u>reticulocyte count</u>; obtain **peripheral blood smear.** Then evaluate as follows:

- **Microcytic (low MCV):** Ferritin, iron, TIBC.
- **Macrocytic (high MCV):** RBC folate, serum B_{12}.
- **Normocytic (normal MCV):** <u>Coombs'</u> test, iron studies, bilirubin.

Obtain serum bilirubin, LDH, and haptoglobin levels if hemolysis is suspected. Consider bone marrow biopsy and immunologic tests; **screen for malignancy.** <u>Right-sided colon cancer</u> can present as a <u>hypochromic</u>, <u>microcytic</u> anemia in an otherwise asymptomatic elderly patient, so perform a hemoccult test to rule out occult GI blood loss.

Decreased serum haptoglobin indicates intravascular hemolysis.

Treatment

- Treat the underlying disease.
- If iron-deficiency anemia, **search for the source** of bleeding (e.g., GI cancer, menstruation, trauma) or the cause of low iron intake (e.g., diet, malabsorption).
- Treat iron-deficiency anemia with oral **<u>ferrous sulfate</u>** or gluconate. Administer <u>monthly B_{12} injections</u> for B_{12} deficiency due to <u>pernicious anemia.</u> Transfuse in the presence of severe symptoms or worsening status. In patients with CAD, there should be a lower threshold for transfusion, as anemia can provoke or worsen myocardial ischemia.
- Anemic patients with <u>renal failure</u> should receive exogenous <u>erythropoietin.</u>

Iron-deficiency anemia in an elderly patient is colon cancer until proven otherwise.

UCV *IM1.42, 43, 48, OB.35, 36*

THALASSEMIA

A group of disorders resulting from reduced synthesis of alpha- or beta-globin protein subunits.

Alpha-globin disorders most frequently affect Asians and blacks and can be classified into the following categories (normal = four alpha-globin alleles):

- **Hydrops fetalis:** All four alpha-globin alleles affected by disease; no alpha-globin chain production. Results in stillborn fetus.
- **Hemoglobin H disease:** Three diseased alpha-globin alleles; minimal alpha-globin production. Associated with **chronic hemolytic anemia, pallor,** and **splenomegaly;** may require occasional transfusion (e.g., during infection).
- **Thalassemia minor:** Two normal alpha-globin alleles; reduced alpha-globin production. Associated with **mild microcytic anemia** and normal life expectancy;
- **Carrier:** Three normal alpha-globin alleles; one diseased allele. Children of carriers are at risk for thalassemia if the other parent is affected or is a carrier.

Beta-globin disorders most frequently affect people of Mediterranean origin, Asians, and blacks and are classified as follows:

- **Thalassemia major:** No beta-globin production (homozygous); presents in the first year of life as HbF expression declines. Characterized by growth retardation, bony deformity/pathologic fracture, hepatosplenomegaly, and jaundice. Symptoms may improve with transfusion therapy, but patients usually die from sequelae of **iron overload** (heart, liver failure) from multiple transfusions. Treat with **transfusions, splenectomy, folic acid,** and **bone marrow transplant** if possible and appropriate (this offers a chance of cure but has a high treatment-associated mortality).
- **Thalassemia minor:** Heterozygote, mild hypochromic/microcytic anemia. Presents similarly to iron deficiency anemia and alpha-thalassemia minor. Treat with **folate, no iron therapy,** and transfusions during severe anemia/pregnancy/stress.

UCV *IM1.53*

Patients with thalassemia major usually die from the sequelae of iron overload.

SICKLE CELL DISEASE

An **autosomal-recessive** disorder due to abnormal hemoglobin. Homozygotes suffer from hematologic/systemic disease, whereas heterozygotes (sickle cell trait) are usually asymptomatic and are less susceptible to malarial infection (balanced polymorphism). **Blacks** are most commonly affected.

History

Acute episodes (vaso-occlusive events) may present with **bone/chest pain and fever** and may be precipitated by infection, dehydration, or hypoxia. Patients may present with **strokes** or **priapism.** Up to 50% of affected children < 3 years old will develop **dactylitis** (painful swelling of the hands and feet). (See complications for other manifestations of sickle cell disease.)

Sickle cell crises are precipitated by infection, dehydration, and hypoxia.

PE

Splenomegaly (in young children), **jaundice,** pallor, fever, and **bone/joint tenderness;** dyspnea/tachypnea with chest pain **(acute chest syndrome).**

Differential

Thalassemia and other hemoglobinopathies, osteomyelitis, pneumonia, rheumatic fever, acute abdomen.

Evaluation

Diagnose by hemoglobin electrophoresis. Obtain CBC (normocytic anemia), reticulocyte count (high), **peripheral blood smear** (sickling; Figure 2.7–5), and CXR (for chest syndrome). **"Fish-mouth vertebrae"** may be seen on radiographs of the lumbar spine.

Treatment

- **Hydration, oxygen,** and **analgesia** during an acute vaso-occlusive attack.
- **Exchange transfusion** or simple transfusion may be necessary for severe attacks or for chest syndrome with respiratory distress.
- Chronic **hydroxyurea** therapy may decrease the frequency of crises.
- **Pneumococcal vaccine** to prevent pneumococcal sepsis; be alert for infection by encapsulated organisms.

Strep. pneu.
H. Inf.
Myelosuppressive agents (bone marrow)

Sickle cell patients are at increased risk of infection by encapsulated organisms due to functional asplenia.

Complications

Hematologic complications include chronic hemolytic anemia, **parvovirus B19 infection** leading to aplastic crisis, high-output cardiac failure, and, in in-

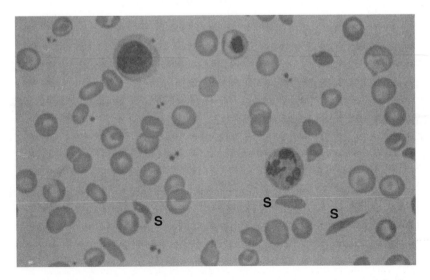

FIGURE 2.7–5. Sickle cells. Sickle-shaped RBCs (S) may appear during infection, dehydration, or hypoxia. Anisocytosis, poikilocytosis, target cells, and nucleated RBCs are also seen in sickle cell disease.

fants and children, splenic sequestration of erythrocytes, leading to massive splenomegaly and a potentially fatal drop in hematocrit. Vaso-occlusive complications include pain crises, widespread organ impairment (retinopathy, splenic infarction, gallbladder disease, chronic renal failure), priapism, stroke, avascular necrosis of the femoral head, and acute chest syndrome. Patients with functional asplenism are susceptible to infection by encapsulated organisms (*Streptococcus pneumoniae*, *Haemophilus influenzae*). Patients are also more susceptible to **osteomyelitis** due to *Salmonella*, although *Staphylococcus aureus* is still the more common cause.

UCV *EM.23, Ped.21*

G6PD DEFICIENCY

An **X-linked recessive** deficiency of the G6PD enzyme that causes episodic hemolytic anemia. **Black males** are most often affected. Mediterranean variants can cause severe hemolytic crises.

History

Exposure to sulfonamides or antimalarial drugs may precipitate a hemolytic crisis in patients with G6PD deficiency.

Usually asymptomatic but may present as acute, self-limited hemolytic anemia (fatigue, **jaundice, dark urine**) with RBC oxidative stress (e.g., from exposure to **fava beans** or to drugs such as dapsone, sulfonamides, quinine/quinidine, and primaquine).

PE

Usually **normal.** Jaundice and signs of anemia (pallor, tachycardia) are found during hemolytic episodes.

Differential

Other causes of hemolytic anemia (e.g., hereditary spherocytosis), drug side effects, sickle cell disease, thalassemia.

Evaluation

During hemolytic episodes, look for a low hematocrit, high reticulocyte count, high indirect bilirubin, low serum haptoglobin, and **Heinz bodies** and "bite" cells on blood smear. A **quantitative G6PD enzyme test** is diagnostic.

Treatment

- Usually **self-limited;** avoid exposure to drugs that can cause hemolytic episodes.
- Transfuse if severe.

POLYCYTHEMIA VERA

A **myeloproliferative disease** marked by increased production of RBCs ± platelets and WBCs. Individuals > 60 years of age are at highest risk; males are affected more frequently than females. The most common cause of erythrocytosis is **chronic hypoxia** secondary to lung disease, not polycythemia vera.

History

Patients can present with malaise, fatigue, **pruritus** (typically after a warm bath), tinnitus, blurred vision, headache, and **epistaxis.** They may also present with signs of vascular sludging, including stroke, angina, and claudication.

PE

Plethora, large retinal veins on funduscopy, and **splenomegaly.**

Polycythemia vera can be distinguished from secondary causes by normal oxygen saturation, low EPO level, and elevated RBC mass.

Differential

Secondary polycythemia due to hypoxia (high altitudes, lung disease), smoking (carboxyhemoglobin), erythropoietin (EPO)-producing renal cyst or mass (e.g., renal cell carcinoma), CML, other myelodysplasias, spurious finding (dehydration).

Evaluation

Assessment should include **RBC mass (increased), hematocrit (> 50%), EPO level (decreased),** WBCs/platelets (normal or increased), peripheral blood smear (normal RBCs; basophilic WBCs), and bone marrow biopsy (hypercellular).

Treatment

- **Serial phlebotomy.**
- Myelosuppressive agents (e.g., **hydroxyurea**) may be used if necessary.
- Daily **aspirin** to prevent thrombotic complications.

Complications

There is a **risk of conversion** to CML, myelofibrosis, or AML.

UCV *IM1.52*

TRANSFUSION REACTIONS

Immunologic reactions to transfused blood, causing hemolysis and systemic symptoms. They may occur as a result of clerical errors, mislabeled specimens, or reactions to antigens not commonly tested. **Viral infections** can also be transmitted through blood transfusions, including hepatitis B and C, HIV, HTLV-I and II, and CMV.

Viruses transmitted through blood transfusions: HBV, HCV, HIV, CMV, HTLV-I and II.

History/PE

Severe chills and **high-grade fever** (chills and low-grade fever are common during transfusions); back, chest, or abdominal pain and **dark urine** (hemoglobinuria). Reactions can progress to vascular collapse with respiratory distress and hypotension.

Differential

Leukoagglutination reaction, anaphylaxis, gram-negative bacterial contamination, MI, **IgA deficiency,** sepsis, abdominal emergency.

Evaluation

Hemoglobinuria may lead to acute tubular necrosis and subsequent renal failure.

Stop the transfusion and **then** investigate; **retype** the patient's blood against that of the donor; follow hematocrit; **assess creatinine** (renal failure); obtain D-dimer/**coagulation studies** (DIC). Culture the blood to rule out bacterial contamination.

Treatment

- **Stop the transfusion** immediately.
- Check for hemoglobinemia (in plasma).
- **IV hydration and mannitol** for renal protection.

THROMBOTIC THROMBOCYTOPENIC PURPURA (TTP)

Features of TTP—

FAT RN
Fever
Anemia
Thrombocytopenia

Renal dysfunction
Neurologic abnormality

Microangiopathic hemolytic anemia, thrombocytopenia, neurologic abnormalities, fever, and **renal dysfunction.** Risk factors include pregnancy, OCP use, and HIV infection; individuals < 50 years of age are at greatest risk. The condition is idiopathic and can be fatal.

History

Patients can present with **fever, symptoms of anemia,** bleeding, **changes in mental status,** headache, aphasia, seizures, and hemiparesis.

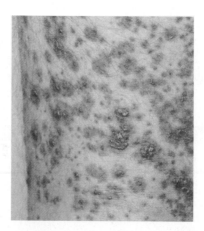

FIGURE 2.7–6. Palpable purpura. Note the round or oval pink to red macules or patches with overlying purple to red papules. Palpable purpura is associated with necrotizing vasculitides, including Henoch–Schönlein purpura, serum sickness, and essential mixed cryoglobulinemia.

| **TABLE 2.7–1. Causes of Microangiopathic Hemolytic Anemia** |

Thrombotic thrombocytopenic purpura
Hemolytic–uremic syndrome
DIC
Prosthetic valve hemolysis
Metastatic adenocarcinoma
Malignant hypertension
Vasculitis

PE

Fever, bleeding, pallor, **purpura/petechiae** (Figure 2.7–6), altered mental status, and splenomegaly.

Differential

DIC, hemolytic–uremic syndrome (HUS), ITP, mechanical hemolysis (e.g., "Waring blender" valve), Evans's syndrome, endocarditis, neoplasm (Table 2.7–1).

Hemolytic–uremic syndrome is TTP without the fever and neurologic abnormalities.

Evaluation

CBC (anemia, thrombocytopenia), peripheral blood smear (**schistocytes;** see Figure 2.7–7), **bilirubin (elevated indirect fraction), LDH (elevated),** Coombs' test (negative), creatinine (may be elevated), and coagulation studies (normal).

Treatment

- Immediate large-volume **plasmapheresis.**
- **Corticosteroids,** antiplatelet agents (aspirin, others), and dextran.
- **Splenectomy** if recurrent or refractory to plasmapheresis and corticosteroids.

UCV *IM1.54*

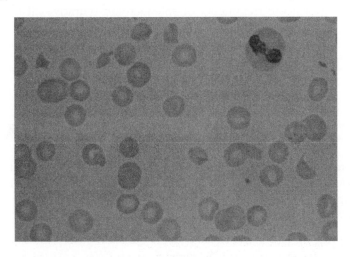

FIGURE 2.7–7. Thrombotic thrombocytopenic purpura (TTP). Note the schistocytes and paucity of platelets.

IDIOPATHIC THROMBOCYTOPENIC PURPURA (ITP)

An **autoimmune** platelet disorder. ITP includes pediatric (postviral, self-limited) and adult (chronic) forms. Females are affected twice as often as males, and individuals < 50 years old are at greatest risk. **Evans's syndrome** is ITP plus autoimmune hemolytic anemia. Diseases that are associated with ITP include Hodgkin's and non-Hodgkin's lymphoma, CLL, HIV, SLE, and RA.

History

Patients are **afebrile** (unlike TTP) and present with **mucosal bleeding** (epistaxis, oral bleeding, menorrhagia), **petechiae/purpura,** and easy bruising.

PE

Petechiae, purpura, ecchymoses, and oral hemorrhagic bullae, but **no splenomegaly** (unlike TTP).

Differential

ALL/CLL, myelodysplastic syndrome, SLE, drug side effects (e.g., ranitidine), DIC, alcoholism, HIV infection, aplastic anemia, TTP.

Evaluation

CBC shows very low platelets and mild or no anemia. Obtain coagulation studies, bleeding time, peripheral blood smear (megathrombocytes, **no schistocytes**), DIC panel, bone marrow aspiration (relatively normal; possibly elevated megakaryocytes), and **platelet-associated IgG test.**

Treatment

Children with ITP usually recover spontaneously, but most adults require treatment.

- In most pediatric patients the condition will resolve **spontaneously,** but the majority of adults require treatment.
- Initial treatment consists of **corticosteroids.**
- **IVIG** (for acute treatment) or **splenectomy** (curative) if refractory to steroids.
- Administer danazol, vincristine/vinblastine, cyclophosphamide, or azathioprine if still refractory.
- Give platelets for severe, uncontrollable bleeding.

UCV *Ped.20*

DISSEMINATED INTRAVASCULAR COAGULATION (DIC)

DIC involves pathologic coagulation and a lack of physiologic coagulation.

A systemic coagulation disorder with pathologic coagulation and a lack of physiologic coagulation. It may occur secondary to **sepsis, transfusion reaction, neoplasia, trauma** (burns and head trauma), and **obstetric complications** (amniotic embolus, septic abortion, retained dead fetus).

History

Patients often present with **bleeding from venipuncture sites or incisional wounds,** epistaxis, hematemesis, and digital gangrene. DIC leads to systemic collapse and death without early identification and institution of supportive measures.

PE

Evidence of diffuse bleeding, digital cyanosis/gangrene, and vascular collapse with hypotension, tachycardia, tachypnea, and respiratory failure.

Differential

Severe liver disease, sepsis without DIC, vitamin K deficiency (normal fibrinogen), TTP.

Evaluation

Evaluation should include **fibrin split products (high),** D-dimer (high), **fibrinogen (low), PT/PTT (may be elevated),** platelets (very low), and hemocrit (low).

DIC causes elevated fibrin split products, low fibrinogen, elevated PT/PTT, and low platelets.

Treatment

- **Treat the underlying disorder** (e.g., infection).
- Transfuse **platelets** if < 30,000–50,000; give **cryoprecipitate** to replenish fibrinogen.
- If refractory, try aminocaproic acid (must be used with heparin) or tranexamic acid.

UCV *IM1.47*

HEMOPHILIA

An **X-linked recessive** (males affected) coagulopathy due to decreased factor VIII (hemophilia A) or factor IX (hemophilia B) activity.

History/PE

Patients may present with **hemarthroses,** intramuscular bleeding, GI bleeding, and excessive **bleeding in response to mild trauma/surgical/dental procedures.**

Hemophilia A and hemophilia B are clinically indistinguishable.

Evaluation

Findings include <u>**prolonged PTT but normal PT,**</u> reduced factor VIII:C with normal vWF, or reduced factor IX levels. <u>**Bleeding time is normal.**</u>

Bleeding time and PT are normal in hemophilia, whereas PTT may be elevated.

Treatment

- **Factor VIII** (hemophilia A) or **factor IX** concentrate (hemophilia B) as needed during bleeding episodes.
- Presupplement with factor VIII or factor IX before surgical and dental procedures.
- Supplement aggressively in the event of trauma.
- In mild hemophilia A, **desmopressin** may be administered before minor surgical procedures to increase endogenous factor VIII production.
- Consider **HIV** testing in older hemophiliacs who received replacement factors in the late 1970s to early 1980s.

UCV *Ped.18*

VON WILLEBRAND'S DISEASE

An **autosomal-dominant** condition resulting in deficient or defective von Willebrand's factor (vWF). vWF, which is produced by megakaryocytes and endothelial cells, is the only clotting factor not synthesized by the liver.

History

Patients often present with **easy bruising** and **mucosal bleeding** (epistaxis, oral bleeding, menorrhagia), GI bleeding, and postincisional bleeding. Symptoms worsen with aspirin use.

PE

Mucosal/GI bleeding and bruises.

Differential

Hemophilia, drug side effects, Glanzmann's thrombasthenia.

Evaluation

See Table 2.7–2 for laboratory findings in von Willebrand's disease.

TABLE 2.7–2. Evaluation of von Willebrand's Disease

Test	Finding with Disease
Bleeding time	↑
Platelet count	normal
PT	normal
PTT	normal/elevated
Factor VIII antigen	↓
Ristocetin platelet study (vWF activity)	↓
vWF	↓

Treatment

- **Desmopressin** is the mainstay of treatment in mild disease (once per 24 hours).
- **Factor VIII concentrate** is given in severe disease or before surgery/dentistry.
- Fresh frozen plasma (FFP) or cryoprecipitate may also be used, but exposure to these is minimized due to risk of viral infection.
- ε-aminocaproic acid may be used to reduce mucosal bleeding.
- Avoid aspirin or aspirin-containing products.

UCV *Ped.22*

MULTIPLE MYELOMA

Primary malignancy of **plasma cell origin.** Risk factors include monoclonal gammopathy of unknown significance (MGUS). Patients > 50 years of age are most commonly affected, and blacks are affected more frequently than whites.

History

Patients can present with **back pain, hypercalcemic symptoms** (weakness, weight loss, altered mental status, constipation), **pathologic bone fractures,** and frequent infections (secondary to dysregulation of antibody production).

PE

Pallor, bone tenderness, bone deformities, and lethargy.

Differential

Metastatic carcinoma, lymphoma, MGUS, Waldenström's macroglobulinemia, primary amyloidosis, hyperparathyroidism.

Evaluation

Obtain CBC (anemia), peripheral smear (plasmacytosis; Figure 2.7–8), SPEP/UPEP (**monoclonal gammopathy, Bence Jones proteinuria),** elec-

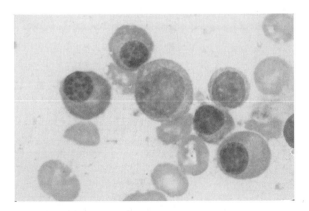

FIGURE 2.7–8. Multiple myeloma. Note the abundance of plasma cells on peripheral blood smear. RBCs will often be in rouleaux formation.

trolytes, BUN/creatinine (renal disease/hypercalcemia), a full-body **skeletal survey** ("**punched-out**" **osteolytic lesions** of the skull and long bones), **bone scan (negative),** and bone marrow biopsy **(plasma cell infiltration).**

Treatment

- Multiple-agent **chemotherapy** (alkylating agents), melphalan, and corticosteroids (prednisone).
- Consider bone marrow/stem cell transplant.
- Patients with multiple osteolytic lesions in a single bone (e.g., femur) may require prophylactic **intramedullary fixation.**
- Pathologic fractures require open reduction–internal fixation.
- The disease usually recurs and carries a poor prognosis.
- Complications include infection, anemia, neurologic disease, and renal failure.

UCV *IM1.50*

LYMPHOMA

Table 2.7–3 summarizes features of non-Hodgkin's and Hodgkin's lymphoma.

UCV *IM1.44, 49, 51*

LEUKEMIAS

Leukemias are the most common type of cancer in children.

Leukemias result from the malignant proliferation of hematopoietic cells and are the most common type of cancer in **children.** Categorization is based on their cellular origin (e.g., promyeloid, myeloid, lymphoid) and level of differentiation of neoplastic cells. **Acute leukemias** are associated with the prolifer-

TABLE 2.7–3. Non-Hodgkin's and Hodgkin's Lymphoma

	Non-Hodgkin's Lymphoma	Hodgkin's Lymphoma
Risk factors	EBV (Burkitt's), HIV infection.	15–45 years (women > men) or > 60 years
Histology	Varies.	**Reed–Sternberg cells.**
Variants	Many; separated into low, intermediate, and high grade.	Nodular sclerosis, mixed cellularity, lymphocyte predominance or lymphocyte depletion.
History	Painless adenopathy, fever, night sweats, other systemic symptoms (malaise, weight loss).	Fever, night sweats, weight loss, pruritus, systemic symptoms.
PE	**Systemic** adenopathy +/– hepatosplenomegaly.	**Regional** adenopathy +/– hepatosplenomegaly.
Differential	Hodgkin's lymphoma, mononucleosis, cat scratch disease, HIV, sarcoid.	Non-Hodgkin's lymphoma, HIV, sarcoid, lymphadenitis, drug reaction.
Evaluation	**Biopsy** for diagnosis followed by CXR, body CT scans, and possibly bone marrow biopsy/LP.	**Biopsy** largest, most central node, then CXR; consider bone marrow biopsy/LP.
Treatment	Radiation + chemotherapy.	Radiation therapy for localized disease, plus chemo for advanced/widespread disease.

ation of minimally differentiated blast cells, while **chronic leukemias** are associated with the proliferation of more mature, differentiated cell forms. Tumor invasion of the bone marrow results in **pancytopenia** (thrombocytopenia, anemia). Thus, the major medical complications of end-stage leukemia are **bleeding** (from thrombocytopenia), **infection,** and anemia.

ACUTE LYMPHOCYTIC LEUKEMIA (ALL)

ALL is most common in children, and whites are affected more frequently than blacks. It is the **most common cancer of childhood.**

History

Patients can present with limp, **bone pain,** refusal to walk, and **fever.**

PE

Physical examination may reveal fever, pallor, widespread **petechiae/purpura,** adenopathy, **hepatosplenomegaly,** easy bruising, and bleeding.

Differential

Aplastic anemia, mononucleosis/other viral infections, rheumatic diseases, other neoplasms.

Evaluation

Look for depression of bone marrow elements (e.g., anemia, severe thrombocytopenia, leukopenia; see Figure 2.7–9), **elevated LDH/uric acid,** and cytogenetic changes. Diagnosis can be made with **bone marrow aspirate.** Obtain CXR (rule out mediastinal involvement), LP (rule out brain metastasis), and CT scan.

Eighty-five percent of children achieve complete remission with chemotherapy.

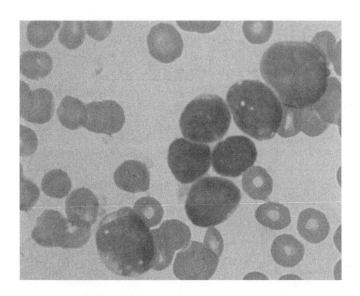

FIGURE 2.7–9. Acute lymphocytic leukemia. Peripheral blood smear reveals numerous large, uniform lymphoblasts with fine granular cytoplasm and faint nucleoli.

Treatment

Good prognosis with **chemotherapy,** with 85% of children achieving long-term survival (30% of adults).

UCV *Ped.16*

ACUTE MYELOGENOUS LEUKEMIA (AML)

Affects children and adults. The adult form increases in incidence with age.

History

The adult form of AML presents as **fatigue, easy bruising, dyspnea, fever,** skin disease (leukemia cutis), CNS symptoms, and a history of **frequent infections.**

PE

Fever, lethargy, bleeding, **purpura/petechiae,** and variable hepatosplenomegaly.

Differential

CML, myelodysplastic syndromes, lymphoma, hairy cell leukemia, mononucleosis.

Evaluation

Bone marrow examination demonstrates depression of all blood cell elements except monocytes (anemia, thrombocytopenia, neutropenia). Blasts are often seen in peripheral blood (Figures 2.7–10 and 2.7–11), and **Auer rods** are pathognomonic. Cytogenic studies provide prognostic information.

Treatment

Treat with intensive multiple-agent **chemotherapy,** transfusions, antibiotics as needed, and allogenic/autologous **bone marrow transplants. Retinoic acid** may induce remission in the promyelocytic form. AML has a moderate prognosis, with 70–80% of adults < 60 years old achieving complete remission.

UCV *IM1.43*

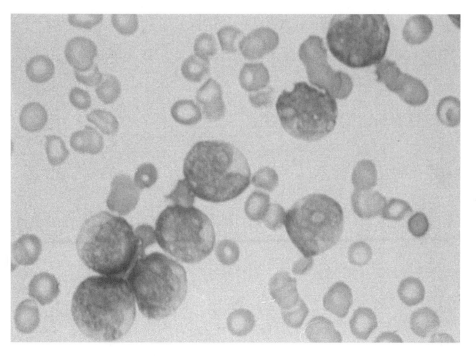

FIGURE 2.7–10. Acute myelogenous leukemia. Large, uniform myeloblasts with notched nuclei and prominent nucleoli are characteristic.

CHRONIC LYMPHOCYTIC LEUKEMIA (CLL)

Primarily affects **patients > 65 years of age.** The disease is slowly progressive and is associated with good short-term and poor long-term survival.

History/PE

Lymphadenopathy, fatigue, and hepatosplenomegaly. This is usually an **indolent disease,** and many patients are diagnosed by incidental lymphocytosis.

CLL is slowly progressive, with good short-term but poor long-term survival.

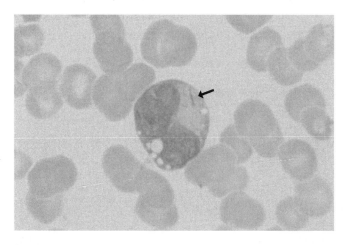

FIGURE 2.7–11. Auer rod in acute myelogenous leukemia. The red rod-shaped structure (arrow) in the cytoplasm of the myeloblast is pathognomonic.

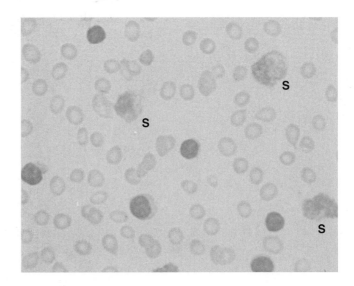

FIGURE 2.7–12. Chronic lymphocytic leukemia. The numerous small, mature lymphocytes and smudge cells (S; fragile malignant lymphocytes are disrupted during blood smear preparation) are characteristic.

Differential

Viral disease, other leukemias, myelodysplastic disorders.

Evaluation

Look for **isolated lymphocytosis** on CBC (hematocrit and platelet count are often normal at presentation; see Figure 2.7–12). Bone marrow will be infiltrated with lymphocytes.

Treatment

CLL may be complicated by autoimmune hemolytic anemia.

Most patients are **managed supportively.** Treatment is usually not instituted until patients develop increasing fatigue or lymphadenopathy, anemia, or thrombocytopenia. Start with chlorambucil or fludarabine; splenectomy and steroids are appropriate for autoimmune hemolytic anemia and thrombocytopenia.

UCV *IM1.45*

CHRONIC MYELOGENOUS LEUKEMIA (CML)

Characterized by overproduction of myeloid cells, this disease is often stable for several years until it transforms into a more overtly malignant form. It is associated with **prior radiation exposure** and most commonly affects patients 40–60 years of age.

History/PE

In its early stages, CML is asymptomatic or presents with mild, nonspecific symptoms (e.g., **fatigue, fever, malaise,** decreased exercise tolerance, weight loss, night sweats). If detected at a later stage, patients present with early satiety, LUQ fullness/pain, splenomegaly, and bleeding. **Blast crisis** (associated with late presentation) presents as fever, bone pain, weight loss, and increasing **splenomegaly**. All patients eventually reach blast crisis with progressive pancytopenia and disseminated disease.

Evaluation

Peripheral blood smear will demonstrate a significantly **elevated WBC** (median of 150,000 at time of diagnosis) and prominent myeloid cells. The leukocyte alkaline phosphatase score is low, and vitamin B_{12} levels are often markedly elevated. Bone marrow biopsy is performed as an adjunct. Definitive diagnosis can be made via cytogenics, which usually reveals the **Philadelphia chromosome** (9,22 translocation) or *bcr-abl* gene fusion product.

The Philadelphia chromosome is the sine qua non of CML.

Treatment

- CML is associated with a poor overall prognosis, with a median survival of 3–4 years.
- Treatment in the chronic phase is **palliative**, using myelosuppressive agents such as alpha-interferon and hydroxyurea.
- Allogenic **bone marrow transplant** is curative in about 60% of cases.
- Blast crisis is difficult to treat and is rapidly terminal in most cases.

CML often terminates in blast crises, which are rapidly fatal in most cases.

UCV *IM1.46*

Four causes of a microcytic anemia.	Thalassemia, iron deficiency, anemia of chronic disease, lead poisoning
An elderly male with hypochromic, microcytic anemia; otherwise asymptomatic. Diagnostic test?	FOBT; suspect right-sided colon cancer
Dietary supplement to give to patients with thalassemia.	Folate but not iron; patients develop iron overload from multiple transfusions
Precipitants of hemolytic crisis in patients with G6PD deficiency.	Sulfonamides, antimalarial drugs, fava beans
How to distinguish polycythemia vera from secondary polycythemia.	Normal oxygen saturation, EPO level, high RBC mass and hematocrit
Treatment for TTP.	Large-volume plasmapheresis; corticosteroids and antiplatelet agents
Treatment for ITP in pediatric population.	Usually resolves spontaneously; may require corticosteroids
Which of the following are elevated in DIC? Fibrin split products, D-dimer, fibrinogen, platelets, hematocrit.	Fibrin split products and D-dimer; the rest are low
A patient presents with excessive bleeding after dental work. Labs show prolonged PTT with normal PT and bleeding time. Most likely diagnosis?	Hemophilia A or B; intrinsic pathway affected
Another patient presents with excessive bleeding after dental work. Labs show normal PT/PTT with prolonged bleeding time. Most likely diagnosis?	von Willebrand's disease
Treatment for vWF.	Desmopressin
Symptoms of sickle cell crisis.	Acute-onset bone/chest pain, fever
Monoclonal gammopathy, Bence Jones proteinuria, "punched-out" lesions in skull and long bones.	Multiple myeloma
Most common cancer of childhood.	Acute lymphocytic leukemia
An elderly patient presents with fatigue, lymphadenopathy, and hepatosplenomegaly. CBC with differential shows an isolated lymphocytosis. Most likely diagnosis?	Chronic lymphocytic leukemia
Late, often life-threatening complication of CML.	Blast crisis (fever, bone pain, splenomegaly with pancytopenia)
Pathognomonic sign is Auer rods on blood smear.	AML
A patient presents with early satiety, LUQ fullness/pain, splenomegaly, bleeding, and diathesis. Cytogenetics show t9,22.	CML, with the Philadelphia chromosome

Questions 1 and 2: Reproduced, with permission, from Berk SL, *PreTest: Medicine*, 9th ed., New York: McGraw-Hill, 2001.
Questions 3 and 4: Reproduced, with permission, from Reteguiz J, *PreTest: Physical Diagnosis*, 4th ed., New York: McGraw-Hill, 2001.

Questions

1. A 52-year-old man presents with a painless neck mass. He states that after he drinks one to two glasses of wine, the neck mass becomes painful. He also complains of intermittent fever, night sweats, pruritus, and a 10-lb weight loss over the last month. On physical examination he has a 3-cm mass in the left anterior cervical lymph node chain that is hard and tender to deep palpation. Several other cervical nodes and a left axillary node are palpable. The liver is enlarged but there is no splenomegaly. Which of the following is the most likely diagnosis?
   a. Non-Hodgkin's lymphoma
   b. Hodgkin's lymphoma
   c. Mononucleosis
   d. Hairy cell leukemia
   e. Sarcoidosis

2. A 62-year-old man presents for his annual health maintenance visit. The review of systems is positive for occasional fatigue and headache. The patient admits to generalized pruritus following a warm bath or shower. He has plethora and engorgement of the retinal veins. A spleen is palpated on abdominal examination. The patient's hematocrit is 63%, and he has a leukocytosis and thrombocytosis. Peripheral blood smear is normal. The patient does not smoke. Which of the following is the most likely diagnosis?
   a. Spurious polycythemia
   b. Essential thrombocytosis
   c. Myelofibrosis
   d. Polycythemia vera
   e. Secondary polycythemia
   f. Chronic myeloid leukemia
   g. Erythropoietin-secreting renal tumor

3. A 42-year-old woman of Italian descent presents for a preemployment physical examination. She has no past medical problems and takes no medications. Her physical examination is normal except for pale conjunctiva. Fecal occult blood test (FOBT) is negative. Her CBC is remarkable for a hemoglobin of 11.4 g/dL, a mean corpuscular volume (MCV) of 60 fL, and a reticulocyte count of 0.6%. Her white blood cell count and platelets are normal. The peripheral smear reveals microcytosis, hypochromia, acanthocytes (cells with irregularly spaced projections), and occasional target cells. Which of the following is the most likely diagnosis?
   a. Iron-deficiency anemia
   b. Sideroblastic anemia
   c. Anemia of chronic disease
   d. Thalassemia trait
   e. Hemolytic anemia

4. A 32-year-old woman presents with the recent onset of petechiae of her lower extremities. She denies menorrhagia and gastrointestinal bleeding.

Encapsulated bacteria	Examples are *Streptococcus pneumoniae* (pneumococcus), *Haemophilus influenzae* (especially b serotype), *Neisseria meningitidis* (meningococcus), and *Klebsiella pneumoniae*. Polysaccharide capsule is an antiphagocytic virulence factor. Positive **Quellung** reaction: if encapsulated bug is present, capsule **swells** when specific anticapsular antisera are added.	IgG_2 necessary for immune response. Capsule serves as antigen in vaccines (Pneumovax, *H. influenzae* b, meningococcal vaccines). **Quellung** = capsular **"swellung."** Pneumococcus associated with "rusty" sputum, sepsis in sickle cell anemia and splenectomy.

Bugs causing watery diarrhea	Include *Vibrio cholerae* (associated with rice-water stools), enterotoxigenic *E. coli*, viruses (e.g., rotaviruses), and protozoans (e.g., *Cryptosporidium* and *Giardia*).
Bugs causing bloody diarrhea	Include *Salmonella, Shigella, Campylobacter jejuni*, enterohemorrhagic/enteroinvasive *E. coli, Yersinia enterocolitica*, and *Entamoeba histolytica* (a protozoan).

Zoonotic bacteria

Species	Disease	Transmission and source	
Borrelia burgdorferi	Lyme disease	Tick bite; *Ixodes* ticks that live on deer and mice	**B**ugs **F**rom **Y**our **P**et
Brucella spp.	Brucellosis/ Undulant fever	Dairy products, contact with animals	**U**ndulates and **U**npasteurized dairy products give you **U**ndulant fever.
Francisella tularensis	Tularemia	Tick bite; rabbits, deer	
Yersinia pestis	Plague	Flea bite; rodents, especially prairie dogs	
Pasteurella multocida	Cellulitis	Animal bite; cats, dogs	

Systemic mycoses

Disease	Endemic location	Notes
Coccidioidomycosis	Southwestern United States, California.	San Joaquin Valley or desert (desert bumps)—"valley fever."
Histoplasmosis	Mississippi and Ohio river valleys	Bird or bat droppings; intracellular (frequently seen inside macrophages).
Paracoccidioidomy-cosis	Rural Latin America	"Captain's wheel" appearance.
Blastomycosis	States east of Mississippi River and Central America	**B**ig, **B**road-**B**ased **B**udding

Broad-based budding

All of the above are caused by **dimorphic** fungi, which are mold in soil (at lower temperature) and yeast in tissue (at higher/body temperature: 37°C) except coccidioidomycosis, which is a spherule in tissue. You can treat with fluconazole or ketoconazole for local infection; amphotericin B for systemic infection.

Cold = Mold.
Heat = Yeast.
Culture on Sabouraud's agar.

Opportunistic fungal infections

Candida albicans	Thrush in immunocompromised (neonates, steroids, diabetes, AIDS), vulvovaginitis (high pH, diabetes, use of antibiotics), disseminated candidiasis (to any organ), chronic mucocutaneous candidiasis.
Aspergillus fumigatus	Ear fungus, lung cavity aspergilloma ("fungus ball"), invasive aspergillosis. **Mold** with septate hyphae that branch at a V-shaped (45°) angle. Not dimorphic.
Cryptococcus neoformans	Cryptococcal meningitis, cryptococcosis. Heavily encapsulated **yeast.** Not dimorphic. Found in soil, pigeon droppings. Culture of Sabouraud's agar. Stains with India ink. Latex agglutination test detects polysaccharide capsular antigen.
Mucor and *Rhizopus* spp.	Mucormycosis. **Mold** with irregular nonseptate hyphae branching at wide angles (≥ 90°). Disease mostly in ketoacidotic diabetic and leukemic patients. Fungi also proliferate in the walls of blood vessels and cause infarction of distal tissue.

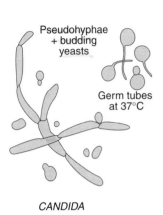

Pseudohyphae + budding yeasts

Germ tubes at 37°C

CANDIDA

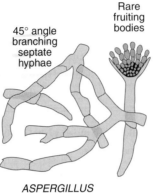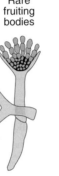

45° angle branching septate hyphae

Rare fruiting bodies

ASPERGILLUS

5-10 μm yeasts with wide capsular halo

Narrow-based unequal budding

CRYPTOCOCCUS

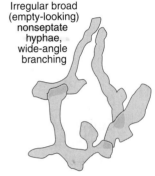

Irregular broad (empty-looking) nonseptate hyphae, wide-angle branching

MUCOR

Time course of HIV infection

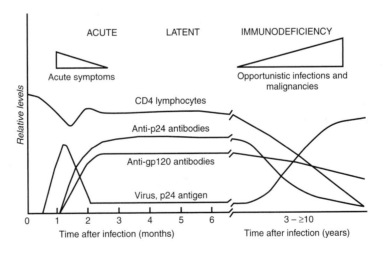

ACUTE   LATENT   IMMUNODEFICIENCY

Acute symptoms

Opportunistic infections and malignancies

Relative levels

CD4 lymphocytes

Anti-p24 antibodies

Anti-gp120 antibodies

Virus, p24 antigen

0 1 2 3 4 5 6

Time after infection (months)

3 – ≥10

Time after infection (years)

(Redrawn, with permission, from Levinson W and Jawetz E, *Medical Microbiology and Immunology: Examination and Board Review,* 6th ed., New York: McGraw-Hill, 2000: p. 276.)

SIRS includes fever or hypothermia, chills, tachypnea, and tachycardia.

Systemic inflammatory response syndrome (SIRS) with a documented infection. Septic shock refers to sepsis-induced hypotension (systolic BP < 90). Gram-positive shock occurs secondary to fluid loss caused by the dissemination of exotoxins; common pathogens include staphylococci and streptococci. Gram-negative shock is caused by vasodilation due to endotoxin (lipopolysaccharide) production by bacteria such as *E. coli*, *Klebsiella*, *Proteus*, and *Pseudomonas*. Other etiologies are as follows:

- **Neonates:** Group B streptococci, *E. coli*, *Klebsiella*.
- **Children:** *H. influenzae*, *Pneumococcus*, *Meningococcus*.
- **Adults:** Gram-positive cocci, aerobic bacilli, anaerobes.
- **IV drug users:** *S. aureus*.
- **Asplenic patients:** *Pneumococcus*, *H. influenzae*, *Meningococcus* (encapsulated organisms).

History

Abrupt onset of fever and chills, often associated with hyperventilation and altered mental status.

PE

Look for **fever** (15% present with hypothermia), **tachycardia,** and tachypnea. **Hypotension** and shock occur in severe cases. Septic shock may start with **warm skin and extremities** (warm shock; peripheral vasodilation) and may then progress to cold shock with **cool skin and extremities** (peripheral vasoconstriction). Petechiae or ecchymoses suggest DIC, which occurs in 2–3% of cases.

— Disseminated Intra vascular coagulation

Evaluation

— lack of
— deficiency

Findings include neutropenia or neutrophilia with increased bands. Thrombocytopenia occurs in 50% of cases. Blood, sputum, and urine cultures may be positive and CXR may show an infiltrate. Obtain coagulation studies and consider a DIC panel (fibrinogen, fibrin split products, D-dimers).

Treatment

Patients often require ICU admission. Treat aggressively with **IV fluids, pressors,** empiric **antibiotics** (Table 2.8–1), and **removal** of predisposing factors (take out Foley catheter, infected IV line, etc.). Patients with severe sepsis (defined as sepsis with at least one acute organ dysfunction) may be candidates for drotrecogin alfa (activated), a form of recombinant human activated protein C.

UCV EM.26

Suspected Diagnosis	Likely Etiology	Drugs of Choice
Meningitis, bacterial	Pneumococcus, meningococcus, *Listeria* (elderly, immuno-compromised)	Ceftriaxone or cefotaxime +/– vancomycin, ampicillin for *Listeria*
Brain abscess	Mixed anaerobes, pneumococci, streptococci	Penicillin G or metronidazole plus cefotaxime or ceftriaxone
Pneumonia, acute, community-acquired, severe	Pneumococci, *M. pneumoniae*, *Legionella*, *C. pneumoniae*	Erythromycin, doxycycline, cefotaxime, or ceftriaxone
Pneumonia, postoperative or nosocomial	*S. aureus*, anaerobes, gram-negative bacilli	Cefotaxime (or ceftriaxone) with gentamicin or tobramycin
Endocarditis, acute (including IV drug user)	*S. aureus*, *E. faecalis*, gram-negative aerobic bacteria, viridans streptococci	Antistaphylococcal penicillin (e.g., nafcillin, oxacillin) plus gentamicin or vancomycin plus gentamicin
Septic thrombophlebitis (e.g., IV tubing, IV shunts)	*S. aureus*, gram-negative aerobic bacteria	Nafcillin, gentamicin
Osteomyelitis	*S. aureus*, *Salmonella* in sickle cell patients	Nafcillin
Septic arthritis	*S. aureus*, *N. gonorrhoeae*	Ceftriaxone
Pyelonephritis with flank pain and fever (recurrent UTI)	*E. coli*, *Klebsiella*, *Enterobacter*, *Pseudomonas*, *Proteus*	Ciprofloxacin or levofloxacin
Intra-abdominal sepsis (e.g., postoperative, peritonitis, cholecystitis)	Gram-negative bacteria, *Bacteroides*, anaerobic bacteria, streptococci, clostridia, *Enterococcus*	Ampicillin plus gentamicin plus metronidazole

(Reproduced, with permission, from Tierney LM, *Current Medical Diagnosis & Treatment*, 39th ed., New York: McGraw-Hill, 2000: p. 1479, Table 37–2.)

FEVER OF UNKNOWN ORIGIN (FUO)

A temperature that exceeds 38.3°C for at least three weeks' duration and remains undiagnosed after three outpatient visits or three days of hospitalization. In adults, **infections** and **cancer** account for > 60% of cases of FUO, while **autoimmune diseases** account for approximately 15%. Causes of FUO include:

- **Infectious:** **TB and endocarditis** (e.g., HACEK organisms) are the most common systemic infections causing FUO, while **occult abscess** is the most common localized infection.
- **Neoplastic:** **Leukemias** and **lymphomas** are the most common neoplasms causing FUO, while **hepatic and renal cell carcinomas** are the most common solid tumors.

213

- **Autoimmune:** Still's disease, SLE, cryoglobulinemia, and polyarteritis nodosa are the most common autoimmune disorders giving rise to FUO, but many rheumatologic/autoimmune diseases can cause FUO.
- **Miscellaneous:** This category includes sarcoidosis, Whipple's disease, recurrent pulmonary emboli, alcoholic hepatitis, drug fever, familial Mediterranean fever, and factitious fever.
- **Undiagnosed** (10–15%).

Evaluation

Evaluation should include serial physical exams, CXR, CBC with differential, ESR, and multiple blood cultures. CT and MRI scans should be done if malignancy or occult abscess is suspected. Specific tests (ANA, RF, viral cultures, viral/fungal antibody/antigen tests) can be obtained if an infectious or autoimmune etiology is suspected.

Treatment

Asymptomatic patients with FUO do not require empiric antibiotic therapy.

Severely ill patients are usually started empirically on broad-spectrum antibiotics until the precise etiology has been determined. However, antibiotics should be stopped if there is no response.

CONGENITAL INFECTIONS

Infections that may occur at any time during pregnancy, labor, and delivery that can have severe consequences after birth. Common sequelae include premature delivery, CNS abnormalities, anemia, jaundice, hepatosplenomegaly, and growth retardation. The most common pathogens can be remembered by the mnemonic **TORCHeS:**

- **T**oxoplasmosis: Transplacental transmission from mom, with primary infection via consumption of **raw meat** or contact with **cat feces.** Specific findings include hydrocephalus, **intracranial calcifications,** and **ring-enhancing lesions** on head CT.
- **O**ther: **HIV,** parvovirus, varicella, *Listeria*, TB, malaria, fungi.
- **R**ubella: Transplacental transmission in the first trimester. Specific findings include a purpuric **"blueberry muffin" rash,** cataracts, hearing loss, and PDA.
- **C**MV (cytomegalovirus): The **most common congenital infection,** primarily transmitted transplacentally. Specific findings include petechial rash (similar to blueberry muffin rash) and **periventricular calcifications.**
- **H**erpes: Intrapartum transmission if mom has **active lesions.** Specific findings include skin, eye, and mouth **vesicles.** Can progress to life-threatening CNS/systemic infection.
- **S**yphilis: Primarily intrapartum transmission. Specific findings include **maculopapular skin rash,** lymphadenopathy, hepatomegaly, **"snuffles"** (mucopurulent rhinitis), and osteitis. In childhood, late congenital syphilis is characterized by saber shins, saddle nose, CNS involvement, and Hutchinson's triad: **peg-shaped upper central incisors, deafness,** and **interstitial keratitis** (photophobia, lacrimation).

Evaluation

Evaluation should include **serologic testing** for rubella, toxoplasmosis, and herpes. Perform urine culture for CMV and dark-field examination of skin lesions/maternal serology for syphilis. Other tests include viral isolation, amniocentesis, and antigen detection. All ill newborns require blood cultures and lumbar puncture.

Treatment

- **Toxoplasmosis:** Pyrimethamine, sulfadiazine, spiramycin.
- **Syphilis:** Penicillin.
- **HSV:** Acyclovir.
- **CMV:** Ganciclovir.

Prevention

- **Toxoplasmosis:** Avoid exposure to cats and cat feces (e.g., changing litter or gardening) during pregnancy; treat women with primary infection with pyrimethamine and sulfadiazine.
- **Rubella:** Immunize before pregnancy; otherwise, consider abortion. Vaccinate the mother after delivery if titers remain negative.
- **Syphilis:** Penicillin in pregnant women.
- **CMV:** Avoid exposure.
- **HSV:** Perform a **C-section** if lesions are present at delivery.
- **HIV:** AZT in pregnant women with HIV; perform C-section.

UCV *OB.48, Ped.32, 34*

MENINGITIS

Infection of the leptomeninges caused by viruses, bacteria, or fungi. Risk factors include recent ear infection, sinusitis, immune deficiencies, recent neurosurgical procedures, and sick contacts.

History/PE

Patients present with **fever,** malaise, **headache, neck stiffness,** photophobia, altered mental status, or seizures. Signs of meningeal irritation (Kernig and Brudzinski) are often absent in infants < 2 years of age.

Evaluation

A high degree of clinical suspicion is required in children < 2 years of age owing to the possible absence of specific meningeal signs. Evaluation should include **LP** (if no papilledema or focal neurologic deficits) and possibly **CT or MRI** to rule out other diagnoses. CBC may reveal leukocytosis. CSF findings vary (see Table 2.8–2).

Treatment

Treat with **antibiotics** (for bacterial infection) and **supportive care.** Viral disease can be treated with supportive care and close follow-up (except herpes meningoencephalitis: treat with acyclovir). The initial choice of antimicro-

TABLE 2.8–2. CSF Findings in Meningitis

Etiology	CSF Findings
Bacterial	Pressure↑, polys↑↑, protein↑, glucose ↓
Viral	Pressure normal/↑, lymphs↑, protein normal/↑, glucose normal
TB/fungal	Pressure↑, lymphs↑, protein↑, glucose ↓

bial agent is based on the most likely organisms involved given the patient's age (Table 2.8–3). Contacts of patients with meningococcal meningitis should receive rifampin prophylaxis.

Complications

- **Hyponatremia:** Administer fluids and monitor sodium concentration.
- **Seizures:** Treat with benzodiazepines and phenytoin.
- **Subdural effusions:** May be seen on CT scan. Occur in 50% of infants with _H. influenzae_ meningitis. No treatment is necessary.
- **Cerebral edema:** Presents with loss of oculocephalic reflex. Treat with IV mannitol.
- **Subdural empyema:** Presents as intractable seizures. Requires surgical evacuation.
- **Brain abscess:** Requires surgical drainage.
- **Ventriculitis:** Presents as worsening clinical picture with improved CSF findings. Requires ventriculostomy and possibly intraventricular antibiotics.

UCV _IM2.24, 40, Neuro.26, 27, Ped.44_

OTITIS EXTERNA

Also known as "swimmer's ear," otitis externa is an inflammation of the skin lining the ear canal and surrounding soft tissue. _Pseudomonas_ (from poorly chlorinated pools) and Enterobacteriaceae are the most common etiologic agents. Both grow in the presence of excess moisture.

TABLE 2.8–3. Treatment of Bacterial Meningitis

Age	Causative Organism	Treatment
< 1 month	Group B strep, _E. coli_, _Listeria_	Cefotaxime + ampicillin
1–3 months	Pneumococci, meningococci, _H. influenzae_	Cefotaxime + vancomycin ± steroids
3 months – adulthood	Pneumococci, meningococci	Ceftriaxone ± vancomycin ± steroids
> 60 years/alcoholism/chronic illness	Pneumococci, gram-negative bacilli, _Listeria_	Ceftriaxone + ampicillin ± steroids

History

Pain, **pruritus,** and a **purulent discharge** from the ear canal.

PE

Pain with movement of the tragus/pinna, an edematous and erythematous ear canal, and purulent discharge.

Otitis media should not cause pain with movement of the tragus/pinna.

Treatment

Eardrops with polymyxin B, neomycin, and hydrocortisone usually suffice. Use **dicloxacillin** for acute disease. **Diabetics** are at risk for malignant otitis externa and osteomyelitis of the skull base and thus require hospitalization and **IV antibiotics.**

UCV *EM.11*

SINUSITIS

Infection of the sinuses due to an undrained collection of pus. Risk factors include barotrauma, allergic rhinitis, viral infection, asthma, smoking, and nasal decongestant overuse.

- Acute sinusitis (symptoms lasting < 1 month) is most commonly associated with **Streptococcus pneumoniae, H. flu, Moraxella catarrhalis,** and viral infection.
- Chronic sinusitis (symptoms persisting > 3 months) is often due to obstruction of sinus drainage and ongoing low-grade anaerobic infections. In diabetic patients, mucormycosis infection may begin in the nose and maxillary sinuses.

The maxillary sinuses are most commonly infected because they drain superiorly against gravity.

History/PE

Fever, facial pain that can **radiate to the upper teeth,** nasal congestion, and **headache. Tenderness,** erythema, swelling over the affected area, and **purulent discharge** may be noted. In chronic sinusitis, pain may be absent but nasal congestion, cough, and purulent drainage continue. Febrile ICU patients may have **occult sinusitis,** especially if they are intubated or have NG tubes.

Always consider occult sinusitis in febrile ICU patients.

Differential

Migraine or cluster headache, dental abscess.

Evaluation

Sinusitis is a **clinical** diagnosis. Culture is generally not required. Clouding of sinuses may be observed on **transillumination** (but the test is difficult to perform and has low sensitivity). Maxillary sinus **radiographs** may be ordered if symptoms persist after therapy and may show air–fluid levels or opacification of the maxillary sinus (Figure 2.8–1). Obtain a coronal CT if complications are suspected.

HIGH-YIELD FACTS

Infectious Disease

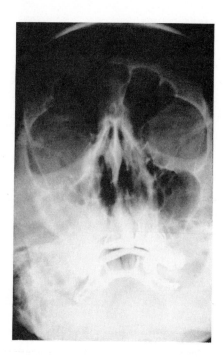

FIGURE 2.8–1. Sinusitis. Compare the opacified right maxillary sinus and normal air-filled left sinus on this sinus x-ray. (Reproduced, with permission, from Saunders CE, *Current Emergency Diagnosis & Treatment,* 4th ed., Stamford, CT: Appleton & Lange, 1992: p. 443, Fig. 26–3.)

Treatment

- **Acute: Amoxicillin** or trimethoprim/sulfamethoxazole for 10 days and symptomatic therapy (e.g., decongestants).
- **Chronic:** 6–12 weeks of PO antibiotic treatment. If medical therapy does not work, treat with surgical drainage and correction of the cause of the obstruction.

Complications

Osteomyelitis of the frontal bone, meningitis, abscess of epidural or subdural spaces, orbital cellulitis, cavernous sinus thrombosis.

PNEUMONIA

An infection of the bronchoalveolar unit with an inflammatory exudate. Causes are often broadly categorized as "typical," caused by bacteria from the nasopharynx, or "atypical," caused by organisms (bacteria, viruses, fungi) inhaled from the environment. Atypical organisms are often difficult to visualize on Gram stain and are not susceptible to antibiotics that act on the cell wall (e.g., beta-lactams).

Rust-colored sputum =
Pneumococcus
Currant jelly sputum =
Klebsiella

History

Classic symptoms are **productive cough** (purulent yellow or green sputum, or hemoptysis), dyspnea, fever/chills, night sweats, and **pleuritic chest pain.** Atypical organisms may present with a more gradual onset, dry cough, headaches, myalgias, sore throat, and pharyngitis.

218

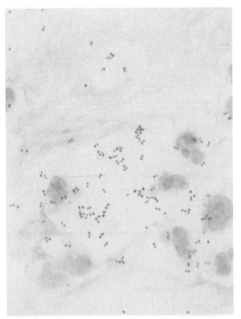

FIGURE 2.8–2. *Staphylococcus aureus.* These clusters of gram-positive cocci were isolated from the sputum of a patient who developed pneumonia while hospitalized.

PE

Decreased or bronchial breath sounds, crackles, wheezing, dullness to percussion, egophony, and tactile fremitus. The elderly and patients with COPD or diabetes may have minimal signs on physical exam.

Evaluation

- **CBC:** <u>Leukocytosis</u> and <u>left shift</u> (bands > 5% and/or immature WBCs).
- **Sputum Gram stain and culture:** Identifies pathogenic organism and the organism's antibiotic susceptibilities (Figures 2.8–2 to 2.8–4). A

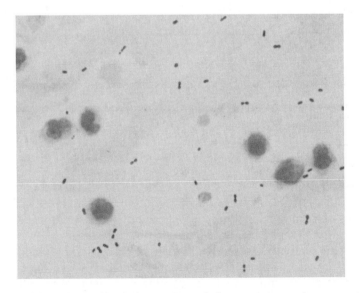

FIGURE 2.8–3. *Streptococcus pneumoniae.* Sputum sample from a patient with pneumonia. Note the characteristic lancet-shaped gram-positive diplococci.

219

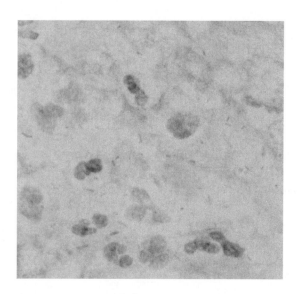

FIGURE 2.8–4. *Pseudomonas.* Sputum sample from a patient with pneumonia revealing gram-negative rods. The large number of neutrophils and relative paucity of epithelial cells indicate that this sample is not contaminated with oropharyngeal flora.

A good sputum sample (i.e., one not contaminated with oropharyngeal flora) has many PMNs and few epithelial cells.

good sputum sample (i.e., one not contaminated by oropharyngeal flora) has many PMNs (> 25 cells/high-power field) and few epithelial cells (< 25 cells/hpf).

- **Blood culture:** If patient appears very ill, suspect sepsis due to pneumonia.
- **ABGs:** Ill patients will have poor oxygen saturation and acid–base disturbances.
- **CXR:** Look for lobar consolidation or patchy or diffuse infiltrates.
- Consider species-specific clues:
  - Rust-colored sputum = pneumococcus.
  - "Currant jelly" sputum = *Klebsiella.*
  - Cold agglutinins = *Mycoplasma.*
  - CD4+ < 200 = PCP.

For persistent recurrent infections, consider the underlying causes of lung injury, obstruction, or decreased immune protection, such as bronchogenic carcinoma, lymphoma, Wegener's, or unusual organisms (TB, *Nocardia, Coxiella burnetii, Aspergillus*).

Treatment

Alcoholics: Klebsiella

Aspiration: anaerobes

COPD: H. flu

Young adults: Mycoplasma

Anyone: S. pneumoniae

Empiric treatment is based on patient demographic and environmental information. Table 2.8–4 summarizes the recommended initial treatment for pneumonia.

- In uncomplicated cases, treat community-acquired pneumonia on an outpatient basis with oral antibiotics (e.g., macrolides).
- Patients > 65 years old as well as those with comorbidity (alcoholism, COPD, diabetes, malnutrition), immunosuppression, unstable vitals or signs of respiratory failure, altered mental status, and/or multilobar involvement require hospitalization with IV antibiotics.
- For patients with obstructive diseases (e.g., cystic fibrosis or bronchiectasis), consider adding pseudomonal coverage.
- Administer the **pneumococcal vaccine** in patients > 65 and those with chronic illnesses, immune compromise, asplenia, and sickle cell disease.

UCV *IM2.23, 25*

TABLE 2.8–4. Initial Antibiotic Treatment of Pneumonia

Category	Suspected Pathogens	Initial (Empiric) Coverage
Outpatient community-acquired pneumonia, < 60 years of age, otherwise healthy	*Streptococcus pneumoniae, Mycoplasma pneumoniae, Chlamydia pneumoniae, H. flu*, viruses	Erythromycin, tetracycline. Consider clarithromycin or azithromycin in smokers to cover *H. flu*.
Greater than 60 or with comorbidity (COPD, heart failure, renal failure, diabetes, liver disease, EtOH abuse)	*S. pneumoniae, H. flu*, aerobic gram-negative rods (GNRs, including *E. coli, Enterobacter, Klebsiella*), *S. aureus, Legionella*, viruses	Second-generation cephalosporin (cefuroxime), TMP-SMX, amoxicillin. Add erythromycin if atypicals (*Legionella, Mycoplasma, Chlamydia*) are suspected.
Community-acquired pneumonia requiring hospitalization	*S. pneumoniae, H. flu*, anaerobes, aerobic GNRs, *Legionella, Chlamydia*	Third-generation cephalosporin (ceftriaxone, cefoperazone). Add erythromycin if atypicals are suspected.
Severe community-acquired pneumonia requiring hospitalization (generally needs ICU care)	*S. pneumoniae, H. flu*, anaerobes, aerobic GNRs, *Mycoplasma, Legionella, Pseudomonas*	Erythromycin and third-generation cephalosporin (ceftriaxone, cefoperazone).
Nosocomial pneumonia—patient hospitalized > 48 hours or in long-term care facility ≥ 14 days	GNR's, including *Pseudomonas, S. aureus, Legionella*, mixed flora	Third-generation cephalosporin and aminoglycoside (gentamicin).

PULMONARY TUBERCULOSIS

Most cases of symptomatic tuberculosis (TB) are due to reactivation of old infection rather than to primary disease and remain confined to the lung. Risk factors include immunosuppression, alcoholism, preexisting lung disease, diabetes, advancing age, homelessness, malnourishment, and crowded living conditions. **Immigrants** from developing nations, healthcare workers, and other persons with "sick contacts" are also at high risk.

History/PE

Cough, hemoptysis, dyspnea, **weight loss,** malaise, **night sweats,** and fever. Pulmonary TB is a common cause of FUO, and the kidney is the most common site of extrapulmonary infection.

TB is a common cause of FUO.

Differential

Pneumonia (bacterial, fungal, viral), other mycobacterial infections, HIV infection, UTI, lung abscess, lung cancer.

Evaluation

- Pulmonary TB is presumptively diagnosed by a **positive sputum acid-fast stain,** since culture may take several weeks (see Clinical Images, p. 13).
- CXR may show **apical fibronodular infiltrates** with or without cavitation.

Immune-compromised individuals with TB may have a negative PPD (check anergy panel).

PPD is injected intradermally on the volar surface of the arm. The transverse length of induration is measured at 48–72 hours. BCG vaccination typically renders a patient PPD positive for at least one year. The size of induration that indicates a positive test is as follows:

- Greater than **5 mm:** HIV or risk factors, close TB contacts, CXR evidence of TB.
- Greater than **10 mm:** Indigent/homeless, developing nations, IVDU, chronic illness, residents of health and correctional institutions.
- Greater than **15 mm:** Everyone else.

A **negative reaction** with negative controls implies anergy from immunosuppression, old age, or malnutrition and thus does not rule out TB.

FIGURE 2.8–5. Purified protein derivative (PPD) placement

- A positive PPD test (see Figure 2.8–5) indicates previous exposure (not necessarily active infection) to *Mycobacterium tuberculosis* and may not be present in immune-compromised individuals.

Treatment

> **Drugs for TB—**
>
> **RESPIre**
> **R**ifampin
> **E**thambutol
> **S**treptomycin
> **P**yrazinamide
> **I**NH

- All cases should be reported to local and state health departments.
- **Institute respiratory isolation** (if TB is suspected) followed by directly observed **multidrug therapy** (usually INH, pyrazinamide, rifampin, and ethambutol). Therapy on at least rifampin and INH should continue for six months.
- Administer **vitamin B$_6$ (pyridoxine)** with INH to prevent peripheral neuritis.
- Initiate **prophylactic therapy** (INH for nine months) for PPD conversion without active symptoms in patients with HIV or other causes of immunosuppression, IV drug users, those age < 35, and those who have had close contact with an infected individual, a CXR suggestive of old TB infection, recent new conversion (< 2 years), poorly controlled diabetes, indigence and malnutrition, or institutional residence.
- Many physicians choose to forgo INH prophylaxis in patients > 35 years old because the risk of INH-induced liver toxicity increases with age.

UCV *IM2.29*

OSTEOMYELITIS

> Osteomyelitis is associated with IV drug use, diabetes, peripheral vascular disease, and penetrating soft tissue injuries.

Bone infection secondary to **direct spread** from a soft tissue infection (80% of cases) or to **hematogenous seeding** (20% of cases). Osteomyelitis secondary to local soft tissue infection is seen in patients with peripheral vascular disease, diabetes (chronic foot ulcers), and penetrating soft tissue injuries. Hematogenous osteomyelitis is most commonly found in children (affecting the metaphyses of the long bones) and IV drug users (affecting the vertebral bodies). **Acute osteomyelitis** is osteomyelitis without a previous bone infection at that site. **Chronic osteomyelitis** occurs when acute osteomyelitis goes untreated or when treatment fails (recurrent infection). Common pathogens responsible for osteomyelitis are listed in Table 2.8–5.

TABLE 2.8–5. Pathogens in Osteomyelitis

If	Think
Most people	S. aureus
IV drug use	S. aureus or Pseudomonas
Sickle cell disease	Salmonella
Hip replacement	S. epidermidis
Foot puncture wound	Pseudomonas
Chronic	S. aureus, Pseudomonas, Enterobacteriaceae

History

Patients present with **fever** and **localized bone pain.**

PE

Localized warmth, tenderness, swelling, erythema, and limited motion of the adjacent joint.

Differential

Cellulitis, soft tissue infection, septic arthritis, rheumatic fever, gout, Ewing's sarcoma, osteoarthritis.

Evaluation

Elevated **WBC** count, **ESR** (>100), and **C-reactive protein** levels. Blood cultures may be positive. Radiographs are often negative on acute presentation; however, radiographic findings **(periosteal elevation)** may be seen 10–14 days later. **Bone scans** are sensitive for osteomyelitis but lack specificity; **indium-labeled leukocyte scanning** is more specific. MRI will show increased signal in the bone marrow consistent with bone marrow edema and may also reveal associated soft tissue infection. Definitive diagnosis is made by **bone aspiration** (Gram stain and culture).

Treatment

Treat with **IV antibiotics** for 4–6 weeks and **surgical debridement** of necrotic, infected bone. Empiric antibiotic selection is based on the suspected organism and Gram stain. Consider oxacillin, nafcillin, a cephalosporin, vancomycin, or quinolone + rifampin if S. aureus is suspected. Empiric gram-negative coverage includes a third-generation cephalosporin, gentamicin, or ciprofloxacin.

Complications

Chronic osteomyelitis, systemic sepsis, soft tissue infection, septic arthritis. Long-standing chronic osteomyelitis with a draining sinus tract may eventually lead to **squamous cell carcinoma.**

UCV Surg.46

Acute or chronic **liver inflammation** due to a variety of agents, most notably viral infection by one of the **hepatitis viruses** or **alcohol** use. Risk factors include IV drug use (hepatitis B/C), alcohol use (alcoholic hepatitis), and travel to developing countries (hepatitis A and E).

> **Hep A** and **E:**
> The vowels hit your bowels.

> **Hep B:**
> **B**lood-borne

> **Hep C:**
> **C**hronic, **C**irrhosis, **C**arcinoma

> **Hep D:**
> **D**efective, **D**ependent on HBV

> **Hep E:**
> **E**nteric, **E**xpectant mothers

- **Hepatitis A virus:** HAV, an RNA picornavirus, can cause **acute hepatitis.** HAV is spread by **fecal–oral** transmission (e.g., contaminated food, water, and **shellfish**) and can lead to epidemics. Acute HAV infection is diagnosed by IgM antibody serology; the presence of IgG antibodies indicates exposure and immunity. It does not cause chronic hepatitis.
- **Hepatitis B virus:** HBV, a DNA hepadnavirus, can cause **acute hepatitis** (1% of patients suffer fulminant or even fatal acute hepatitis) or **chronic hepatitis** (frequently with neonatal infection) and is a major cause of **hepatocellular carcinoma** worldwide. HBV is spread by **blood and other body fluids, including saliva.** HBsAg is present before and during clinical disease, whereas anti-HBs antibodies indicate disease resolution or vaccination. **Anti-HBc antibodies are never seen after vaccination** (Table 2.8–6).
- **Hepatitis C virus:** HCV, an RNA virus similar to flavivirus, causes **acute** or **chronic** hepatitis. It is a major cause of cirrhosis and a major cause of **post-transfusion hepatitis.** It is often associated with IV drug abuse and is spread by **blood-borne** transmission. It can also lead to hepatocellular carcinoma.
- **Hepatitis D virus:** HDV causes disease only in association with HBV (coinfection or superinfection). HDV can cause **acute** or **chronic** (often severe) hepatitis and is spread by **blood-borne** transmission.
- **Hepatitis E virus:** HEV, an RNA virus, normally causes self-limited disease but can be severe (fatal) in **pregnant** women. It is commonly seen in Asia and third-world countries and is spread by fecal–oral (especially water-borne) transmission.
- **Alcoholic hepatitis:** Acute or chronic disease secondary to years of alcohol use; varies in severity.
- **Autoimmune hepatitis:** Usually causes chronic hepatitis in young women and can lead to cirrhosis requiring transplantation. Treat with prednisone +/– azathioprine.
- **Granulomatous hepatitis:** May be caused by TB, fungal infections, sarcoidosis, and other granulomatous disease. Diagnose with liver biopsy and treat with antibiotics and with prednisone for sarcoidosis.

TABLE 2.8–6. Common Serologic Patterns in Hepatitis B Virus Infection

HBsAg	Anti-HBs	Anti-HBc	HBeAg	Anti-HBe	Interpretation
+	–	IgM	+	–	Acute hepatitis B
–	–	IgM	+/–	–	Acute hepatitis B, window period
+	–	IgG	+ *viral replication*	–	Chronic hepatitis B with active viral replication
+	–	IgG	–	+	Chronic hepatitis B with low viral replication
+	+	IgG	+/–	+/–	Chronic hepatitis B with heterotypic anti-HBs (10% of cases)
–	+	IgG	–	+/–	Recovery from hepatitis B (immunity)
–	+	–	–	–	Vaccination (immunity)

ACUTE HEPATITIS

History

Acute hepatitis often starts with a viral prodrome of nonspecific symptoms (**malaise,** joint pain, fatigue, URI symptoms, **nausea, vomiting,** changes in bowel habits) followed by **jaundice,** fatigue, and other symptoms. There is then a convalescent period followed by recovery.

PE

Jaundice, scleral icterus, **tender hepatomegaly,** possible splenomegaly, and lymphadenopathy.

Differential

Mononucleosis and other systemic viral illnesses (CMV), toxoplasmosis, rickettsial diseases (Q fever, Rocky Mountain spotted fever), drug-induced hepatitis, autoimmune hepatitis, "shock liver" secondary to hypoperfusion (e.g., MI or trauma), neoplasm, alcohol use.

Evaluation

Normal WBC (with relative lymphocytosis), dramatically **elevated ALT/ AST,** and elevated bilirubin/alkaline phosphatase. Diagnosis is made on the basis of **hepatitis serology.** Liver biopsy may be performed in severe cases.

An AST:ALT > 2 suggests alcoholic hepatitis.

Treatment

- Rest and wait for resolution of symptoms.
- **Look for sick contacts.**
- Administer **alpha-interferon for HBV and HCV** to decrease the likelihood of chronic hepatitis.
- **Steroids** for severe alcoholic hepatitis.
- Hospitalization for fulminant hepatic failure (development of encephalopathy and coagulopathy).

CHRONIC HEPATITIS

History/PE

Chronic hepatitis usually gives rise to symptoms indicative of chronic liver disease (jaundice, cirrhosis). At least 80% of those infected with HCV and 10% of those with HBV will develop chronic hepatitis.

Eighty percent of patients infected with HCV will develop chronic hepatitis.

Etiologies

HBV, HCV, HDV, autoimmune hepatitis, alcoholic hepatitis (IM1.38), drug-induced disease (INH or methyldopa), Wilson's disease, hemochromatosis, alpha-1-antitrypsin deficiency, neoplasms.

Evaluation

Findings include an **elevated ALT/AST** lasting > 6 months and a rise in bilirubin/alkaline phosphatase. In severe cases, PT will be prolonged (most clotting factors are produced by the liver). Diagnosis is made on the basis of **hepatitis serologies** and **liver biopsy,** which may show inflammation, fibrosis, and necrosis involving hepatocytes. Additional evaluation may include ANA (autoimmune hepatitis) and antimitochondrial antibody.

Treatment

- For autoimmune hepatitis, **immunosuppression** with steroids and other agents (azathioprine) is standard of care. **Alpha-interferon** and lamivudine (3TC) have proven efficacy in chronic HBV infection. Treat HCV infection with **alpha-interferon** and ribavirin.
- **Liver transplantation** (if available) is the treatment of choice for patients with end-stage liver failure.

Complications

> *Sequelae of chronic hepatitis include cirrhosis, liver failure, and hepatocellular carcinoma.*

Chronic HBV infection carries a risk of **cirrhosis (40%),** liver failure, and **hepatocellular carcinoma (3–5%),** and about half of patients die within five years of onset of symptoms. Chronic HCV infection is more indolent and subclinical but can also lead to eventual cirrhosis (30%) or **hepatocellular carcinoma.**

UCV *IM1.35*

URINARY TRACT INFECTION (UTI)

Includes cystitis, pyelonephritis, and urosepsis. UTIs affect women more frequently than men, and positive *E. coli* cultures are obtained in 80% of cases. Other pathogens include *Staphylococcus saprophyticus, Klebsiella, Proteus,* and *Enterococcus.* Risk factors include use of a **Foley catheter** or other urologic instrumentation, anatomic abnormalities (e.g., BPH, vesicoureteral reflux), a history of previous UTIs or acute pyelonephritis, **diabetes mellitus,** recent antibiotic use, immunosuppression, and **pregnancy.**

> *Urosepsis must be considered in any elderly patient with altered mental status.*

History/PE

Patients complain of **urinary frequency, dysuria,** and **urgency.** Acute pyelonephritis may present with nausea, vomiting, **fever,** and **back/flank pain.** Children often present with **bedwetting,** and infants can present with poor feeding, recurrent febrile episodes, and foul-smelling urine.

> **UTI bugs—**
>
> **SEEKS PP**
> **S.** saprophyticus
> **E.** coli
> **E**nterobacter
> **K**lebsiella
> **S**erratia
>
> **P**roteus
> **P**seudomonas

Evaluation

Urine dipstick may reveal **increased leukocyte esterase** (75% sensitive for WBCs), **elevated nitrites** (low sensitivity; false positives with bacterial contamination), elevated urine pH (characteristic of *Proteus* infections), or hematuria (seen with cystitis). Microscopic analysis may show > **5 leukocytes/hpf** (indicative of GU infection) and a bacterial pathogen. WBC casts on UA indicate acute pyelonephritis. The gold standard is a clean-catch urine culture with > 10^5 **bacteria/mL** (diagnosis is often made on the basis of the dipstick alone).

Treatment

Treat healthy young females on an outpatient basis with oral **TMP-SMX** or **ciprofloxacin** for three days. Elderly patients, those with comorbid diseases, or those with acute toxicity in the setting of acute pyelonephritis should be hospitalized and treated with **IV antibiotics** (ciprofloxacin or ampicillin and gentamicin to cover enterococcus). **Prophylactic antibiotics** may be given to those with recurrent UTIs.

UCV *IM2.31*

SEXUALLY TRANSMITTED DISEASES

STDs are among the most common outpatient/ER gynecologic complaints. All sexually active patients should be screened for STDs. Risk factors include multiple sexual partners, unprotected sexual intercourse, high frequency of sexual intercourse, high-risk behavior, young age at first intercourse, and unusual sexual practices. Twenty-five to fifty percent of patients with STDs have multiple genital tract infections.

Up to 50% of patients with STDs have multiple genital tract infections.

SYPHILIS

Syphilis is caused by *Treponema pallidum*, a spirochete.

History/PE

- **Primary** (10–60 days after infection): A **painless ulcer (chancre)** is found on or near the area of contact (Figure 2.8–6). The lesion often goes unnoticed and heals spontaneously in 3–9 weeks.
- **Secondary** (4–8 weeks after appearance of chancre): Patients present with low-grade **fever,** headache, malaise, anorexia, and generalized **lymphadenopathy** and with a diffuse, symmetric, asymptomatic **maculopapular rash on the soles and palms.** Meningitis, hepatitis, and nephritis may also be seen. Highly infective secondary eruptions (mucous patches) can coalesce, forming condylomata lata; lesions heal spontaneously in 2–6 weeks.
- **Early latent:** No symptoms, positive serology, first year of infection.
- **Late latent:** No symptoms, positive or negative serology, > 1 year of infection. One-third will progress to tertiary syphilis.

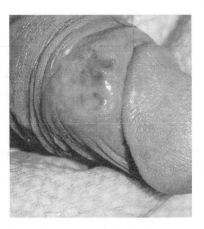

FIGURE 2.8–6. Primary syphilis. The chancre, which appears at the site of infection, is an ulcerated papule with a smooth, clean base; raised, indurated borders; and scant discharge.

TABLE 2.8–7. Diagnostic Test for Syphilis

Test	Comments
Dark-field microscopy	Identifies motile spirochetes (only on primary or secondary lesions).
VDRL/RPR _+ secondary_	Rapid and cheap, but sensitivity is only 60–75% in primary disease; nonspecific. Reverts to negative with treatment.
FTA-ABS	Sensitive, specific. Used as a secondary diagnostic test. Positive for life.

- **Tertiary** (1–20 years after initial infection): Destructive, granulomatous **gummas** can severely damage the skin, bones, and liver. Neurologic findings include **tabes dorsalis** (posterior column degeneration) and **Argyll–Robertson pupil** (small, irregular pupil that accommodates but does not react to light). Cardiovascular findings include aortitis, aortic root aneurysms, and aortic regurgitation.

Evaluation

Evaluation (see Table 2.8–7) consists of **dark-field microscopy** (motile spirochetes) of primary or secondary lesions, **VDRL/RPR** (a rapid, nonspecific screening test), and **FTA-ABS/MHA-TP** (specific, diagnostic).

Treatment

Treat with **penicillin.** Tetracycline or doxycycline can be used in patients with penicillin allergies. Neurosyphilis should be treated with IV penicillin; penicillin-allergic patients should be desensitized prior to therapy.
UCV _IM2.27, 28_

CHLAMYDIA TRACHOMATIS

C. trachomatis, a sexually transmitted disease, often coexists with or mimics *N. gonorrhoeae* infection. Patients should be tested for both at the same time.

History/PE

Vertical transmission causes ocular infections in the newborn. In adults, it may present asymptomatically or as cervicitis, urethritis, salpingitis, or pelvic inflammatory disease (PID), with mucopurulent discharge and cervical or adnexal pain. In men, chlamydia is a common cause of nongonococcal and postgonococcal urethritis. The L type causes lymphogranuloma venereum, a rare systemic disease occurring in three stages: (1) painless genital ulcers followed by (2) painful lymphadenopathy (buboes) and nonspecific systemic symptoms and (3) a tertiary stage with suppuration of buboes, formation of anal and rectal fistulas, and elephantiasis.

Evaluation

The diagnosis is usually made on clinical grounds, as culture is difficult and takes 48–72 hours; immunoassays of cervical specimens may help confirm suspicions.

Treatment may induce a Jarisch–Herxheimer reaction with fever and flulike symptoms due to massive destruction of spirochetes.

Treatment

- Doxycycline or azithromycin.
- In pregnant patients, erythromycin.
- Also treat for presumptive gonorrhea coinfection (with ceftriaxone).

Complications

Chronic infection and pelvic pain, infertility, Fitz-Hugh–Curtis syndrome (perihepatic inflammation and fibrosis).

Neisseria gonorrhoeae

Gram-negative diplococci that can infect the pharynx and almost any site in the female reproductive tract, including Bartholin's ducts as well as the urethra, vagina, cervix, ovaries, fallopian tubes, and anus. Mucopurulent cervicitis and PID are the most common concerns. Infection in men tends to be limited to the urethra.

Gonorrhea is very easily transmitted to women during sexual intercourse; 80–90% of women who have a single encounter with an infected individual contract the disease, while males become infected only 20–25% of the time after sex with an infected female.

History/PE

Presents in women as a greenish-yellow cervical discharge, pelvic or adnexal pain, swollen Bartholin's glands, PID, salpingitis, and tubo-ovarian abscess (TOA). Infection may be indistinguishable from chlamydial disease; patients may be treated for both infections at once. Men experience purulent urethral discharge, dysuria, and erythema of the urethral meatus.

Diagnosis

Swab the pharynx, cervix, urethra, or anus as appropriate for culture on Thayer–Martin medium (80–95% sensitivity). Gram stain of cervical discharge showing gram-negative intracellular diplococci may provide confirmatory diagnosis.

Treatment/Prevention

- IM ceftriaxone.
- Also treat for presumptive chlamydia coinfection (doxycycline or macrolide).
- Condoms are effective prophylaxis.

Complications

Persistent infection with pain, infertility, TOA with rupture.

UCV *IM2.18, OB.7*

Genital Lesions

See Table 2.8–8.

UCV *IM2.19, OB.5, 11*

TABLE 2.8–8. Sexually Transmitted Genital Lesions

Syphillis

	Calymmato-bacterium granulomatis	_H. ducreyi (chancroid)_	_Herpes simplex virus 1 or 2*_	_Human papillo-mavirus**_	_Treponema pallidum_
Lesion	Papule	Papule or pustule (chancroid)	Vesicle	Papule (condylomata acuminata: warts)	Papule (chancre)
Appearance	Raised, red lesions	Irregular, deep, well demarcated	Regular, red, shallow	Irregular, pink or white, raised; cauliflower	Regular, red, round, raised
Number	1 or multiple	1–3	Multiple	Multiple	Single
Size	5–10 mm	10–20 mm	1–3 mm	1–5 mm	1 cm
Pain	No	Yes	Yes	No	No
Concurrent signs and symptoms	Granulomatous ulcers	Inguinal lymphadenop-athy	Vulvar pain and pruritus	Pruritus	Regional adenopathy
Diagnosis	Clinical exam, visualize with smear	Difficult to culture; diagnosis made on clinical grounds	Tzanck smear or viral cultures	Clinical exam; biopsy for confirmation	Spirochetes seen under dark-field microscopy; _T. pallidum_ identified by serum antibody test
Treatment	Doxycycline (100 mg BID × 3 weeks)	Ceftriaxone, erythromycin, or ciprofloxacin	Acyclovir for primary infection	Cryotherapy, topical agents such as podo-phyllin, trichloroacetic acid, or 5-fluorouracil cream	Penicillin

* 85% of genital herpes lesions are caused by HSV-2.
** HPV serotypes 6 and 11 are associated with genital warts; types 16, 18, and 31 are associated with cervical cancer.

HUMAN IMMUNODEFICIENCY VIRUS (HIV)

CD4 count is a marker for the extent of disease, while viral load indicates rate of disease progression.

A retrovirus that targets and destroys CD4 lymphocytes, leading to AIDS. Risk factors include unprotected sexual intercourse, IV drug abuse, maternal HIV infection, needle sticks and mucocutaneous exposures, and receipt of blood products. Infection is characterized by a high rate of viral replication leading to a progressive decline in the CD4 count. Broadly stated, the **CD4**

TABLE 2.8–9. HIV Complications

CD4 Count | Associated Complications

CD4 Count	Associated Complications
> 500	Lymphadenopathy, recurrent vaginal candidiasis.
200–500	Pneumococcal pneumonia, pulmonary TB, shingles, oral candidiasis (thrush), cervical intraepithelial neoplasia, anemia, Kaposi's sarcoma, non-Hodgkin's lymphoma, histoplasmosis, coccidioidomycosis.
100–200	*Pneumocystis carinii* pneumonia, AIDS dementia complex, wasting syndrome.
50–100	Toxoplasmosis, cryptococcosis.
< 50	CMV retinitis *(IM2.12)*, MAC, cryptosporidiosis, PML, primary CNS lymphoma.

count is a surrogate marker for the **extent** of disease progression, while the **viral load** is an indicator of the **rate** of disease progression.

History/PE

Primary HIV infection is often **asymptomatic;** patients may present with **flu-like symptoms,** e.g., generalized malaise, fever, generalized lymphadenopathy, rash, or even viral meningitis. Later, HIV may present as night sweats, weight loss, and cachexia. Complications correlate with CD4 count, as indicated in Table 2.8–9.

Evaluation

The **ELISA test (high sensitivity, moderate specificity)** detects anti-HIV antibodies in the bloodstream (which can take up to six months to appear after exposure). Confirm a positive ELISA with a **Western blot (low sensitivity, high specificity).** If the patient is HIV positive, then check viral load, PPD with anergy panel, VDRL, and CMV and toxoplasmosis serologies.

A positive ELISA must be confirmed with a Western blot.

Treatment

Management is evolving rapidly. Currently, **antiretroviral therapy** is initiated for patients with CD4 counts < 500 or with a detectable viral load. Start patients on two **nucleoside analogs** (e.g., AZT, ddI, 3TC, D4T). Non-nucleoside reverse transcriptase inhibitors and **protease inhibitors** (e.g., saquinavir, ritonavir, indinavir) are added depending on drug–drug interactions, drug tolerance, and patient compliance. **Prophylaxis** for *Pneumocystis carinii* pneumonia and toxoplasmosis (TMP-SMX) is started in patients with CD4 counts < 200. Prophylaxis for MAC (clarithromycin or azithromycin) is started in patients with CD4 counts < 100. Opportunistic infections are treated as they arise (Table 2.8–10).

UCV *Ped.26*

TABLE 2.8–10. Opportunistic Infections in HIV

Disease	Treatment
CMV	Ganciclovir, foscarnet
Esophageal candidiasis	Fluconazole, ketoconazole
Cryptococcal meningitis	Amphotericin B, fluconazole
HSV	Acyclovir, foscarnet
Herpes zoster	Acyclovir, foscarnet
Kaposi's sarcoma	Cutaneous—observation, intralesional vinblastine; severe cutaneous—systemic chemotherapy, alpha-interferon, radiation; visceral disease—combination chemotherapy
Lymphoma	Combination chemotherapy, radiation therapy with dexamethasone (if CNS lymphoma)
MAC	Clarithromycin, azithromycin, ethambutol, rifabutin
Mycobacterium tuberculosis	Multiagent therapy (INH, rifampin, pyrazinamide, ethambutol, streptomycin)
Pneumocystis carinii pneumonia	TMP-SMX ± steroids, atovaquone, pentamidine
Toxoplasmosis	Pyrimethamine, sulfadiazine, clindamycin

IM2.7

LYME DISEASE

A tick-borne disease caused by the spirochete *Borrelia burgdorferi*. Lyme disease is usually seen during the summer months and is carried by *Ixodes* ticks; it is endemic to the Northeast, northern Midwest, and Pacific coast. It is the most common vector-borne disease in North America.

History

Fever, malaise, and rash are characteristic of primary Lyme disease.

PE

Erythema migrans begins as a small erythematous macule or papule **found at the tick-feeding site** and expands slowly over days to weeks. The border may be macular or raised, and **central clearing** is often present ("bull's eye"). Median lesion width is 15 cm. Primary Lyme disease may be followed by secondary Lyme disease, which is characterized by **arthralgias, migratory polyarthropathies,** neurologic phenomena (e.g., **Bell's palsy**), meningitis, and/or **myocarditis** (presents as conduction abnormalities). Tertiary Lyme disease is characterized by arthritis and subacute encephalitis (memory loss and mood change).

Lyme disease is the most common vector-borne disease in North America.

Differential

- **Early:** Viral exanthem.
- **Later:** Collagen vascular disease, chronic fatigue syndrome, other causes of neuropathies, encephalitis, aseptic meningitis, myocarditis.

Evaluation

Diagnosis is based on clinical and laboratory findings (ELISA and Western blot). Use Western blot to confirm a positive or indeterminate ELISA. A positive ELISA denotes **exposure** and is not specific for active disease (culture/molecular tests are currently under development).

Treatment

Treat with **doxycycline** or **ceftriaxone.** Consider empiric therapy for patients with characteristic rash, arthralgias, or a tick bite acquired in an endemic area. Vaccines are available but are < 75% effective.

UCV *Ped.29*

ROCKY MOUNTAIN SPOTTED FEVER

A tick-borne rickettsial disease caused by *Rickettsia rickettsii*, Rocky Mountain spotted fever is carried by the *Dermacentor tick.* The organism invades the endothelial lining of capillaries and leads to **small vessel vasculitis.**

History

Patients present with **headache, fever,** malaise, and a **rash.**

PE

The rash characteristic of Rocky Mountain spotted fever is initially macular (beginning on the **palms** and **soles**) but becomes petechial/purpuric as it spreads centrally. Altered mental status or DIC may develop in severe cases.

Syst Coagulation disorder

Differential

Meningococcemia, Lyme disease, measles, typhoid, endocarditis, hemorrhagic fevers (Ebola, Hanta), vasculitis, other rickettsial diseases (e.g., ehrlichiosis).

Evaluation

This is a **clinical diagnosis** that is confirmed retrospectively with acute and convalescent antibody titers utilizing complement fixation or the Weil–Felix test (antigen cross-reactivity with *Proteus* antigens).

HIGH-YIELD FACTS

Infectious Disease

Treatment

Treat with **doxycycline;** use chloramphenicol in children and pregnant women. The condition can be rapidly fatal if left untreated.

UCV *Ped.31*

FOOD-BORNE ILLNESSES

Table 2.8–11 summarizes the major pathogens in food-borne illnesses.

	TABLE 2.8–11. Food-Borne Illnesses	
Pathogen	**Source**	**Signs/Symptoms/Treatment**
Staphylococcus aureus	Meats, **dairy** (mayonnaise). Pre-formed toxin.	Abrupt, intense vomiting within 1–8 hours. Self-limited.
Bacillus cereus	Reheated fried **rice.** Pre-formed toxin.	Abrupt vomiting (within 1–8 hours) followed by watery diarrhea (8–16 hours). Self-limited.
Clostridium perfringens	Rewarmed meat. Pre-formed toxin.	Abrupt, profuse, watery diarrhea (within 8–16 hours).
Clostridium botulinum	Home-canned food (ingestion of toxin). Honey.	**Flaccid paralysis.** Onset in 1–4 days. May also occur in infants who are fed honey (ingest spores). Treat with IV antitoxin.
E. coli	Uncooked foods, fecal contamination.	Abrupt diarrhea; vomiting rare. "Traveler's diarrhea."
Vibrio cholera	Endemic areas. Toxin-mediated.	Severe, voluminous, **"rice water" diarrhea.** Treat with vigorous fluid and electrolyte replacement.
Vibrio parahaemolyticus	Contaminated **seafood.**	Self-limited unless immune compromised.
Campylobacter jejuni	Contaminated food, milk, and water.	Fever and inflammatory diarrhea (blood, pus). Usually self-limited. Ciprofloxacin if severe.
Shigella	Transmission by **F**ood, **F**lies, **F**ingers, **F**eces.	Abrupt inflammatory diarrhea, often with blood and mucus, lower abdominal cramps. Ciprofloxacin if severe.
Salmonella	Raw/undercooked chicken.	Fever and inflammatory diarrhea, nausea/vomiting. Usually self-limited. Antibiotics may prolong carrier state and increase relapse rate.
Yersinia enterocolitica	Raw/undercooked pork.	Fever, abdominal pain, inflammatory diarrhea. Ciprofloxacin if severe.

Meningitis in neonates.	Group B strep, *E. coli*, *Listeria*
Meningitis in infants.	Pneumococcus, meningococcus, *H. influenzae*
Asplenic patients are particularly susceptible to these organisms.	Encapsulated organisms—pneumococcus, meningococcus, *H. influenzae*, *Klebsiella*
Begin PCP prophylaxis in HIV+ patient at what CD4+ cell count? MAC prophylaxis?	< 200 for PCP (with Bactrim); < 100 for MAC (with clarithromycin/azithromycin)
Primary lesion of syphilis.	Painless chancre
Neurologic findings in tertiary syphilis.	Tabes dorsalis, Argyll–Robertson pupil
Fever and flulike symptoms upon initiation of penicillin in patient with syphilis.	Jarisch–Herxheimer reaction
Three most common causes of fever of unknown origin (FUO).	Infection, cancer, and autoimmune disease
Treatment for herpes meningitis.	Acyclovir
Organism responsible for 80% of UTIs.	*E. coli*
Number of bacteria on clean-catch specimen that is diagnostic of UTI.	10^5 bacteria/mL
Hepatitis serology shows: 1. Positive HBsAg and HBeAg; IgM anti-HBc; negative for anti-HBs and anti-HBe. 2. Positive anti-HBs; negative HBsAg, HBeAg, anti-HBc, or anti-HBe. 3. Positive HBsAg, IgG anti-HBc, HBeAg; negative anti-HBs or anti-HBe.	1. Acute hepatitis B infection 2. Vaccination (+) IgG anti-HBc 3. Chronic hepatitis B with active viral replication (+) HBe Ag
Erythema migrans.	Lesion of primary Lyme disease
Characteristics of secondary Lyme disease.	Arthralgias, migratory polyarthropathies, Bell's palsy, myocarditis
Antigen test used to confirm diagnosis of Rocky Mountain spotted fever rickettsial disease.	Weil–Felix test
"Blueberry muffin" rash is characteristic of what congenital infection?	Rubella
Initial test for HIV, with high sensitivity but only moderate specificity.	ELISA

Questions 1 and 2: Reproduced, with permission, from Reteguiz J, *PreTest: Physical Diagnosis*, 4th ed., New York: McGraw-Hill, 2001.

Questions 3 and 4: Reproduced, with permission, from Elkind MSV, *PreTest: Neurology*, 4th ed., New York: McGraw-Hill, 2001.

Questions 5 and 6: Reproduced, with permission, from Berk SL, *PreTest: Medicine*, 9th ed., New York: McGraw-Hill, 2001.

Questions

1. A 46-year-old woman with a history of sinusitis presents with a severe headache. She complains of neck stiffness and photophobia. On physical examination she has a temperature of 103.4°F. Blood pressure is normal and heart rate is 110/min. She has a normal funduscopic examination and no focal neurologic deficit. She has nuchal rigidity. Brudzinski and Kernig signs are positive. Which of the following is the most likely diagnosis?
   a. Migraine headache
   b. Cluster headache
   c. Torticollis
   d. Bacterial meningitis
   e. Cysticercosis
   f. Fever of unknown origin

2. A 41-year-old woman develops abdominal cramps and diarrhea two hours after eating fried rice. Physical examination is normal except for some mild abdominal tenderness with palpation. Examination of the stool reveals no fecal leukocytes. Which of the following is the most likely etiology for the symptoms?
   a. *Shigella*
   b. *Salmonella*
   c. *Vibrio cholerae*
   d. *Bacillus cereus*
   e. *Staphylococcus aureus*
   f. *Vibrio parahaemolyticus*

DIRECTIONS: The question below consists of lettered options followed by numbered items. For each numbered item, select the single most appropriate lettered option. Each lettered option may be used once, more than once, or not at all. **Choose exactly the number of options indicated following each item.**

Items 3–4

Select from the following list the condition that best fits each clinical scenario.
   a. Subacute HIV encephalomyelitis (AIDS encephalopathy)
   b. Subacute sclerosing panencephalitis (SSPE)
   c. Progressive multifocal leukoencephalitis (PML)
   d. Rabies encephalitis
   e. Guillain–Barré syndrome
   f. Tabes dorsalis
   g. Neurocysticercosis

3. A 27-year-old man developed recurrent episodes of involuntary movements. He had abused intravenous drugs for several years and had several admissions for recurrent infections, including subacute bacterial endocarditis. His invol-

untary movements were largely restricted to the right side of his body. Associated with this problem were hoarseness and difficulty swallowing. He had suffered a weight loss of 40 lb over the preceding four months. Examination revealed diffuse lymphadenopathy and right-sided hypertonia. His CSF was normal except for a slight increase in the protein content. Computed tomography revealed a large area of decreased density on the left side of the cerebrum. The EEG revealed diffuse slowing over the left side of the head. Biopsy of this lesion revealed oligodendrocytes with abnormally large nuclei that contained darkly staining inclusions. There was extensive demyelination and there were giant astrocytes in the lesion. Over the course of one month, this man exhibited increasing ataxia. Within two months, he had evidence of mild dementia and seizures. Within three months of presentation, his dementia was profound and he had bladder and bowel incontinence. Over the course of a few days he became obtunded and died. **(SELECT ONE CONDITION)**

4. A 50-year-old immigrant from eastern Europe developed problems with bladder control, an unsteady gait, and pain in his legs over the course of six months. On examination, it was determined that he had absent deep tendon reflexes in his legs, markedly impaired vibration sense in his feet, and a positive Romberg sign. Despite his complaint of unsteady gait, he had no problems with rapid alternating movement of the feet and no tremors were evident. He had normal leg strength. The pain in his legs was sharp, stabbing, and paroxysmal. His serum glucose and glycohemoglobin levels were normal. **(SELECT ONE CONDITION)**

Items 5–6

A 25-year-old male student presents with a chief complaint of rash. There is no headache, fever, or myalgia. A slightly pruritic maculopapular rash is noted over the abdomen, trunk, palms of hands, and soles of feet. Inguinal, occipital, and cervical lymphadenopathy is also noted. Hypertrophic, flat, wartlike lesions are noted around the anal area. Laboratory studies show the following:

Hct: 40%
Hgb: 14 g/dL
WBC: 13,000/mm^3
Differential:
  Segmented neutrophils 50%
  Lymphocytes 50%

5. The most useful laboratory test in this patient is
   a. Weil–Felix titer
   b. Venereal Disease Research Laboratory (VDRL) test
   c. *Chlamydia* titer
   d. Blood cultures

6. The treatment of choice for this patient would be
   a. Penicillin
   b. Ceftriaxone
   c. Tetracycline *or doxycycline if allergic w penicilline*
   d. Interferon alpha
   e. Erythromycin

1. **The answer is d.** The patient is demonstrating signs of meningeal irritation. She has nuchal rigidity, a positive **Brudzinski sign** (involuntary flexion of the hips and knees when flexing the neck), and a positive **Kernig sign** (flexing the hip and knee when the patient is supine, then straightening out the leg, causes resistance and back pain). Other signs of meningitis include headache, photophobia, seizures, and altered mental status. Patients with meningitis (< 1%) rarely have papilledema secondary to increased intracranial pressure. Risk factors for meningitis include sinusitis, ear infection, and sick contacts. Fever of unknown origin **(FUO)** is defined as a fever of > 101°F for three weeks that remains undiagnosed after one week of aggressive investigation.

2. **The answer is d.** The incubation period for both *S. aureus* and *B. cereus* is 1–2 hours after eating. *B. cereus* toxicity is often due to eating fried (the toxin is heat-stable) or uncooked rice. *S. aureus* toxicity is usually due to eating ham, poultry, potato or egg salad, mayonnaise, or cream pastries. All the other organisms require an incubation period of > 16 hours. *V. cholerae* toxicity is due to eating shellfish and causes an inflammatory (presence of fecal leukocytes) diarrhea. *V. parahaemolyticus* toxicity is due to eating mollusks and crustaceans and causes dysentery (production of cytotoxins, bacterial invasion, and destruction of intestinal mucosal cells). *Salmonella* toxicity is due to eating beef, poultry, eggs, or dairy products and causes a watery diarrhea. *Shigella* causes dysentery and can be present in potato or egg salad, lettuce, or raw vegetables.

3. **The answer is c.** This patient probably had AIDS with PML as a complication of that disease. The inclusion bodies in the oligodendrocyte nuclei are JC virus, a papillomavirus. Primary infection with JC virus is universal and asymptomatic. Immunosuppression leads to reactivation of the virus. Diagnosis is typically made by MRI, which shows multiple, focal, well-defined white matter lesions that do not enhance or have mass effect. Cerebrospinal fluid PCR for JC virus is also available, obviating the need for brain biopsy in most cases. Treatment with cytarabine arabinoside has not been shown to be effective in clinical trials. Less than 10% of patients may experience spontaneous remission. PML may also develop with lymphomas, leukemias, or sarcoid, but the incidence of this disease in the U.S. population has expanded greatly since the dissemination of HIV in the population.

4. **The answer is f.** Tabes dorsalis is caused by *Treponema pallidum*, the agent responsible for all types of neurosyphilis, but it is a disease entity distinct from general paresis, the form of neurosyphilis in which personality changes and dementia do occur. With tabes dorsalis, the patient develops a leptomeningitis. The posterior columns of the spinal cord and the dorsal root ganglia are hit especially hard by degenerative changes associated with this form of neurosyphilis.

5–6. **The answers are 5-b, 6-a.** The diffuse rash involving palms and soles would in itself suggest the possibility of secondary syphilis. The hypertrophic, wartlike lesions around the anal area are called *condylomata lata*, which are specific for secondary syphilis. The VDRL slide test will be positive in all patients with secondary syphilis. The Weil–Felix titer has been used as a screening test for rickettsial infection. In this patient, who has condyloma and no systemic symptoms, Rocky Mountain spotted fever would be unlikely. No chlamydial infection would present in this way. Blood cultures might be drawn to rule out bacterial infection such as chronic meningococcemia; however, the clinical picture is not consistent with a systemic bacterial infection. Penicillin is the drug of choice for secondary syphilis. Ceftriaxone and tetracycline are usually considered to be alternative therapies. Interferon alpha has been used in the treatment of condyloma acuminatum, a lesion that can be mistaken for syphilitic condyloma.

Musculoskeletal

Brachial plexus

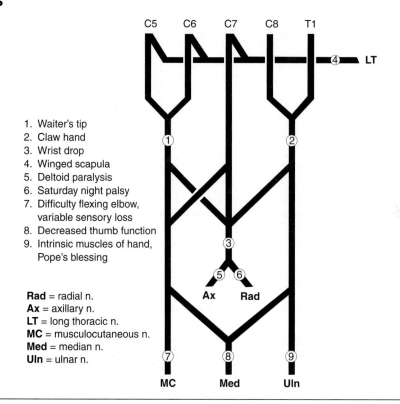

1. Waiter's tip
2. Claw hand
3. Wrist drop
4. Winged scapula
5. Deltoid paralysis
6. Saturday night palsy
7. Difficulty flexing elbow, variable sensory loss
8. Decreased thumb function
9. Intrinsic muscles of hand, Pope's blessing

Rad = radial n.
Ax = axillary n.
LT = long thoracic n.
MC = musculocutaneous n.
Med = median n.
Uln = ulnar n.

COX-2 inhibitors (celecoxib, rofecoxib)

Mechanism	Selectively inhibit cyclooxygenase (COX) isoform 2, which is found in inflammatory cells and mediates inflammation and pain; spares COX-1, which helps maintain the gastric mucosa. Thus, should not have the corrosive effects of other NSAIDs on the GI lining.
Clinical use	Rheumatoid arthritis and osteoarthritis.
Toxicity	Similar to other NSAIDs; may have less toxicity to GI mucosa (i.e., lower incidence of ulcers, bleeding).

An exceedingly common pain complex that may arise from paraspinous muscles, ligaments, facet joints, or disk or nerve roots. Strains refer to muscular injuries, whereas sprains refer to ligamentous injuries.

History/PE

Low back pain is associated with the following manifestations and conditions:

- Paraspinous muscular pain/spasm suggest a back sprain/strain.
- Pain radiating to the posterior thigh and exacerbated by coughing or straining implies a herniated disk with nerve root impingement.
- **Positive straight leg raise** favors nerve **root impingement** most commonly due to a herniated disk (see Table 2.9–1).
- Pain with walking or prolonged standing **(pseudoclaudication)** and hyperextension suggests **spinal stenosis.**
- Pain that worsens with rest and improves with activity is typical of ankylosing spondylitis.
- Pain that worsens at night and is unrelieved by rest or positional changes suggests malignancy.
- Point tenderness over a particular vertebral body suggests vertebral osteomyelitis, fracture, or malignancy.
- **Bowel or bladder dysfunction** and **saddle-area anesthesia** are consistent with **cauda equina syndrome.**

Cauda equina syndrome is a surgical emergency.

Differential

Herniation, strain, sprain, fracture, spondylolisthesis, degenerative arthritis. Rule out infection, cancer, cauda equina syndrome, ankylosing spondylitis, and aortic aneurysm.

Evaluation

Diagnosis is primarily **clinical.** X-rays may reveal evidence of osteomyelitis, cancer (pathologic vertebral fractures, punched-out or sclerotic lesions), frac-

TABLE 2.9–1. Motor and Sensory Deficit in Back Pain

Root	Associated Deficits
L4	Motor: Foot dorsiflexion (tibialis anterior). Reflex: Patellar. Sensory: Medial aspect of the leg.
L5	Motor: Big toe dorsiflexion (extensor hallucis longus). Reflex: None. Sensory: Medial forefoot and lateral aspect of the leg.
S1	Motor: Foot eversion (peroneus longus/brevis). Reflex: Achilles. Sensory: Lateral foot.

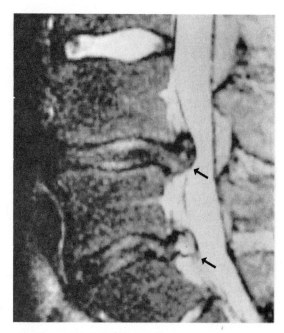

FIGURE 2.9–1. Disk herniation. MRI reveals herniations of L4–L5 and L5–S1 (arrows). (Reproduced, with permission, from Skinner HB, *Current Diagnosis & Treatment in Orthopedics*, 1st ed., Stamford, CT: Appleton & Lange, 1995: p. 186, Fig. 5–10.)

tures, or ankylosing spondylitis. MRI scans as well as electrodiagnostic studies (e.g., nerve conduction velocity testing) are used to evaluate persistent radiculopathy or myelopathy (Figure 2.9–1).

The majority of patients with low back pain recover spontaneously within six weeks.

Treatment

For sprains and strains, **NSAIDs**, physical therapy, and continuation of ordinary activities as tolerated are recommended. **Rest for more than 1–3 days is considered unnecessary.** Ninety percent of patients recover spontaneously within six weeks. Surgery (laminectomy, diskectomy) is indicated for patients with correctable spinal disease. Cauda equina syndrome is a surgical emergency requiring immediate decompression with laminectomy.

UCV *Surg.48*

HERNIATED DISK

A condition in which the nucleus pulposus herniates posteriorly, resulting in nerve root or cord compression with neck/back pain and sensory and motor deficits. Causes include degenerative changes, trauma, or neck/back strain/sprain. Disk herniations occur most frequently in middle-aged and older men and often follow strenuous activity. Herniation is most common in the lumbar region.

History/PE

Severe low back pain made worse by straining and coughing and characterized by **sciatica** (pain radiating down the leg in an L4–S3 distribution). Associated symptoms include tingling or numbness in a lower extremity, muscle weakness, atrophy, contractions, or spasms. **Passive straight leg** lifts increase pain. Large midline herniation may result in **cauda equina syndrome** with urinary and/or bowel incontinence and sensory/motor deficits in the lower extremities.

Evaluation

MRI is used to show disk herniation.

Treatment

Bed rest, NSAIDs, physical therapy, and local heat lead to resolution within 2–3 weeks in the majority of patients. Patients with persistent or disabling symptoms may require surgical removal of the disk.

SPINAL STENOSIS

A narrowing of the lumbar or cervical spinal canal that may cause compression of the nerve roots, most commonly due to degenerative joint disease. It is seen primarily in middle-aged or elderly people.

History/PE

Patients may complain of neck pain, back pain that radiates to the buttocks and legs, or leg numbness and weakness. Leg cramping may occur at rest **and** with walking **(pseudoclaudication).**

Evaluation

X-ray of the spine shows degenerative changes and a narrowed spinal canal. MRI or CT shows spinal stenosis.

Treatment

Mild to moderate cases may be treated conservatively with NSAIDs and abdominal muscle strengthening. Epidural steroid injections can provide relief in advanced cases. When these measures fail, surgical laminectomy can be used to achieve significant short-term success, although many patients will have a recurrence of symptoms.

CARPAL TUNNEL SYNDROME

Results from compression of the median nerve at the wrist. It is most commonly seen in women aged 30–55. Risk factors include pregnancy, rheumatoid arthritis, diabetes, acromegaly, hypothyroidism, obesity, and work-related or athletic activity requiring repetitive movements of the wrist.

History/PE

Presents with wrist pain that may radiate up the arm and is exacerbated by activities that involve flexion of the hand, as well as difficulty holding a cup or opening a jar. Examination reveals weak grip and decreased thumb opposition together with numbness and tingling in the thumb and in the first and middle digits. Diminished two-point sensation in all but the radial aspect of the palm (innervated by a branch that does not pass through the tunnel) is also seen. Thenar muscle atrophy may occur in severe cases.

Evaluation

Tapping on the palmaris longus tendon at the wrist over the median nerve elicits a tingling sensation radiating into the thumb and fingers (Tinel's sign). In Phalen's sign, the dorsal aspects of the hands are placed together with the wrists flexed at 90°; the onset of symptoms within one minute supports the diagnosis. Electromyography and nerve conduction studies are used to evaluate the degree of neural and motor compromise.

Treatment

Treat with wrist splints, modification of behaviors involving repetitive wrist motions, and NSAIDs to reduce inflammation. Corticosteroids injected into the carpal space may diminish symptoms. If symptoms persist, surgical diversion of the transverse carpal ligament is indicated.

OSTEOPOROSIS

Obesity is protective against osteoporosis.

A common metabolic bone disease characterized by **osteopenia with normal bone mineralization.** Osteoporosis most often affects **thin, Caucasian, postmenopausal women.** Bone mass peaks at age 30–35 and then progressively declines. **Smoking** and long-term administration of heparin and glucocorticoids are associated with an increased risk of osteoporosis.

History/PE

Commonly asymptomatic. Patients often present with **hip fractures, vertebral compression fractures,** or **distal radius fractures** after minimal trauma. Loss of height may result from progressive thoracic kyphosis secondary to multiple vertebral compression fractures.

Differential

Osteomalacia, hyperparathyroidism, multiple myeloma, metastatic carcinoma (pathologic fracture).

Evaluation

Laboratory tests are all normal in osteoporosis, and radiographic changes are apparent only after significant osteopenia has developed.

Laboratory tests are normal; radiographs show global demineralization after > 30% of bone density is lost. Dual-energy x-ray absorptiometry (DEXA) scanning may show significant osteopenia, most commonly in the vertebral bodies, proximal femur, and distal radius.

Treatment

Prevention is key; **hormone replacement therapy (HRT)** is the most effective means of preventing bone loss in perimenopausal women. **Calcium supplementation with vitamin D** should be taken throughout adulthood to maintain bone density. **Smoking cessation** and weight-bearing exercises help maintain bone density, while **alendronate** and intranasal calcitonin can increase bone density.

Complications

Fractures of the proximal femur, distal radius, and vertebrae.

GOUT

A metabolic condition causing recurrent attacks of **acute monoarticular arthritis.** Gout results from the intra-articular deposition of monosodium urate crystals and is especially common in **men** (90%) and Pacific Islanders. Most patients have hyperuricemia secondary to uric acid underexcretion. Other causes include Lesch–Nyhan syndrome, diuretic use, cyclosporine use, malignancies, and hemoglobinopathies.

History

The patient is typically awakened from sleep with excruciating joint pain.

PE

Gout most commonly affects the **first metatarsophalangeal joint** (podagra), midfoot, knees, ankles, and wrists and spares the hips and shoulders. Joints are erythematous, swollen, and exquisitely tender. Patients with long-standing disease may develop **tophi,** deposits of urate crystals that lead to deformed joints.

Differential

Pseudogout (positively birefringent rhomboid crystals in aspirate; most commonly affects the knee), cellulitis, septic joint, trauma, foreign body synovitis, avascular necrosis, malignancy.

Pseudogout is often less severe than gout.

Evaluation

Joint fluid aspiration may reveal **needle-shaped, negatively birefringent** (yellow when parallel to the condenser) **crystals** (see Clinical Images, p. 16) and an elevated WBC. In many cases, serum uric acid > 7.5, but some patients have normal uric acid levels. Radiographs show no changes in early gout. Characteristic punched-out erosions with overhanging cortical bone ("rat bite") are seen in more advanced gout.

The presence of gout crystals on joint fluid aspiration confirms the diagnosis.

Treatment

Administer IV colchicine, **NSAIDs** (e.g., indomethacin), or steroids for acute attacks. **Allopurinol** and **probenecid** can be given for **maintenance** therapy. Avoid use of thiazide/loop diuretics (worsen hyperuricemia). The most frequent adverse effect of allopurinol is the precipitation of an acute gouty attack.

Allopurinol is contraindicated in acute attacks.

UCV *IM2.52*

A poorly characterized disease with excessive bone turnover. Paget's disease is frequently associated with paramyxovirus infection.

History/PE

Patients with Paget's disease may complain that their hats no longer fit.

The condition is often asymptomatic, although patients may complain of deep bone pain. Bone softening results in tibial bowing, kyphosis, and frequent fractures. It is also associated with an increase in cranial diameter (frontal bossing). Deafness may occur in advanced cases.

Evaluation

Alkaline phosphatase and urinary hydroxyproline are elevated. Serum Ca^{2+} and phosphate are normal. X-rays show a **markedly expanded bony cortex** of increased density, thickened bony trabeculae, and bowing of the long bones (Figure 2.9–2).

Treatment

Treat symptomatic patients with **alendronate.** Calcitonin is used in some cases.

Complications

Fractures, vertebral collapse leading to spinal cord compression, high-output cardiac failure, arthritis, deafness, **osteosarcoma.**

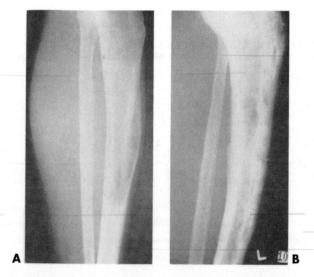

FIGURE 2.9–2. Paget's disease. (A) 45 years old. There are lytic changes in the proximal tibia associated with bulging of the anterior cortex. (B) 65 years old. There is increased cortical density of the tibia in this x-ray taken 20 years later. (Reproduced, with permission, from Way L, *Current Surgical Diagnosis & Treatment*, 10th ed., Stamford, CT: Appleton & Lange, 1994: p. 317, Fig. 6–87A and B.)

A multisystem autoimmune disorder that most frequently affects women (90%), especially **black women.** Its pathogenesis is related to antibody-mediated cellular attack and the deposition of antigen–antibody complexes. Drugs, including hydralazine and procainamide, may produce a lupus-like syndrome that resolves when the drug is discontinued.

History

Fever, anorexia, weight loss, **joint pain, photosensitivity,** and oral ulcers.

PE

Malar rash (see Clinical Image, plate 4), **joint tenderness and inflammation,** pericarditis, pleuritis, and neurologic, renal, and hematologic abnormalities (Figure 2.9–3).

Evaluation

A positive ANA is sensitive but not specific. **Anti-DNA** and **anti-SM antibodies** are very specific but not as sensitive.

Treatment

Treat with **NSAIDs** initially. **Steroids** are used for **acute exacerbations.** Steroids, hydroxychloroquine, cyclophosphamide, and azathioprine are used in progressive or refractory cases. Patients should **avoid sun exposure.**

Complications

Progressive impairment of the lung, heart, brain, or kidneys; opportunistic infections.

UCV *IM2.56*

Criteria for SLE—

4 RASHNIA
4 rashes
 • Malar rash
 • Discoid rash
 • Photosensitivity
 • Oral ulcers
Renal—proteinuria
Arthritis
Serositis
Hematologic—
  hemolytic anemia,
  leukopenia, thrombocytopenia
Neurologic—
  psychosis, seizures
Immunologic—anti-dsDNA, anti-SmAb, false positive VDRL
ANA

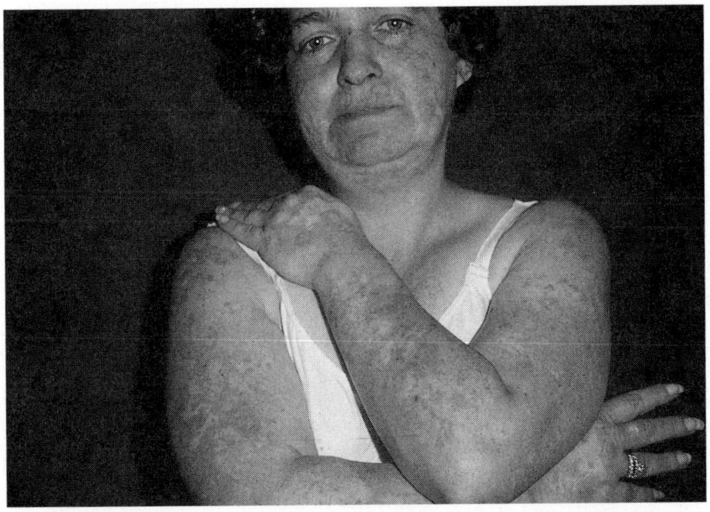

HIGH-YIELD FACTS

Musculoskeletal

FIGURE 2.9–3. SLE. Erythematous patches and plaques of SLE, predominantly in sun-exposed areas. Note the malar rash across the bridge of the nose. (Reproduced, with permission, from Hurwitz RM, *Pathology of the Skin: Atlas of Clinical–Pathological Correlation,* 2nd ed., Stamford, CT: Appleton & Lange, 1998: p. 39, Fig. 2–41A.)

A chronic, destructive, systemic inflammatory arthritis characterized by **symmetric** involvement of both large and small joints. RA causes synovial hypertrophy and pannus formation with resultant erosion of adjacent cartilage, bone, and tendons. It is most common in **females 20–40 years old.** There is a high incidence in patients with the HLA-DR4 serotype.

Distal interphalangeal (DIP) joints are spared in RA.

History

Insidious onset of **morning stiffness, pain, warmth,** boggy swelling, and decreased mobility that affects numerous joints (polyarthropathy) and is associated with fatigue, **malaise,** anorexia, and weight loss.

PE

The most commonly involved joints are the **wrists, metacarpophalangeal (MCP)** and **proximal interphalangeal (PIP) joints,** ankles, knees, shoulders, hips, elbows, and cervical spine. Ulnar deviation of the fingers with MCP joint hypertrophy is a common finding in RA (Figure 2.9–4). Extra-articular manifestations include **subcutaneous nodules,** vasculitis, and carpal tunnel syndrome.

Evaluation

Rheumatoid factor (anti-F$_c$ IgG antibody) is elevated in > 75% of cases but is not specific for RA. ESR is also elevated. Synovial fluid aspiration reveals slightly turbid fluid with decreased viscosity and a WBC count of 3000–50,000. Early in the course of the disease, radiographs show soft tissue swelling and juxta-articular demineralization. Later findings include joint space narrowing and erosions.

Treatment

Treat with **NSAIDs.** Severe cases are treated with corticosteroids, methotrexate, hydroxychloroquine sulfate, gold, and azathioprine. Be aware of the po-

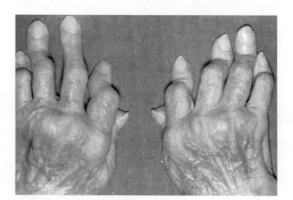

FIGURE 2.9–4. Rheumatoid arthritis. Note the boutonnière deformities of the digits, ulnar deviation of the fingers, MCP joint hypertrophy, and severe involvement of the proximal interphalangeal joints. (Reproduced, with permission, from Chandrasoma D, *Concise Pathology*, 3rd ed., Stamford, CT: Appleton & Lange, 1998: p. 978, Fig. 68–2.)

tential complications associated with NSAIDs, corticosteroids, and other therapies for this disease. Operative therapy may be necessary in advanced cases.

UCV *IM2.55*

JUVENILE RHEUMATOID ARTHRITIS (JRA)

A nonmigratory mono/polyarthropathy that occurs during childhood and lasts for at least three months. In 95% of cases, the disease resolves by puberty. It can be classified into three subtypes: systemic, polyarticular, and pauciarticular.

History/PE

- **Systemic acute febrile:** High fevers, an **evanescent salmon-colored rash,** arthritis, and hepatosplenomegaly.
- **Polyarticular:** Multiple, inflamed, symmetrically involved joints (resembles adult RA). Systemic features are less prominent; patients may develop iridocyclitis.
- **Pauciarticular:** Chronic arthritis frequently involving weight-bearing joints. Up to 30% will develop insidious **iridocyclitis,** which may cause blindness if untreated.
- All three patterns may be accompanied by **fever, nodules, erythematous rashes, pericarditis,** and **fatigue.**

Differential

Trauma, reactive arthritis, septic arthritis.

Evaluation

There is no diagnostic test for JRA. Rheumatoid factor is positive in 15% of cases. A normal ESR does not exclude the diagnosis. Imaging may show soft tissue swelling and regional osteoporosis.

Treatment

Treat with **NSAIDs** or corticosteroids and range-of-motion and **strengthening exercises.** Methotrexate is used as a second-line agent. Monitor for iridocyclitis with routine ophthalmologic examinations.

Complications

Iridocyclitis (most commonly seen in pauciarticular JRA) may lead to blindness if left untreated.

UCV *Ped.55*

POLYMYOSITIS

A progressive, systemic connective tissue disease characterized by muscle inflammation, polymyositis is thought to be an autoimmune disease, but its specific etiology is poorly understood. One-third of patients have **dermatomyosi-**

tis with coexisting cutaneous involvement (a red heliotropic rash over the face, upper extremities, chest, and back). Patients may also develop myocarditis, cardiac conduction deficits, or malignancy. The condition may affect the young (5–15 years) but is most commonly seen in older people (50–70 years). Women are twice as likely to be affected as men.

History/PE

Symmetric, progressive, proximal (shoulder, hips) muscle weakness and pain. Patients classically complain of difficulty rising from a chair. They may eventually have difficulty breathing or swallowing.

Evaluation

Elevated serum creatine, aldolase, and CPK. Electromyography shows fibrillations. Muscle biopsy shows inflammatory cells and muscle degeneration.

Management

High-dose corticosteroids generally result in improved muscle strength in 4–6 weeks and can be tapered to a lower dose for maintenance therapy. If the patient is unresponsive to initial treatment, immunosuppressive medication may be used. Monitor for malignancy.

TEMPORAL ARTERITIS

Always assess for temporal arteritis in patients with PMR.

Generally not seen before age 50, temporal arteritis (or giant cell arteritis) affects twice as many women as men. It is often due to subacute granulomatous inflammation of the external carotid (especially the temporal branch) and vertebral arteries. The most feared complication of temporal arteritis is **blindness** secondary to occlusion of the central retinal artery (a branch of the internal carotid artery). Half of all patients also have polymyalgia rheumatica (PMR).

History/PE

Don't wait for biopsy results before starting high-dose prednisone.

A new headache that is unilateral or bilateral and associated with scalp pain, **temporal tenderness, jaw claudication,** and transient or permanent **monocular blindness.** It is also associated with weight loss, myalgias/arthralgias, and fever.

Evaluation

Obtain **ESR** (> 50, usually > 100), ophthalmologic evaluation, and **temporal artery biopsy.** On biopsy, look for inflammation in the media and adventitia with lymphocytes, plasma cells, and giant cells.

Treatment

Treat immediately with **prednisone** 60 mg daily for 1–2 months before tapering. Since blindness may be permanent, do not wait for biopsy results to initiate treatment. Continue to follow eye exam for improvements or changes.

UCV *Neuro.47*

A rheumatologic disorder most commonly seen in **elderly females.** Polymyalgia rheumatica is considered to be part of the same spectrum of diseases as **temporal arteritis** (same HLA haplotypes), and the two frequently coexist.

PMR is rarely seen in patients < 55.

History

Pain and stiffness of the shoulder and pelvic girdle area, often associated with **fever,** malaise, weight loss, and minimal joint swelling. Patients classically have great difficulty getting out of a chair or lifting their arms above their heads.

PE

Although patients often complain of leg and shoulder weakness, weakness is not appreciated on physical exam.

Evaluation

Evaluation is primarily clinical. **Anemia** and markedly **elevated ESR** are almost always present.

Treatment

Low-dose prednisone (5–20 mg/day) works in almost all cases.

FIBROMYALGIA

A common connective tissue disorder characterized by myalgias and weakness in the absence of signs of inflammation. The etiology is unknown. Associated conditions include depression, anxiety, and irritable bowel syndrome. It is most common in women aged 20–50 years.

History/PE

Multiple (at least 11 of 18) diffuse tender areas and standard "trigger areas" that, when palpated, reproduce the pain. Body aches, fatigue, and sleep disorders may also be present.

Evaluation

A diagnosis of exclusion. The presence of fewer than 11 of 18 tender points or specific regional tender points is known as myofascial pain syndrome.

Treatment

Treat with supportive measures such as stretching and application of heat to painful areas. Hydrotherapy as well as a transcutaneous electrical nerve stimulation (TENS) unit can also provide relief of symptoms. Reassurance about the benign nature of the disease, patient education, stress reduction, psychotherapy, and low-dose antidepressants may also help.

HIGH-YIELD FACTS

Musculoskeletal

251

DUCHENNE MUSCULAR DYSTROPHY (DMD)

An **X-linked disorder** that results from a deficiency of **dystrophin** (Becker muscular dystrophy results from abnormal-sized dystrophin), a subsarcolemmal cytoskeletal protein. DMD is the most common and most lethal muscular dystrophy. Its usual onset is between 2 and 6 years of age, and death occurs by age 20 secondary to respiratory complications.

History

Progressive **clumsiness, fatigability,** difficulty standing or walking, difficulty walking on toes (due to calf muscle shortening), and waddling gait. **Gowers' maneuver**—pushing off with the hands when rising from the floor—indicates proximal muscle weakness. Patients are usually wheelchair-bound by age 13.

PE

Pseudohypertrophy of the calf muscles and possibly mental retardation. DMD affects the axial and proximal muscles before the distal muscles.

Differential

Other muscular dystrophies (facioscapulohumeral, limb-girdle, myotonic, Becker), myasthenia gravis, metabolic myopathies.

Evaluation

CK is consistently elevated. EMG shows polyphasic potentials and increased recruitment. **Muscle biopsy** shows degeneration and variation in fiber size with fibrosis and basophilic fibers. Immunostaining for dystrophin expression (absent) is diagnostic. DNA analysis may reveal the dystrophin mutation (but does not rule out Becker dystrophy).

Treatment

Institute **physical therapy** to maintain ambulation and prevent contractures. Perform Achilles tendon release as necessary.

UCV *Ped.49*

ANKYLOSING SPONDYLITIS

A chronic inflammatory disease of the spine and pelvis that eventually causes fusion of the affected joints. Age of onset is typically between 20 and 40 years. It is strongly associated with HLA-B27. Risk factors include a positive family history and male gender.

History/PE

Intermittent hip or lower back pain typically worsens with inactivity and early in the morning, improving over the course of the day. Limited low back motion, hip pain and stiffness, and limited chest expansion may be present. Kyphosis occurs with pain that is eased by bending forward; the patient may chronically stoop.

Evaluation

HLA-B27 testing. Spine and pelvic x-rays may show characteristic findings (fused **"bamboo spine"** and fusion of the sacroiliac joints) late in the course of the disease. ESR may be elevated; RF and ANA are both negative.

Treatment

The goal of treatment is to minimize joint pain with NSAIDs and to maximize exercises to improve posture and breathing.

OSTEOARTHRITIS (OA)

A chronic, noninflammatory arthritis of movable joints that is also known as degenerative joint disease (DJD). OA has **no systemic manifestations** and is characterized by deterioration of the articular cartilage and osteophyte formation at joint surfaces. Risk factors for OA include family history, **obesity,** and previous joint trauma (particularly previous intra-articular fractures).

History

Joint pain, crepitus, decreased range of motion of the affected joint, insidious onset of joint stiffness and pain that is **worsened by activity and weight bearing and relieved by rest.**

OA typically has an asymmetric pattern.

PE

OA most commonly involves the **weight-bearing joints** (hip, knee, and lumbar spine) but may also involve the **DIP** joints (Heberden's nodes), PIP joints **(Bouchard's nodes),** metatarsophalangeal joint of the big toe, and cervical spine. Physical examination usually reveals stiffness and marked **crepitus** of the affected joint.

> **Nodes in OA—**
> **"HO DIP and BO PIP"**
> **H**eberden's nodes = **DIP**
> **B**ouchard's nodes = **PIP**

Evaluation

Laboratory values are normal. Radiographs show irregular <u>joint space narrowing,</u> osteophytes, and dense subchondral bone. ESR is normal. Synovial fluid aspiration reveals <u>straw-colored,</u> normal-viscosity fluid with a WBC count < 3000.

The ESR is normal in osteoarthritis.

Treatment

Treat mild cases with **physical therapy, weight reduction,** and **NSAIDs.** Intra-articular corticosteroid injection may also provide temporary relief of symptoms. **Elective joint replacement** (e.g., total hip/knee arthroplasty) may be necessary when symptoms significantly interfere with activities of daily living.

UCV *Surg.44*

Table 2.9–2 summarizes the major adult orthopedic injuries.

TABLE 2.9–2. Common Adult Orthopedic Injuries

Injury	Mechanics	Treatment
Shoulder dislocation Surg.47	Most commonly anteriorly dislocated. Axillary artery and nerve are at risk for injury. Posterior shoulder dislocations are associated with seizures and electrical shocks.	Closed reduction followed by sling and swathe.
Hip dislocation Surg.42	Most commonly posteriorly dislocated via a posteriorly directed force on **internally rotated, flexed,** adducted hip ("dashboard injury").	Closed reduction followed by abduction pillow/bracing.
Colles' fracture Surg.49	**Most common wrist fracture.** Involves the distal radius and commonly results from a **fall onto an outstretched hand,** resulting in a dorsally displaced, dorsally angulated fracture. Commonly seen in the **elderly** (osteoporosis) as well as in children.	Closed reduction followed by application of long arm cast.
Scaphoid (carpal navicular) fracture	**Most commonly fractured** carpal bone. May take 1–2 weeks for radiographs to show the fracture; thus, a high index of suspicion is necessary. Assume there is a fracture if there is **tenderness in the anatomical snuff box.**	Thumb spica cast. With proximal third scaphoid fractures, **avascular necrosis** may result from disruption of blood flow (vessel enters at the distal portion of the bone).
Boxer's fracture	Fracture of the fifth metacarpal neck. Often results from forward trauma of **closed fist** (e.g., punching a wall, an individual's jaw, or another fixed object).	Closed reduction and ulnar gutter splint. Percutaneous pinning if fracture angulation is excessive. If skin is broken, assume infection by human oral pathogens **("fight bite"),** and treat with surgical irrigation, debridement, and IV antibiotics.
Humerus fracture	Direct trauma, radial nerve at risk (travels in spiral groove of the humerus). Signs of radial nerve palsy include wrist drop and loss of thumb abduction (see Figure 2.9–5).	Hanging arm cast vs. coaptation splint and sling. Functional bracing.
Monteggia's fracture	Dislocation of the radial head with diaphyseal fracture of the ulna. Also known as **"nightstick fracture"** (self-defense with arm against a blunt instrument).	Closed reduction of the radial head and open reduction/internal fixation (ORIF) of the ulna.

TABLE 2.9–2 (continued). Common Adult Orthopedic Injuries

Injury	Mechanics	Treatment
Galeazzi's fracture	Dislocation of the distal radioulnar joint with fracture of the diaphysis of the radius.	ORIF of the radius with casting of the forearm in supination to reduce the distal radioulnar joint.
Hip fracture *Surg.43*	Falls, common in **osteoporotic women.** Patients are **at risk for subsequent DVT.** Patients present with the affected leg **shortened** and **externally rotated.** Displaced femoral neck fractures are associated with a high risk of avascular necrosis and fracture nonunion.	ORIF with parallel pinning of the femoral neck. Displaced fractures in elderly patients (> 80 years old) may require hemiarthroplasty. **Anticoagulate** to prevent DVT.
Femur fracture	Direct trauma (motor vehicle accident). Beware of fat emboli syndrome (presents with fever, scleral petechiae, confusion, dyspnea, and hypoxia).	Intramedullary nailing of the femur. Open fractures also require thorough irrigation and debridement.
Tibial fracture	Direct trauma (car + pedestrian bumper injury).	Casting vs. intramedullary nailing. Be aware of **compartment syndrome** (swelling in a confined space causes pain on passive extension of the toes, sensory/motor deficits, etc.).
Ankle fracture	Supination/external rotation injury resulting in fractures of medial and lateral malleoli (see Figure 2.9–6).	ORIF.

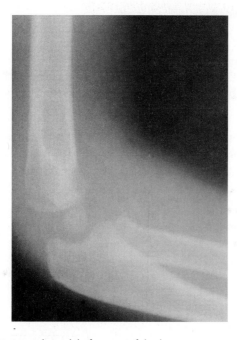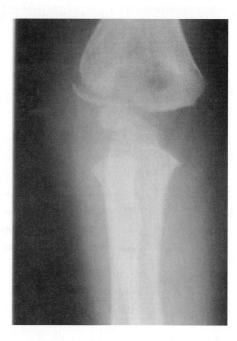

FIGURE 2.9–5. Lateral condyle fracture of the humerus. (Reproduced, with permission, from Skinner HB, *Current Diagnosis & Treatment in Orthopedics,* 2nd ed., Stamford, CT: Appleton & Lange, 2000: p. 572, Fig. 11–45.)

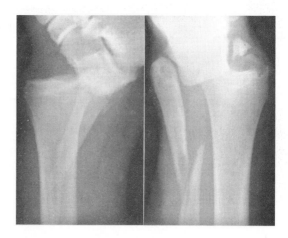

FIGURE 2.9–6. Fracture–dislocation of the ankle. (Reproduced, with permission, from Saunders CE, *Current Emergency Diagnosis & Treatment,* 4th ed., Stamford, CT: Appleton & Lange, 1992: p. 348, Fig. 22–26.)

Table 2.9–3 describes common pediatric orthopedic injuries.

TABLE 2.9–3. Orthopedic Injuries in Children

Fracture	Characteristics	Treatment
Clavicular fracture	The most frequently fractured long bone in children. Often occurs during athletic activity. May be birth related (especially in large infants) and can be associated with brachial nerve palsies. Fractures usually involve the **middle third of the clavicle,** with the proximal fracture end displaced superiorly due to pull of the sterno-cleidomastoid muscle.	Figure-of-eight sling vs. arm sling.
Greenstick fracture	Incomplete fracture involving the cortex of only one side of a bone.	Reduction with casting. Films should be obtained at 7–10 days to assess for adequate reduction.
Nursemaid's elbow	Radial head subluxation. Typically occurs as a result of being **pulled or lifted by the hand.** The child complains of pain and **will not bend the elbow.**	**Manual reduction by gentle supination of the elbow at 90° of flexion.** No immobilization is necessary.
Torus fracture	Buckling of the cortex of a long bone secondary to trauma. Usually occurs in the distal radius or ulna.	Cast immobilization for 3–5 weeks.
Supracondylar humeral fracture	Tends to occur between the ages of 5 and 8. Dangerous because of proximity to **brachial artery.**	Closed reduction with percutaneous pinning. Beware of **Volkmann's ischemic contracture** (compartment syndrome of the forearm).

A spectrum of conditions characterized by varying displacement of the proximal femur from the acetabulum. Congenital hip dislocations are seen more often in **females, firstborn children,** and **breech presentations.** The hip may be subluxed, dislocatable, or dislocated. Dislocations typically result from poor development of the acetabulum and hip due to **excessive uterine packing** (e.g., breech presentation), which causes excessive stretching of the posterior hip capsule and adductor muscle contracture. The deformity will progress if it is not corrected.

History/PE

- **Barlow's maneuver:** Pressure is placed on the inner aspect of the thigh while the hip is abducted, causing posterior dislocation.

Perform Ortolani's and Barlow's maneuvers on all newborns.

HIGH-YIELD FACTS

Musculoskeletal

257

- **Ortolani's maneuver:** The thighs are gently abducted from the midline with anterior pressure on the greater trochanter. The greater trochanter is displaced anteriorly and produces a **soft click.**
- **Allis' (Galeazzi's) sign:** The knees are at unequal heights when the hips and knees are flexed (the dislocated side is lower).
- **Trendelenburg's sign:** A dip of the pelvis to the opposite side when the patient stands on the affected leg. With bilateral involvement, the patient may have a waddling gait.

Additional signs include asymmetric skin folds and limited abduction of the affected hip secondary to adductor contracture.

Evaluation

Evaluation is clinical, although ultrasound may help. X-rays are unreliable until the patient is at least 4 months old.

Treatment

Splint with a **Pavlik harness** (maintains hip flexed and abducted) within the first four months of life. Delayed treatment is possible before 2 years of age by closed or open reduction of the hip, but the benefits of treatment diminish with time.

Complications

Joint contractures, dysplasia of the femoral head and acetabulum.

UCV *Ped.51*

SLIPPED CAPITAL FEMORAL EPIPHYSIS (SCFE)

Separation of the proximal femoral epiphysis through the growth plate such that the femoral head is displaced medially and posteriorly to the femoral neck. SCFE occurs most commonly in **adolescent** (11- to 13-year-old), **obese African-American males.** Its etiology is not known. The condition is bilateral in about 30% of cases.

History

Thigh or **knee pain** and a **limp.**

PE

Limitation of internal rotation and abduction of the hip along with hip tenderness. Flexion of the hip leads to an **obligatory external rotation** secondary to physical displacement.

Evaluation

Radiographs of both hips in anteroposterior and frog-leg lateral views show **posterior and medial displacement** of the femoral head (Figure 2.9–7).

Treat congenital hip dislocation early for the best results.

Patients may complain of knee and thigh pain instead of hip pain.

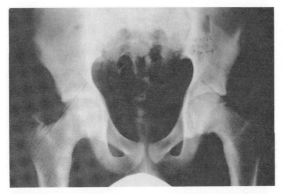

A

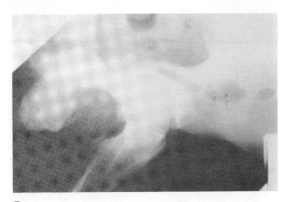

B

FIGURE 2.9–7. Slipped capital femoral epiphysis. (A) Anteroposterior x-ray. The medial displacement of the left femoral epiphysis is best seen with a line drawn up the lateral femoral neck. The abnormal epiphysis does not protrude beyond this line. (B) Frog-leg lateral x-ray. Posterior displacement of the femoral epiphysis is characteristic. (Reproduced, with permission, from Skinner HB, *Current Diagnosis & Treatment in Orthopedics,* 2nd ed., Stamford, CT: Appleton & Lange, 2000: p. 546, Fig. 11–13A and B.)

Treatment

- Patients should not bear any weight on the affected limb until the slip is surgically stabilized.
- Prompt **surgical treatment** is warranted with fixing of the slip into the correct anatomic position (in situ screw fixation).
- **Gentle closed reduction** is warranted only in acute slips.
- Avascular necrosis results in 30% of uncorrected cases.
- Patients are at risk of developing premature degenerative arthritis.

OSTEOSARCOMA

The most common primary malignant tumor of bone. Osteosarcoma tends to occur in the distal femur, proximal tibia, and proximal humerus and metastasizes to the lungs. It is usually diagnosed during adolescence, with boys more commonly affected than girls.

History/PE

Patients generally present with bony pain; later, a mass near a major joint may be detected.

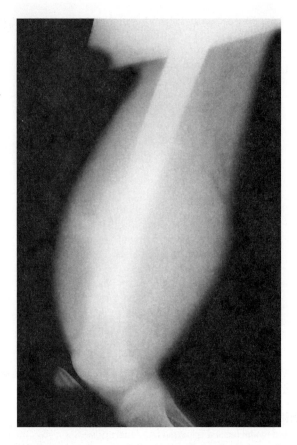

FIGURE 2.9–8. Osteosarcoma. "Sunburst" appearance of neoplastic bone formation in the femur of a 15-year-old girl. Amputation was required owing to the size of the tumor. (Reproduced, with permission, from Skinner HB, *Current Diagnosis & Treatment in Orthopedics*, 2nd ed., Stamford, CT: Appleton & Lange, 2000: p. 272, Fig. 6–26.)

Evaluation

X-ray may show a classic "sunburst" pattern of neoplastic bone (see Figure 2.9–8) or Codman's triangle (periosteal new bone formation at the diaphyseal end of the lesion). MRI should be conducted to determine the extent of the tumor and to plan for surgery.

Treatment

Treat with limb-sparing surgical removal followed by adjuvant chemotherapy (e.g., methotrexate, doxorubicin, cisplatin, ifosfamide) and amputation for large tumors. The five-year prognosis is 60%.

UCV *Surg.45*

Joints in the hand affected in rheumatoid arthritis.	MCP and PIP; DIP joints are spared
Joint pain and stiffness that worsen over the course of the day and are relieved by rest.	Osteoarthritis
Hip and back pain along with stiffness that improves with activity over the course of the day and worsens at rest.	Ankylosing spondylitis
Sudden-onset, excruciating monoarticular joint pain. Needle-shaped negatively birefringent crystals are seen on joint fluid aspirate.	Gout
Recurrent attacks of monoarticular pain; rhomboid-shaped positively birefringent crystals on joint fluid aspirate.	Pseudogout
Patient complains of bony pain; he mentions that his favorite hat no longer fits.	Paget's disease with frontal bossing
Elderly female patient presents with pain and stiffness of shoulders and hips; she cannot lift her arms above her head. Labs show anemia and elevated ESR.	Polymyalgia rheumatica
Bone fractured in fall on outstretched hand.	Distal radius (Colles' fracture)
Complication of scaphoid fracture.	Avascular necrosis
Signs suggesting radial nerve damage with humeral fracture.	Wrist drop, loss of thumb abduction
Patient presents with proximal muscle weakness, waddling gait, and pronounced calf muscles.	Duchenne muscular dystrophy
Radiographic evaluation for slipped capital femoral head.	Anteroposterior and frog-leg lateral view
Most common primary malignant tumor of bone.	Osteosarcoma *[handwritten: M/c primary bone tumor → Multiple myelomas]*
Imaging modality used to diagnose herniated disk.	MRI
Diffuse myalgias in stereotypical "trigger areas."	Fibromyalgia
Symmetric progressive proximal weakness and pain. Muscle biopsy shows inflammation and degeneration.	Polymyositis

HIGH-YIELD FACTS

Musculoskeletal

The following clinical questions and accompanying answers are reproduced, with permission, from Reteguiz J, *PreTest: Physical Diagnosis*, 4th ed., New York, McGraw-Hill, 2001.

Questions

For each patient in questions 1 and 2, choose among the following:
   a. Dermatomyositis
   b. Polymyositis
   c. Polymyalgia rheumatica
   d. Felty syndrome
   e. Scleroderma

1. A 75-year-old woman presents with malaise and myalgias for the last several months. She is chronically tired and has one hour of morning stiffness in the cervical, shoulder, and hip areas. She often has a low-grade temperature and has lost approximately 8 lb during this period. Neurologic exam reveals normal sensation, strength, and reflexes. **(CHOOSE ONE DIAGNOSIS)**

2. A 53-year-old woman presents with a two-month history of difficulty climbing stairs and rising from the seated position. On physical examination, she has a purplish discoloration of the skin over the forehead, eyelids, and cheeks. She has tenderness of the quadriceps muscles on palpation. **(CHOOSE ONE DIAGNOSIS)**

3. A 7-year-old boy presents with a one-year history of pain of the left anterior thigh. He has no history of trauma. On physical examination, he has limited hip motion, especially with abduction and internal rotation. A slight limp is noticeable with ambulation. Pain is brought on by activity and improves with rest. Which of the following is the most likely diagnosis?
   a. Legg–Calvé–Perthes disease
   b. Osgood–Schlatter's disease
   c. Muscular dystrophy
   d. Rickets
   e. Juvenile rheumatoid arthritis

4. An 81-year-old woman has recurrent back pain in her lumbar area. The pain radiates to her buttocks but is worse on the right side than the left side. Both sitting and walking aggravate the pain. She denies bladder dysfunction. On physical examination, the patient has diminished sensation and decreased reflexes of the right lower limb. Straight-leg raising and cross-leg raising tests are positive for reproduction of right lower limb symptoms. The patient has no spinal deformities. Which of the following is the most likely diagnosis?
   a. Sciatica
   b. Osteomyelitis
   c. Cauda equina syndrome
   d. Kyphosis
   e. Epidural abscess

Answers

1–2. The answers are 1-c, 2-a. Polymyalgia rheumatica affects older patients. They present with weight loss, profound fatigue, and pain and stiffness of the neck, shoulders, thighs, and hips. Physical examination is typically normal. **Temporal arteritis** may be seen in patients with polymyalgia rheumatica and must always be ruled out. **Dermatomyositis** is an autoimmune disease that causes proximal muscle weakness that involves the skin; **polymyositis** spares the skin. Patients with rheumatoid arthritis who develop splenomegaly and neutropenia are said to have **Felty syndrome.**

3. The answer is a. Legg–Calvé–Perthes disease (osteochondrosis) is an uncommon disorder that affects boys more than girls between the ages of 2 and 12. The hallmark is avascular necrosis of the capital femoral epiphysis, which has the potential to regenerate new bone. Consequently, children with Legg–Calvé–Perthes disease are of short stature and present with a "painless limp." **Osgood–Schlatter's disease** occurs in adolescence and is usually self-limiting. It is due to patellar tendon stress, which causes pain in the region of the tibial tuberosity especially when the patient extends the knee against resistance. **Rickets** is attributed to vitamin D deficiency and is manifested by bowing of the long bones, enlargement of the epiphyses of the long bones, delayed closure of the fontanelles, and enlargement of the costochondral junctions of the ribs (rachitic rosary). **Juvenile rheumatoid arthritis** is an inflammatory disorder that begins in childhood and may produce extraarticular symptoms, including iridocyclitis, fever, rash, anemia, and pericarditis. Muscular dystrophy is characterized by progressive weakness and muscle atrophy.

4. The answer is a. The sciatic nerve is located between the ischial tuberosity and the greater trochanter; tenderness over the nerve indicates irritation of the nerve roots forming the nerve. **The most common cause of sciatica is a herniated disk** usually occurring at the L4–L5 or L5–S1 levels. The **straight-leg raising test** is usually positive in sciatic nerve irritation (pain is produced with elevation of < 70° and worsened with dorsiflexion of foot or **Lasègue's sign**). A pulling or tight sensation in the hamstring is not a positive straight-leg raising test. **Cross-leg raising test** (elevation of unaffected leg causes pain in affected leg) may also be positive. Osteomyelitis and epidural abscesses are usually accompanied by systemic symptoms (i.e., fever) and are found in patients who are immunocompromised. The typical presentation for **cauda equina syndrome** is progressive weakness and numbness of the lower extremities bilaterally with urinary retention. There is perineal and perianal sensory loss (**"saddle anesthesia"**) and a lax anal sphincter. The cauda equina syndrome is a true surgical emergency. Kyphosis ("hunchback") is a smooth and rounded backward convexity of the thoracic region.

Neurology

Extraocular muscles and nerves

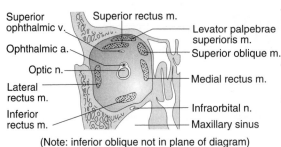

Superior ophthalmic v.
Ophthalmic a.
Optic n.
Lateral rectus m.
Inferior rectus m.
Superior rectus m.
Levator palpebrae superioris m.
Superior oblique m.
Medial rectus m.
Infraorbital n.
Maxillary sinus

(Note: inferior oblique not in plane of diagram)

Lateral **R**ectus is CN VI,
Superior **O**blique is CN IV,
the **R**est are CN III.
The "chemical formula"
$LR_6SO_4R_3$
The superior oblique **a**bducts, **i**ntroverts, **d**epresses.

Visual field defects

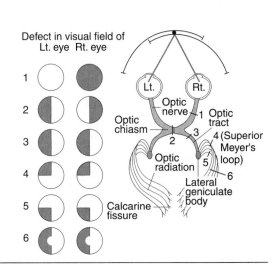

1. Right anopsia
2. Bitemporal hemianopsia
3. Left homonymous hemianopsia
4. Left upper quadrantic anopsia (right temporal lesion)
5. Left lower quadrantic anopsia (right parietal lesion)
6. Left hemianopsia with macular sparing

Defect in visual field of Lt. eye Rt. eye

Optic nerve
Optic chiasm
Optic tract
(Superior Meyer's loop)
Optic radiation
Lateral geniculate body
Calcarine fissure

Circle of Willis

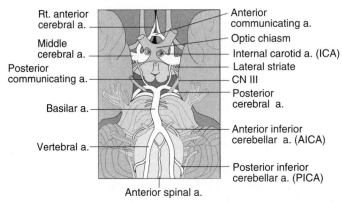

Rt. anterior cerebral a.
Middle cerebral a.
Posterior communicating a.
Basilar a.
Vertebral a.
Anterior spinal a.
Anterior communicating a.
Optic chiasm
Internal carotid a. (ICA)
Lateral striate
CN III
Posterior cerebral a.
Anterior inferior cerebellar a. (AICA)
Posterior inferior cerebellar a. (PICA)

Anterior cerebral artery—supplies medial surface of the brain, leg–foot area of motor and sensory cortices.
Middle cerebral artery—supplies lateral aspect of brain, Broca's and Wernicke's speech areas.
Anterior communicating artery—most common circle of Willis aneurysm; may cause visual field defects.
Posterior communicating artery—common area of aneurysm; causes CN III palsy.
Lateral striate—"arteries of stroke"; supply internal capsule, caudate, putamen, globus pallidus.
In general, stroke of anterior circle → general sensory and motor dysfunction, aphasia;
    stroke of posterior circle → vertigo, ataxia, visual deficits, coma.

Spinal cord and associated tracts

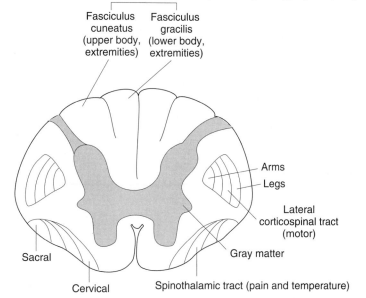

Dorsal columns (pressure, vibration, touch, proprioception)

Fasciculus cuneatus (upper body, extremities)

Fasciculus gracilis (lower body, extremities)

Arms

Legs

Lateral corticospinal tract (motor)

Gray matter

Sacral

Cervical

Spinothalamic tract (pain and temperature)

Spinal cord lesions

Poliomyelitis/Werdnig–Hoffmann disease: lower motor neuron lesions only, flaccid paralysis

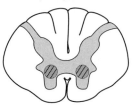

Multiple sclerosis: mostly white matter of cervical region; random and asymmetric lesions

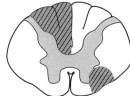

ALS: combined upper and lower motor neuron deficits with no sensory deficit

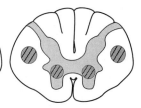

Complete occlusion of ventral artery; spares dorsal columns

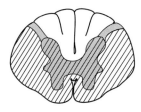

Tabes dorsalis: impaired proprioception and locomotor ataxia resulting from tertiary syphilis

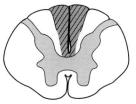

Syringomyelia: ventral white commissure and ventral horns

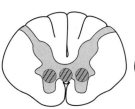

Vitamin B$_{12}$ neuropathy/ Friedreich's ataxia: dorsal columns, lateral corticospinal tracts and spinocerebellar tracts

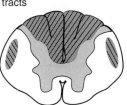

Dorsal column organization

In dorsal columns, lower limbs are inside to avoid crossing the upper limbs on the outside.
Fasciculus gracilis = legs.
Fasciculus cuneatus = arms.

Dorsal column is organized like you are, with hands at sides—arms outside and legs inside.

Epilepsy drugs

	PARTIAL		GENERALIZED			Notes
	Simple	Complex	Tonic–Clonic	Absence	Status	
Phenytoin	✓	✓	✓		✓	Also a Class IB antiarrhythmic
Carbamazepine	✓	✓	✓			Monitor LFTs weekly
Lamotrigine	✓	✓	✓			
Gabapentin	✓	✓	✓			Adjunct in refractory seizures. Renal excretion.
Topiramate	✓	✓				Adjunct use
Phenobarbital			✓			Safer in pregnant women Crigler–Najjar II
Valproate			✓	✓		
Ethosuximide				✓		
Benzodiazepines (diazepam or lorazepam)					✓	

Primary headache is generally classified into three categories: migraine, tension, and cluster.

Approach

- Note whether the headache is new or old. Recent or sudden-onset, severe headaches (such as headaches that awaken the patient in the middle of the night) warrant immediate workup (for SAH, tumor, temporal arteritis, meningitis, etc.). An old headache also requires prompt evaluation if there has been a change in character or intensity.
- Note the **characteristics** of the headache, including its intensity, quality, location, and duration.
- Look for **associated symptoms**—e.g., jaw claudication, fever, nausea, vomiting, weight loss.
- Evaluate **neurologic symptoms**—e.g., paresthesias, numbness, ataxia, visual disturbances, photophobia, neck stiffness. Focal neurologic defects and papilledema warrant immediate workup.
- If an SAH is suspected with a negative head CT, an LP is mandatory.

Recent-onset headaches warrant immediate workup.

Additional Studies

Obtain CBC, ESR, and CT/MRI in patients suspected of having SAH or elevated ICP, or if a patient has **focal neurologic findings.** CT without contrast is the preferred study for an acute hemorrhage.

CT without contrast is the preferred study for an acute hemorrhage.

Differential

- **Acute: SAH,** hemorrhagic stroke, meningitis, seizure, acutely elevated ICP, **hypertensive encephalopathy,** post-LP, ocular disease (glaucoma, iritis), new migraine headache.
- **Subacute: Temporal arteritis,** intracranial **tumor,** subdural hematoma, pseudotumor cerebri, trigeminal/glossopharyngeal neuralgia *(Neuro.52)*, postherpetic neuralgia, hypertension.
- **Chronic/episodic:** Migraine, cluster headache, tension headache *(Neuro.51)*, sinusitis, dental disease, neck pain.

Glioblastoma multiforme is the most common primary brain tumor.

MIGRAINE HEADACHE

Most commonly affects **women** < 30 years of age and those with a **family history.** Its etiology is not fully understood; **vascular abnormalities** due to abnormalities in brain neurotransmitters (serotonin) may be responsible. Migraines are often precipitated by certain foods (e.g., chocolate), fasting, stress, menses, OCPs, and bright light.

History/PE

Throbbing headache that lasts > 2 hours but usually < 24 hours. Headaches are typically associated with **nausea and vomiting, photophobia,** and noise

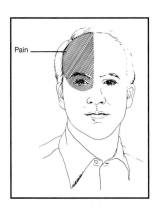

FIGURE 2.10–1. Distribution of pain in migraine headache. Pain is most commonly hemicranial but may be holocephalic, bifrontal, or unilateral frontal. (Reproduced, with permission, from Aminoff MJ, *Clinical Neurology*, 3rd ed., Stamford, CT: Appleton & Lange, 1996: p. 91, Fig. 3–13.)

sensitivity. **Classic migraines** are commonly **unilateral,** associated with **aura,** and preceded by **visual symptoms** such as scintillating lights, scotomas, and field defects. Migraines more commonly present without these associated symptoms and may be bilateral and periorbital.

Evaluation

Consider CT or MRI on first presentation, especially if there are focal neurologic findings (migraine itself can be associated with transient focal neurologic deficits). Rule out meningitis or SAH with an LP if symptoms are acute in onset.

Treatment

Avoid known triggers. **Abortive therapy** includes aspirin/NSAIDs, sumatriptan (a $5HT_1$ agonist), ergots (partial $5HT_1$ agonists), isometheptene, and opiates. **Prophylaxis** for patients with frequent/severe migraines includes beta-blockers (propranolol), ergots, tricyclic antidepressants (amitriptyline), calcium channel blockers, and valproic acid. Narcotics should not be used prophylactically.

UCV *Neuro.28*

TENSION HEADACHE

Tension headaches are chronic headaches that do not share the specific symptomatology of migraine headaches but are thought to have similar pathophysiology and respond to the same treatments. Tension headaches are the **most common type** of headache diagnosed in adults.

History/PE

Patients complain of a **vise-like** or **tight** pain that is exacerbated by noise, bright lights, fatigue, and stress. Patients also report other nonspecific symptoms such as anxiety, poor concentration, and difficulty sleeping. Headaches are generalized but may be most intense in the **occipital and neck region.** Surrounding musculature may also be tightly contracted.

Evaluation

A diagnosis of exclusion; other causes of headache must be considered first. There are no focal neurologic signs in tension headache.

Treatment

Relaxation, massage, hot baths, and avoidance of exacerbating factors may alleviate symptoms. As with migraine, abortive medications (NSAIDs, sumatriptan, ergots) and prophylactic treatment (calcium channel blockers, beta-blockers, tricyclic antidepressants) may be useful.

UCV *Neuro.48*

CLUSTER HEADACHE

Affects **men** more often than women, with an average age of onset of 25.

History

A **brief,** severe, **unilateral periorbital headache** (Figure 2.10–2). Attacks tend to occur in clusters, affecting the same part of the head and taking place at the same time of day (usually at night) and at the same time of the year. Headaches may be precipitated by the use of alcohol or vasodilating drugs.

PE

Ipsilateral tearing of the eye, **conjunctival injection, Horner's syndrome,** and **nasal stuffiness.**

Evaluation

Classic presentations require no evaluation.

Treatment

Institute acute therapy with **high-flow oxygen** (100% nonrebreather oxygen), ergots, or sumatriptan. Prophylactic therapy includes ergots, calcium channel blockers, prednisone, lithium, valproic acid, and topiramate.

UCV *Neuro.6*

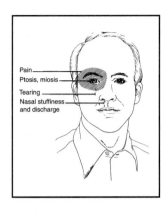

FIGURE 2.10–2. Distribution of pain in cluster headache. Pain is commonly associated with ipsilateral conjunctival injection, tearing, nasal stuffiness, and Horner's syndrome. (Reproduced, with permission, from Aminoff MJ, *Clinical Neurology,* 3rd ed., Stamford, CT: Appleton & Lange, 1996: p. 92, Fig. 3–14.)

SEIZURES/EPILEPSY

Seizures occur when excessive discharge by cortical neurons results in focal and/or general neurologic symptoms. Epilepsy is the predisposition to recurrent, unprovoked seizures. Patients with a first seizure should be evaluated prior to the initiation of treatment. An **aura,** which is a subjective sensation/feeling preceding the onset of a seizure, is experienced by 50–60% of patients with epilepsy. The **EEG is the most important diagnostic test** used in the workup of seizures. Common etiologies of seizures according to age are listed in Table 2.10–1.

Evaluate patients after their first seizure (for mass lesions, etc.) before initiating treatment for epilepsy.

TABLE 2.10–1. Causes of Seizures

Infant	Child (2–10)	Adolescent	Adult (18–35)	Adult (35+)
Perinatal injury	Idiopathic	Idiopathic	Trauma	Trauma
Infection	Infection	Trauma	Alcoholism	Stroke
Metabolic	Trauma	Drug withdrawal	Brain tumor	Metabolic disorder
Congenital	Febrile seizure	AVM		Alcoholism
				Brain tumor

FOCAL (PARTIAL) SEIZURES

Focal (partial) seizures arise from a discrete region in one of the cerebral hemispheres and do **not** lead to loss of consciousness unless they secondarily generalize.

History/PE

Manifestations of focal seizures depend on the region of the cortex that is affected. **Simple partial seizures** may involve motor (e.g., jacksonian march, the progressive jerking of successive body regions), sensory (parietal lobe), or autonomic functions **without alteration of consciousness.** Postictally, there may be a focal neurologic deficit (**Todd's paralysis**) that resolves within 1–2 days.

Complex partial seizures typically involve the **temporal lobe** (70–80%) and are characterized by **impaired level of consciousness,** auditory or visual hallucinations, déjà vu, automatisms (e.g., lip smacking, chewing, or even walking), and **postictal confusion**/disorientation and amnesia. Symptoms may mimic schizophrenia or acute psychosis.

Evaluation

Perform a careful neurologic exam. Rule out systemic causes with CBC, electrolytes, calcium, fasting glucose, LFTs, renal panel, RPR, ESR, and toxicology screen. Perform an **EEG** to look for epileptiform waveforms. A focal seizure implies a focal brain lesion. Rule out a mass by MRI or CT with contrast.

Treatment

Treat the underlying cause if possible. For recurrent partial seizures, phenytoin, carbamazepine, and phenobarbital are first-line anticonvulsants.

UCV *Neuro.41*

GENERALIZED SEIZURES

Generalized seizures involve both cerebral hemispheres and lead to a **sudden loss of consciousness,** usually without aura, followed by a period of **postictal confusion.** The two most common types of generalized seizures are absence (petit mal) and tonic–clonic (grand mal).

TONIC–CLONIC (GRAND MAL) SEIZURES

History/PE

In patients with loss of consciousness, always differentiate between seizure and syncope.

Tonic–clonic (grand mal) seizures begin with loss of consciousness and tonic extension of the back and extremities, followed by 1–2 minutes of repetitive, symmetric clonic movements. **Cyanosis** (secondary to limited respiratory function) and **incontinence** may occur during the seizure. Consciousness slowly returns in the postictal period. Patients may then complain of muscle aches and headache. The serum prolactin level is usually elevated during the

TABLE 2.10–2. Seizure Versus Syncope

	Tonic–Clonic Seizure	**Syncope**
Onset	Sudden onset without prodrome. Focal sensory or motor phenomena. Sensation of fear, smell, memory.	Progressive lightheadedness. Dimming of vision, faintness.
Course	Sudden LOC with tonic–clonic activity. May last 1–2 minutes. May see tongue laceration, head trauma, and bowel/urinary incontinence.	Gradual LOC, limp or with jerking. Rarely lasts longer than 15 seconds. Less commonly injured.
Recovery	Postictal confusion and disorientation.	Typically immediate return to lucidity.

postictal period and can be used to distinguish a seizure from a pseudoseizure. Generalized seizure must be differentiated from syncope (Table 2.10–2). Examine the patient for tongue lacerations, head injuries, and shoulder dislocations (typically posterior).

Treatment

Phenytoin, carbamazepine, or phenobarbital (in children) are first-line agents for recurrent grand mal seizures. Treat any underlying cause.

UCV *Neuro.43*

ABSENCE (PETIT MAL) SEIZURES

Absence (**petit mal**) seizures begin in childhood, subside before adulthood, and are often familial.

History/PE

Brief, often unnoticeable episodes of impaired consciousness lasting only **5–10 seconds** and occurring up to hundreds of times per day. Patients are amnestic during and immediately after seizures. Classically, a teacher may observe a child "daydreaming" or "staring" in class. No loss of muscle tone. Eye fluttering or lip smacking during absence seizures is common.

Children with absence seizures often get into trouble for daydreaming in class.

Evaluation

EEG shows classic **three-per-second spike-and-wave** discharges.

Treatment

Ethosuximide and valproate are first-line agents.

UCV *Neuro.40*

STATUS EPILEPTICUS

Status epilepticus, a medical emergency, consists of prolonged (> 30 minutes) or repetitive seizures without a return to baseline consciousness. Common causes include anticonvulsant withdrawal/noncompliance, anoxic brain injury, **EtOH/sedative withdrawal** or other drug intoxication, **metabolic disturbances** (e.g., hyponatremia), trauma, and infection. Status epilepticus is associated with a 20% mortality rate.

Status epilepticus is a medical emergency associated with a 20% mortality rate.

History/PE

Continuous seizure activity or multiple episodes of seizure activity occurring without return to consciousness.

Evaluation

Determine the underlying cause with pulse oximetry, CBC, electrolytes, calcium, glucose, ABGs, LFTs, BUN/creatinine, ESR, and toxicology screen. Defer EEG and brain imaging until the patient is stabilized. Perform LP in the setting of fever or meningeal signs.

Treatment

Maintain airway, breathing, and circulation **(ABCs).** Consider rapid intubation for airway protection. Administer an IV **benzodiazepine** such as lorazepam or diazepam and a loading dose of **phenytoin.** If seizures continue, intubate and load with phenobarbital. Consider an IV sedative such as midazolam or pentobarbital if seizures continue. Glucose, thiamine, and naloxone may also be given to presumptively treat other potential etiologies.

UCV *EM.34*

STROKE

Acute onset of **focal neurologic deficits** resulting from diminished blood flow **(ischemic stroke)** or hemorrhage **(hemorrhagic stroke).** Nonmodifiable risk factors are age, male gender, genetics, and race. Modifiable risk factors include obesity, diabetes, hypertension, smoking, and atrial fibrillation. The most common etiology is atherosclerosis of the extracranial vessels (internal and common carotids, basilar, and vertebral arteries). **Lacunar infarcts** occur in regions supplied by small perforating vessels and result from atherosclerosis, hypertension, or diabetes.

History/PE

- **Middle cerebral artery (MCA):** Aphasia (dominant hemisphere), neglect (nondominant hemisphere), contralateral hemiparesis, gaze preference, and homonymous hemianopsia (Figure 2.10–3).
- **Anterior cerebral artery:** Leg paresis, amnesia, personality changes, foot drop, gait dysfunction, and cognitive changes.
- **Posterior cerebral artery:** Homonymous hemianopsia, memory deficits, and dyslexia/alexia.
- **Basilar artery:** Coma, cranial nerve palsies, apnea, visual symptoms, drop attacks, and dysphagia.

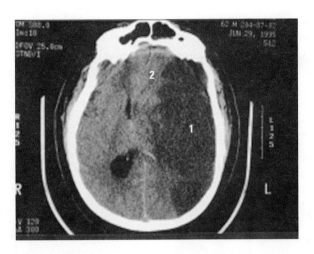

FIGURE 2.10–3. Left MCA stroke. Note the ischemic brain parenchyma (1), subtle midline shift to the right (2), and left lateral ventricles obliterated by edema. There is no visible hemorrhage. (Reproduced, with permission, from Bhushan V, *First Aid for the USMLE Step 1*, 1st ed., Stamford, CT: Appleton & Lange, 2001.)

- **Lacunar stroke:** Pure motor or sensory stroke, dysarthria–clumsy hand syndrome, ataxic hemiparesis.
- **TIA:** Transient neurologic deficit that lasts < 24 hours (although most last < 1 hour). *(EM.34)*.

Differential

Brain tumor, subdural or epidural hematoma, brain abscess, endocarditis, multiple sclerosis, metabolic abnormalities (hypoglycemia), neurosyphilis.

Evaluation

Evaluation should include:

- CT without contrast (to differentiate ischemic from hemorrhagic stroke).
- MRI (to identify early ischemic changes and neoplasms and to adequately image the brainstem/posterior fossa).
- CBC, glucose, coagulation panel, lipid evaluation, ESR, and hemoglobin A_{1c}.
- EKG and an echocardiogram if embolic stroke is suspected (transesophageal echo is most sensitive for mural thrombus).
- **Vascular studies** for extracranial disease (carotid ultrasound, MRA or traditional angiography) and for intracranial disease (transcranial doppler or MRA). See Figure 2.10–4A.
- Screen for hypercoagulable states (if history of bleeding, first stroke, or < 50 years of age).

Rule out hemorrhage before administering heparin.

Treatment

- Antiplatelet agents such as aspirin, clopidogrel, and dipyridamole/aspirin are the mainstays of treatment for ischemic stroke.
- **Heparin** and **coumadin** are used primarily for cardioembolic strokes.
- Maintain vigilance for signs and symptoms of brain swelling, increased ICP, and herniation, which occur in large hemispheric strokes.

Allow BP to rise up to 200/100 to maintain cerebral perfusion.

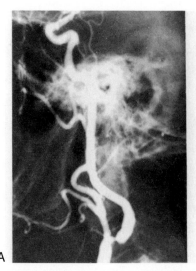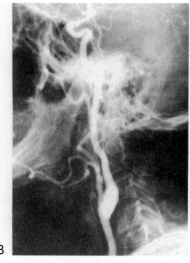

FIGURE 2.10–4. (A) Carotid arteriogram showing stenosis of the proximal internal carotid artery. (B) Postoperative arteriogram with restoration of the normal lumenal size following endarterectomy. (From Way LW, *Current Diagnosis & Treatment*, 10th ed., Stamford, CT: Appleton & Lange, 1994: p. 763, Fig. 35–11.)

- TPA (tissue plasminogen activator) is indicated for ischemic stroke if administered within three hours of onset of symptoms.
- **Neuroprotective agents** are investigational medical interventions.
- **Do not overtreat hypertension** (may diminish cerebral perfusion).
- Treat aspiration pneumonia, UTI, or DVT, the main causes of morbidity and mortality following stroke.

Prevention

Preventive and long-term treatment should consist of the following:

- **Aspirin** or clopidogrel if stroke is secondary to small vessel disease or thrombosis or if anticoagulation is contraindicated.
- **Carotid endarterectomy** if stenosis is > 70% (endarterectomy is contraindicated in vessels that are 100% occluded). See Figure 2.10–4B.
- **Anticoagulation** (heparin initially, then warfarin) in cases of cardiac emboli, new atrial fibrillation, or hypercoagulable states.
- Management of hypertension (including isolated systolic hypertension).
- Treatment of high cholesterol and diabetes.

UCV *Neuro.9, 11, 12, 13, 14*

WERNICKE'S APHASIA

A disorder in the comprehension of language—an expressive (fluent) aphasia. Features are as follows:

Wernicke's is **W**ordy but makes no sense.

- Etiology is usually embolic.
- **Fluent, expressive speech** that is empty of meaning.
- **Comprehension, naming, and repetition of language are impaired;** marked neologisms and paraphasic errors.
- Hemiparesis is mild or absent.
- No dysarthria.
- The patient is often unaware of his deficit.
- The lesion is frequently in the left posterior superior temporal lobe (Sylvian fissure) secondary to a **left inferior MCA** stroke.

Treatment

Institute speech therapy. Patients have a wide range of outcomes, and prognosis is intermediate.

UCV *Neuro.16*

BROCA'S APHASIA

A disorder in the production of language—a nonfluent aphasia. Features are as follows:

- **Speech is nonfluent** with decreased rate and short phrase length, and **impaired speech articulation.**
- **Comprehension is intact.**
- Associated with face and arm hemiparesis, hemisensory loss, and apraxia of oral muscles.
- The patient is often frustrated by the deficit.
- The lesion is frequently in the left superior temporal gyrus in the inferior frontal lobe secondary to a **superior MCA stroke.**

> **B**roca's is
> **B**roken speech.

Treatment

Institute speech therapy. Patients have a wide range of outcomes, and prognosis is intermediate.

UCV *Neuro.10*

SUBARACHNOID HEMORRHAGE (SAH)

Commonly caused by a ruptured aneurysm (e.g., congenital berry), AVM, or trauma to the circle of Willis (often at the MCA). **Berry aneurysms are the most common cause** and are associated with polycystic kidney disease and coarctation of the aorta. SAH typically occurs at 50–60 years of age and has a high mortality rate (35%).

History/PE

A **sudden-onset, intensely painful** headache, often with **neck stiffness** and other signs of meningeal irritation, fever, nausea/vomiting, and a fluctuating level of consciousness. SAH may be heralded by milder **sentinel headaches** in preceding weeks. Seizure may result from blood irritating the cerebral cortex. Third-nerve palsy with pupil involvement is associated with berry aneurysms.

SAH will give the patient "the worst headache of my life."

Differential

Hemorrhagic stroke, trauma, meningitis, migraine headache.

Evaluation

Immediate **head CT** without contrast (Figure 2.10–5) to look for blood in the subarachnoid space (contrast can trigger a seizure if leaks occur beyond the blood-brain barrier). Obtain an immediate **LP if CT is negative** to look for red cells, **xanthochromia** (yellowish CSF due to breakdown of red blood

With a bloody CSF, xanthochromia indicates SAH rather than traumatic LP.

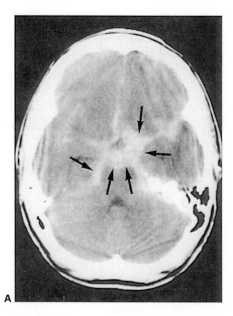
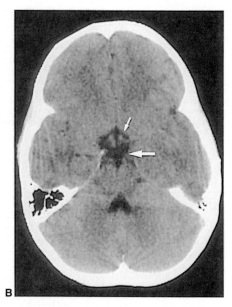

FIGURE 2.10–5. Subarachnoid hemorrhage. (A) CT scan without contrast reveals blood in the subarachnoid space at the base of the brain (arrows). (B) A normal CT scan without contrast shows no density in this region (arrows). (Reproduced, with permission, from Aminoff MJ, *Clinical Neurology,* 3rd ed., Stamford, CT: Appleton & Lange, 1996: p. 78, Fig. 3–6A and B.)

cells), and elevated ICP. Four-vessel angiography should be performed once SAH is confirmed.

Treatment

Focus on **lowering ICP** by raising the head of the bed, administering IV fluids to prevent vasospasm, treating hypertension, and administering calcium channel blockers **(nimodipine)** and antiseizure medications **(phenytoin).** Surgical treatment involves open or interventional radiologic clipping or coiling of an aneurysm or AVM.

Complications

Rebleeding (more common with aneurysm than with AVM), extension into the brain parenchyma (more common with AVM), arterial vasospasm (occurs in one-third of aneurysmal SAHs) and obstructive hydrocephalus.

UCV *Neuro.15*

PARENCHYMAL HEMORRHAGE

A hemorrhage within the brain parenchyma. Etiologies include hypertension, tumor, amyloid angiopathy (seen in the elderly), and vascular malformations (AVMs, cavernous hemangiomas).

History

Lethargy and **headache.**

PE

Focal motor and sensory deficits. Patients may have some degree of obtundation.

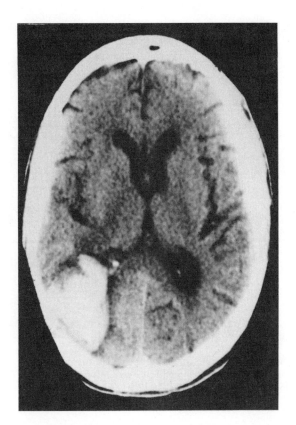

FIGURE 2.10–6. Intracerebral hematoma. Head CT without contrast reveals the irregularly shaped hyperdensity with midline shift of the choroid plexus. (Reproduced, with permission, from Saunders C, *Current Emergency Diagnosis & Treatment,* 4th ed., Stamford, CT: Appleton & Lange, 1992: p. 248, Fig. 16–5.)

Evaluation

Immediate head CT reveals an intraparenchymal hemorrhage (Figure 2.10–6). Look for mass effect or edema that may predict herniation.

Treatment

Treatment is similar to that for SAH: raise the head of the bed and institute antiseizure prophylaxis. Surgical evacuation may be necessary.

EPIDURAL HEMATOMA

A traumatic intracranial hemorrhage of arterial origin that is commonly due to a lateral skull fracture (blunt trauma), with resultant tear of the **middle meningeal artery.**

History/PE

Patients present with a **lucid interval** ranging from several minutes to hours followed by the onset of headache, progressive obtundation, and hemiparesis. Ultimately epidural bleeding may lead to a "blown pupil" (fixed and dilated pupil; usually occurs secondary to uncal herniation).

With an epidural hematoma, mental status changes occur within minutes to hours.

279

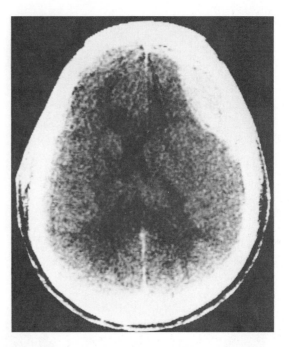

FIGURE 2.10–7. Epidural hematoma. CT scan without contrast reveals a convex, lens-shaped hyperdensity. (Reproduced, with permission, from Saunders C, *Current Emergency Diagnosis & Treatment,* 4th ed., Stamford, CT: Appleton & Lange, 1992: p. 247, Fig. 16–3.)

Evaluation

CT shows a **lens-shaped, convex hyperdensity** that may cross the midline (see Figure 2.10–7). Patients require close observation and serial neurologic examinations before surgery.

Treatment

Emergent neurosurgical evacuation.

UCV *Surg.40*

SUBDURAL HEMATOMA

An intracranial hemorrhage that typically occurs after head trauma with resultant rupture of the **bridging veins** (especially in the **elderly** and **alcoholics**).

History/PE

With a subdural hematoma, mental status changes can occur within days to weeks.

Headache, changes in mental status, contralateral hemiparesis, or other focal changes. In contrast to epidural hematoma, changes can be **subacute** or **chronic** and may present as **dementia,** especially in the elderly. There may be a **remote history of a fall.**

Evaluation

CT demonstrates a **crescent-shaped, concave hyperdensity** that does not cross the midline (see Figure 2.10–8).

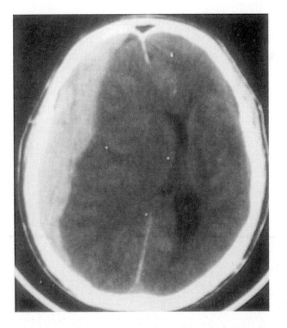

FIGURE 2.10–8. Subdural hematoma. CT scan without contrast reveals a concave, crescent-shaped hyperdensity with compression of the left lateral ventricle and midline shift of the cortex. (Reproduced, with permission, from Aminoff MJ, *Clinical Neurology*, 3rd ed., Stamford, CT: Appleton & Lange, 1996: p. 296, Fig. 11–6A.)

Treatment

Surgical evacuation if symptomatic.

UCV *EM.35*

INTRACRANIAL NEOPLASMS

Brain tumors are very common and are found in approximately 2% of all routine autopsies.

- Primary tumors present most often in early adult or middle life. Symptomatology is due to local growth and resulting mass effect, cerebral edema, **increased ICP,** and ventricular obstruction. Adult tumors tend to be supratentorial, whereas childhood tumors are mainly infratentorial. Primary tumors rarely spread beyond the CNS (see Table 2.10–3).
- Metastatic tumors (more common) are most often from primary **lung,** breast, kidney, and GI tract neoplasms and melanoma. Metastatic tumors most often occur **supratentorially** and are characterized by rapid growth, invasiveness, necrosis, and neovascularization.

History/PE

Symptoms usually develop gradually. Patients often complain of persistent **vomiting and headache** or focal neurologic defects. Other common symptoms are personality changes, lethargy, intellectual decline, **seizures,** and mood swings.

Evaluation

CT with contrast and MRI with gadolinium are used to locate the lesion. Histologic diagnosis may be obtained via CT-guided biopsy or during surgical tu-

Table 2.10–3. Most Common Primary Neoplasms

Tumor	Presentation	Treatment
Astrocytoma *Neuro.2*	Presents with headache and increased ICP May cause unilateral paralysis in 5th–7th and 10th cranial nerves Slow, **protracted course** Prognosis much better than glioblastoma multiforme	Resection if possible Radiation
Glioblastoma multiforme (grade IV astrocytoma) *Neuro.19*	Most common primary brain tumor Often presents with headache and increased ICP Progresses rapidly **Poor prognosis** (<1 year from the time of prognosis)	Surgical removal/resection Radiation and chemotherapy have variable results
Meningioma	Originates from **dura mater or arachnoid** Good prognosis Incidence increases with age	Surgical resection Radiation for unresectable tumors
Acoustic neuroma (schwannoma) *Neuro.32*	Presents with ipsilateral hearing loss, tinnitus, vertigo, and signs of cerebellar dysfunction Derived from **Schwann cells**	Surgical removal
Medulloblastoma *Neuro.24*	**Common in children** Arises from fourth ventricle and leads to increased ICP Highly malignant; may seed subarachnoid space	Surgical resection coupled with radiation and chemotherapy
Ependymoma	Common in children May arise from ependyma of a ventricle (commonly the fourth) or the spinal cord; may lead to hydrocephalus	Surgical resection Radiation

mor debulking. Look for a primary source if metastasis is suspected. LP is rarely indicated owing to possible herniation.

Treatment

Resection (if possible), radiation, and chemotherapy. The type of therapy is highly dependent on the type of tumor and its histology, progression, and site (see Table 2.10–3). Management is often palliative.

A slowly progressive degenerative brain disease that is the **most common cause of dementia**. Age is the most important risk factor. Other risk factors include female gender, family history, Down's syndrome, and low educational level. Pathology includes neurofibrillary tangles, neuritic plaques with amyloid deposition, amyloid angiopathy, and neuronal loss.

History/PE

Memory impairment is usually the first presenting sign, followed by language deficits, acalculia, depression, agitation, and apraxia (inability to perform skilled movements). Death occurs within 5–10 years after the onset of symptoms and is usually secondary to aspiration pneumonia or other infections.

Differential

The two most common causes of dementia are Alzheimer's disease and multi-infarct dementia. Depression may also cause pseudodementia. (For a more complete workup of dementia, see entry in Psychiatry section, page 389.)

Evaluation

AD is a **diagnosis of exclusion.** MRI or CT may show atrophy and can rule out multi-infarct dementia, normal pressure hydrocephalus, subdural hemorrhage, abscess, or tumor. Other tests include CBC, B_{12}, glucose, electrolytes, calcium, TSH, ESR, and RPR. Neuropsychological testing helps distinguish between dementia and depression.

Treatment

Institute supportive therapy. Donepezil or tacrine may temporarily slow disease progression.

UCV *Psych.2*

Parkinson's disease is an idiopathic disorder that occurs in all ethnic groups and usually begins after 50 years of age. Parkinson's is due to **dopamine depletion** in the substantia nigra.

History/PE

Begins with **resting tremor, bradykinesia,** stiffness, and fatigue. Symptoms progress variably to a very typical presentation of sloped posture, **cogwheel rigidity,** shuffling steps, and festinating gait (an unwanted acceleration of gait once commenced). Other common manifestations include masked facies, memory loss, micrographia, and **postural instability.**

The four cardinal features of Parkinson's are resting tremor, bradykinesia, rigidity, and postural instability.

Differential

Patients presenting with the same constellation of symptoms may have one of the **Parkinsonian syndromes,** which include Wilson's disease, **Huntington's disease,** progressive supranuclear palsy (PSP), Shy–Drager syndrome, Creutzfeldt–Jakob disease, **toxin-induced** parkinsonism (manganese dust, CO, cyanide), or **drug-induced** parkinsonism (neuroleptics, metoclopramide). Clues to nonidiopathic Parkinson's are younger age of onset, lack of response to levodopa, and **rapid** progression of disease.

Treatment

Diagnosis is made strictly on a clinical basis. Long-term treatment is directed at dopamine replacement. Medications used are levodopa/carbidopa, dopamine agonists (bromocriptine), amantadine, selegiline, and anticholinergics. SSRIs can be used to treat associated depression. Surgery has had limited success in ameliorating symptoms.

UCV *Neuro.34*

HUNTINGTON'S DISEASE

A rare autosomal-dominant disease involving multiple abnormal triple CAG repeats on **chromosome 4.** The disease is invariably fatal, with death often occurring within 20 years of diagnosis.

History/PE

Huntington's presents in patients 30–50 years of age with a gradual onset of chorea, altered behavior, and **dementia.** Early motor symptoms of rigidity and stiffness give way to prominent **choreiform activity.** Dementia begins as irritability, moodiness, and antisocial behavior. This develops into **schizophreniform illness** and depression.

Differential

Gilles de la Tourette's syndrome, senile chorea, hemiballismus, Wilson's disease, Parkinson's disease.

Evaluation

Diagnosis is made on a clinical basis. CT scan shows cerebral atrophy (especially of the putamen and caudate).

Treatment

There is **no cure,** and progression of the disease cannot be halted. Treatment is targeted directly at ameliorating symptoms. Haloperidol can be used for treatment of psychosis, and reserpine can minimize unwanted movements. **Genetic counseling** should be offered to offspring.

UCV *Neuro.23*

AMYOTROPHIC LATERAL SCLEROSIS (ALS)

A chronic, progressive degenerative disease of unknown etiology characterized by loss of motor neurons within the spinal cord, brainstem, and motor cortex. ALS almost always progresses to respiratory failure and death.

History

Asymmetric, slowly progressive weakness affecting the arms, legs, and cranial nerves. Some patients initially complain of fasciculations.

PE

Upper motor neuron signs (spasticity, increased DTRs, upward-going toes) and/or **lower motor neuron signs** (flaccid paralysis, loss of DTRs, fasciculations, downward-going toes, **tongue fasciculations**).

A combination of upper and lower motor neuron signs in three or more extremities is diagnostic of ALS.

Differential

Spondylitic cervical myopathy, syringomyelia, neoplasms, demyelinating diseases, benign fasciculations, polio, hypothyroidism, hyperparathyroidism, dysproteinemia, lymphoma, heavy metal poisoning, postradiation effects, Guillain–Barré syndrome.

Evaluation

EMG/nerve conduction studies reveal **widespread denervation and fibrillation potentials.** Obtain CT/MRI of the cervical spine to exclude structural lesions. Rule out systemic causes with CBC, TSH, SPEP, UPEP, Ca^{2+}, PTH, urine for heavy metals (if history of exposure), and PFTs. Clinical presentation is most often diagnostic.

Treatment

Supportive measures, patient education, and aggressive pulmonary toilet. Riluzole, which reduces presynaptic glutamate release, may slow disease progression.

UCV *Neuro.1*

MULTIPLE SCLEROSIS (MS)

An acquired demyelinating disease of the CNS that may have a T-cell-mediated **autoimmune pathogenesis** (involving both environmental and genetic components). MS is twice as common in **women** as in men and has a peak incidence at **20–40 years of age.** It is generally a disorder of **temperate climates.** Subtypes are relapsing, remitting, secondary progressive, and primary progressive.

History/PE

Patients present with neurologic complaints that are **separated in time and space** and cannot be explained by a single lesion. The most common present-

The classic triad in MS is scanning speech, intranuclear ophthalmoplegia, and nystagmus.

285

ing complaints include **limb weakness, optic neuritis, paresthesias, diplopia, urinary retention,** and **vertigo.** Neurologic symptoms can wax and wane or be progressive. Exacerbating factors include infection, heat, trauma, pregnancy, and vigorous activity.

Differential

CNS tumors or trauma, vasculitis, vitamin B_{12} deficiency, CNS infections (Lyme disease, neurosyphilis), sarcoidosis.

Evaluation

MRI reveals **multiple, asymmetric, often periventricular lesions** in white matter. Active lesions enhance with gadolinium on MRI. CSF analysis may show **mononuclear pleocytosis** (> 5 cells/µL) in 25% of cases, elevated CSF IgG in 80% of cases, and/or **oligoclonal bands** (nonspecific).

Treatment

Steroids should be given during acute exacerbations. **Prophylactic immunosuppressants or beta-interferon** may decrease the number and severity of relapses.

UCV *Neuro.29*

MYASTHENIA GRAVIS

An autoimmune disease caused by circulating **antibodies that bind to postsynaptic acetylcholine receptors** (as opposed to Lambert–Eaton syndrome, which is characterized by autoantibodies to presynaptic Ca^{2+} channels). Myasthenia gravis occurs at all ages (most often in young adulthood and women) and can be associated with thyrotoxicosis, thymoma, and autoimmune disorders such as rheumatoid arthritis or SLE.

History/PE

Patients most often present with fluctuating fatigable **ptosis** or double vision. Difficulty swallowing and proximal muscle weakness can also be present. **Symptoms typically worsen throughout the day.** Respiratory compromise and aspiration are rare but potentially lethal complications and are termed "myasthenic crisis."

Differential

Neurasthenia, Lambert–Eaton myasthenic syndrome (associated with small cell carcinoma of the lung), **botulism,** tick paralysis, and drug-induced myasthenic syndrome (aminoglycosides).

Evaluation

Diagnosis is often made on a clinical basis. **Edrophonium testing** is diagnostic; in a symptomatic patient, IV injection of the anticholinesterase agent leads to rapid amelioration of clinical symptoms. EMG testing can give additional confirmation. An assay for **level of circulating acetylcholine receptor antibodies** is being increasingly used.

Treatment

- Anticholinesterase drugs such as neostigmine and pyridostigmine are symptomatic therapies.
- Prednisone and other immunosuppressants are the mainstays of treatment.
- In severe cases, **plasmapheresis** or IV immunoglobulin may provide temporary relief (days to weeks).
- Resection of thymoma can be curative.

UCV *Neuro.30*

GUILLAIN-BARRÉ SYNDROME (GBS)

An **acute, acquired demyelinating autoimmune disorder** of the peripheral nerves resulting in weakness. GBS is associated with recent *Campylobacter jejuni* infection, preceding viral infection, and recent vaccination.

History

Rapidly progressive weakness that **begins distally** and progresses proximally to involve the trunk, diaphragm, and cranial nerves **(ascending paralysis).** It is often accompanied by a history of **recent viral infection, diarrhea,** or **immunization.** Autonomic symptoms may be present as well.

PE

Weakness with **areflexia.** Dysesthesias may also be present.

Differential

Myasthenia gravis, multiple sclerosis, chronic inflammatory demyelinating polyneuropathy, ALS, poliomyelitis, porphyria, heavy metal poisoning, botulism, transverse myelitis, diphtheric neuropathy, tick paralysis.

Closely monitor respiratory function in patients with GBS.

Evaluation

Findings include evidence of **diffuse demyelination** on EMG and nerve conduction studies. Diagnosis is supported by a **CSF protein level > 55 mg/dL** with little or no pleocytosis (albuminocytologic dissociation).

Treatment

Plasmapheresis or **IV immunoglobulin** with close monitoring of respiratory function (intubation may be necessary). Most patients will regain premorbid function, but depending on the degree of weakness, it may take up to a year to regain full strength.

UCV *Neuro.20*

MÉNIÈRE'S DISEASE (ENDOLYMPHATIC HYDROPS)

A form of **peripheral vertigo** that results from distention of the endolymphatic compartment of the inner ear. Causes include head trauma and syphilis.

History/PE

Episodic vertigo associated with nausea, vomiting, **ear fullness, hearing loss,** and **tinnitus.** Episodes resolve within hours to days. Significant permanent hearing loss can occur over a period of years.

Differential

Hypothyroidism, aminoglycoside or furosemide toxicity, stroke, trauma, benign paroxysmal positional vertigo, labyrinthitis, acoustic neuroma.

Evaluation

Audiometry shows **low-frequency pure-tone hearing loss** that fluctuates in severity.

Treatment

Treat with a **low-salt diet** and **acetazolamide.** Antihistamines, antiemetics, and benzodiazepines may be given for acute attacks. Surgical decompression may be necessary in refractory cases.

UCV *Neuro.25*

BENIGN PAROXYSMAL POSITIONAL VERTIGO (BPPV)

A common form of **peripheral** (i.e., end-organ) vertigo. BPPV results from a dislodged otolith that causes disturbances in the semicircular canals.

History/PE

Transient, episodic vertigo (lasting less than one minute) and nystagmus with specific head postures (classically **while turning in bed or getting up in the morning**), together with **nausea and vomiting.** Dizziness is usually exacerbated by changes in position. BPPV is also characterized by **habituation** of vertigo/nystagmus (they decrease with repetitive testing). **Recent trauma** is the most common identifiable etiology. Table 2.10–4 summarizes the different signs and symptoms of central and peripheral vertigo.

Differential

Hypothyroidism, aminoglycoside or furosemide toxicity, stroke, trauma, Ménière's syndrome, labyrinthitis, acoustic neuroma.

Evaluation

Peripheral causes of vertigo always produce horizontal nystagmus, whereas vertical nystagmus indicates a central lesion.

Evaluation should include the Nylen–Bárány maneuver, i.e., having the patient go from a sitting to a supine position while quickly turning the head to the side. If vertigo and/or nystagmus is reproduced, BPPV is the likely diagnosis. Other studies can include CT/MRI (with attention to the posterior fossa and temporal bone to rule out cerebellopontine-angle lesions), an audiogram to rule out Ménière's disease, and TSH.

TABLE 2.10–4. Etiologies of Peripheral and Central Dysequilibrium

Peripheral Vestibular Disorders	Acute Central Ataxias	Chronic Central Ataxias
Benign positional vertigo	Drug intoxication (EtOH, benzodiazepines, barbiturates, hallucinogens, anticonvulsants)	Multiple sclerosis
Ménière's disease		Cerebellar degeneration
Acute peripheral vestibulopathy	Wernicke's encephalopathy	Hypothyroidism
Otosclerosis	Vertebrobasilar ischemia	Wilson's disease, CJD
Cerebellopontine-angle tumor	Vertebrobasilar infarction	Posterior fossa masses
Vestibulopathy/acoustic neuropathy	Inflammatory disorders (viral encephalitis, bacterial infections)	Ataxia–telangiectasia
Toxin-induced (EtOH, aminoglycosides, salicylates)	Cerebellar hemorrhage	

Treatment

Treat with **repositioning exercises.** BPPV usually subsides in weeks or months but may recur.

CLOSED-ANGLE GLAUCOMA

This medical emergency occurs most often in older patients and in Asians. The cause is an **acute** closure of a narrow anterior chamber angle (usually unilateral). This type of injury generally occurs with **pupillary dilation** (prolonged time in a darkened area, stress, medications), anterior uveitis, or dislocation of the lens.

History/PE

Patients present with great **pain** and blurred vision. The eye is hard and red, and the pupil is dilated and nonreactive to light. Nausea and vomiting are not uncommon. Intraocular pressure is elevated.

Do not dilate the pupil in suspected closed-angle glaucoma.

Differential

Conjunctivitis, uveitis, corneal trauma, and infectious processes.

Treatment

- **Lower intraocular pressure** with acetazolamide.
- Once pressure drops, use pilocarpine.
- **Laser iridotomy** is curative.

UCV *EM.10*

HIGH-YIELD FACTS

Neurology

OPEN-ANGLE GLAUCOMA

Open-angle glaucoma is the most common form of glaucoma and is almost always bilateral. It occurs most often in individuals > 40 and in those with a **family history. African-Americans,** diabetics, and those with myopia are also at increased risk. In open-angle glaucoma, intraocular pressure becomes elevated secondary to a diseased trabecular meshwork that obstructs proper drainage of the eye. The pressure rises **gradually,** causing progressive vision loss. The eye appears structurally normal. Vision loss begins **peripherally** and moves centrally, ultimately resulting in blindness.

History/PE

Patients are initially asymptomatic. However, glaucoma should be suspected in patients > 35 who need **frequent lens changes** and have mild headaches, visual disturbances, and impaired adaptation to darkness. The earliest visual defect is seen in the peripheral nasal fields. **Cupping** of the optic disk may be seen on funduscopic examination.

Evaluation

Tonometry, ophthalmoscopic visualization of the optic nerve, and central field testing are the most important examinations in evaluating glaucoma. All examinations must be evaluated on a **long-term basis** owing to wide variations in intraocular pressure. Because of its insidious nature, glaucoma can be difficult to diagnose until its advanced stages.

Treatment

Prevention is the most important treatment available. All people over age 40 should visit an ophthalmologist every 3–5 years. Annual examinations are recommended for individuals with increased risk factors. Most cases can be controlled with topical beta-blockers (timolol, betaxolol), which decrease aqueous humor production, or pilocarpine, which increases aqueous outflow. Carbonic anhydrase inhibitors are used when eyedrops do not adequately control intraocular pressure. If medication fails, laser trabeculoplasty can be performed to improve aqueous drainage.

MACULAR DEGENERATION

In the United States, macular degeneration is the leading cause of **permanent, bilateral visual loss** in the elderly. There is a higher incidence of macular degeneration in Caucasians, females, smokers, and those with a family history. Vision loss occurs centrally; patients do not lose their peripheral vision and ability to move around safely.

- **Atrophic macular degeneration:** Causes gradual vision loss.
- **Exudative macular degeneration:** Causes more rapid and severe vision damage.

History/PE

Painless loss of central vision. Funduscopy reveals pigmentary or hemorrhagic disturbance in the macular region.

Treatment

Treatment is greatly limited. **Laser photocoagulation** may delay loss of central vision in exudative macular disease.

RETINAL OCCLUSION

Retinal occlusion can be arterial or venous.

History/PE

- **Central retinal artery occlusion:** Sudden, painless, **unilateral blindness.** The pupil accommodates but is sluggishly reactive to direct light. On funduscopic exam, there may be a **cherry-red spot** on the fovea (see Clinical Images, p. 7), arteries may appear bloodless, and retinal swelling may be present.
- **Central retinal vein occlusion:** Rapid, painless, **vision loss.** Retinal hemorrhage, cotton wool spots, and edema of the fundus may be seen on funduscopic exam. Occurs in **elderly patients** and is often idiopathic. Results in macular disease and glaucoma.

Treatment

- **Central retinal artery occlusion: Thrombolysis** of the ophthalmic artery within eight hours of onset of symptoms. Reduction of intraocular pressure through drainage of the anterior chamber, IV acetazolamide may also improve perfusion of the retina. If treatment is not instituted immediately, retinal infarction and permanent blindness may result.
- **Central retinal vein occlusion:** Laser photocoagulation has variable results.

UCV *Neuro.47*

Unilateral, severe periorbital headache with tearing and conjunctival erythema.	Cluster headache
Prophylactic treatment for migraine.	Includes beta-blockers, calcium channel blockers, TCAs
Most common cause of subarachnoid hemorrhage.	Trauma; second most common is berry aneurysm
Crescent-shaped hyperdensity on CT that does not cross the midline.	Subdural
CSF findings with subarachnoid hemorrhage.	Elevated ICP, red cells, xanthochromia
Most common primary sources of mets to the brain.	Lung, breast, kidney, GI tract
Most frequent presentation of intracranial neoplasm.	Headache
Most common cause of seizures in children (age 2–10 years).	Infection, febrile seizures, trauma, idiopathic
Most common cause of seizures in young adults (18–35 years).	Trauma, alcohol withdrawal, brain tumor
Mainstay of treatment for myasthenia gravis.	Immunosuppressants (e.g., prednisone)
First-line medication for status epilepticus.	IV benzodiazepine
Location of lesion with development of Broca's aphasia.	MCA distribution: left superior temporal gyrus, inferior frontal lobe
What % lesion is an indication for carotid endarterectomy?	70%, if stenosis is symptomatic
Most common causes of dementia.	Alzheimer's and multi-infarct
Patient complains of gradually worsening weakness and spasms in both legs and the right arm.	ALS
Rigidity and stiffness, with resting tremor and masked facies.	Parkinson's disease
Treatment for Guillain–Barré syndrome.	Plasmapheresis or IV Ig
Rigidity and stiffness that progress to choreiform movements, accompanied by moodiness and antisocial behavior.	Huntington's disease
Administer to symptomatic patient to diagnose myasthenia gravis.	Edrophonium

The following clinical questions and accompanying answers are reproduced, with permission, from Elkind MSV, *PreTest: Neurology*, 9th ed., New York: McGraw-Hill, 2001.

Questions

A 73-year-old man with a history of hypertension complains of a ten-minute episode of left-sided weakness and slurred speech. On further questioning, he relates three brief episodes in the last month of sudden impairment of vision affecting the right eye. His examination now is normal.

1. Which of the following would be the most appropriate next diagnostic test?
   a. Creatine phosphokinase (CPK)
   b. Holter monitor
   c. Visual evoked responses
   d. Carotid artery Doppler ultrasound
   e. Conventional cerebral angiography

2. The episodes of visual loss are most likely related to
   a. Retinal vein thrombosis
   b. Central retinal artery ischemia
   c. Posterior cerebral artery ischemia
   d. Middle cerebral artery ischemia
   e. Posterior ciliary artery ischemia

3. A 23-year-old woman complained of two days of visual loss associated with discomfort in the right eye. She appeared otherwise healthy, but her family reported recurrent problems with bladder control over the prior two years, which the patient was reluctant to discuss. On neurologic examination, this young woman exhibited dysmetria in her right arm, a plantar extensor response of the left foot, and slurred speech. The most informative ancillary test would be expected to be
   a. Visual evoked response (VER) testing
   b. Sural nerve biopsy
   c. Electroencephalography (EEG)
   d. Magnetic resonance imaging (MRI)
   e. Computed tomography (CT)

4. For the following clinical scenario, pick the most likely diagnosis.
   a. Hepatolenticular degeneration
   b. Hyperparathyroidism
   c. Central pontine myelinolysis
   d. Akinetic mutism
   e. MPTP poisoning
   f. Locked-in syndrome
   g. Postencephalitic parkinsonism
   h. Neuroleptic effect
   i. Essential tremor
   j. Vegetative state
   k. Hypermagnesemia
   l. Rhombencephalitis

A 19-year-old woman developed auditory hallucinations and persecutory delusions over the course of three days. She was hospitalized and started on haloperidol (Haldol), 2 mg three times daily. Within a week of treatment, she developed stooped posture and a shuffling gait. Her head was slightly tremulous and her movements were generally slowed. Her medication was changed to thioridazine (Mellaril), and trihexyphenidyl (Artane) was added. Over the next two weeks, she became much more animated and reported no recurrence of her hallucinations. (SELECT ONE DIAGNOSIS)

Answers

1. **The answer is d.** This patient is experiencing the classical symptoms of extracranial internal carotid artery disease, which include episodes of ipsilateral transient monocular blindness, or amaurosis fugax, and contralateral transient ischemic attacks consisting of motor weakness. Patients with symptomatic extracranial carotid artery disease have a high likelihood of going on to develop strokes (approximately 26% over two years on medical therapy). The appropriate test to confirm the suspicion of carotid stenosis is a Doppler ultrasound test of the carotid arteries. This test utilizes the fact that sound waves will bounce back from particles moving in the bloodstream, primarily red blood cells, at a different frequency, depending upon the velocity and direction of the blood flow. A great deal of important information about the structure of the blood vessel can be obtained in this way. Although angiography can also provide this information, it is invasive, carries a risk of causing a stroke, and is more expensive.

2. **The answer is b.** The presumed mechanism of transient monocular blindness in carotid artery disease is embolism to the central retinal artery or one of its branches. Although classic teaching has emphasized the role that cholesterol emboli play in causing this blindness, it has been noted that cholesterol emboli (Hollenhorst plaques) may be seen on funduscopic examination even of asymptomatic individuals. Retinal vein thrombosis may produce a rapidly progressive loss of vision, with hemorrhages in the retina, but would not be associated with the transient ischemic attacks (TIAs) described here. Although both posterior and middle cerebral artery ischemia can cause visual loss, they would not be expected to cause the monocular blindness described here. Posterior ciliary artery ischemia can cause ischemic optic neuropathy, but this is usually acute, painless, and not associated with preceding transient monocular blindness or TIAs.

3. **The answer is d.** This young woman almost certainly has MS. Her visual loss can be explained by optic neuritis. Her bladder problems may be from demyelination of corticospinal tract fibers. Many patients are reluctant to discuss minor problems with bladder, bowel, or sexual function with a physician of the opposite sex. The positive Babinski sign, focal dysmetria, and apparent dysarthria all support the diagnosis of a multifocal CNS lesion. Multiple lesions disseminated in time and space are typical of MS. With MRI, the multifocal areas of demyelination should be apparent. Many more lesions may be evident on MRI than are suggested by the physical examination.

4. **The answer is h.** Butyrophenones, the most commonly prescribed of which is haloperidol, routinely produce some signs of parkinsonism if they are used at high doses for more than a few days. This psychotic young woman proved to be less sensitive to the parkinsonian effects of the phenothiazine thioridazine than she was to haloperidol. Adding the anticholinergic trihexyphenidyl may also have helped to reduce the patient's parkinsonism. Another commonly used medication that can cause parkinsonism, in addition to tardive dyskinesia, is metoclopramide hydrochloride (Reglan).

HIGH-YIELD FACTS

Neurology

Obstetrics

Estrogen

Source	Ovary (estradiol), placenta (estriol), blood (aromatization), testes.	Potency: estradiol > estrone > estriol
Function	1. Growth of follicle	Estrogen hormone replacement therapy after menopause: decreased risk of heart disease, decreased hot flashes, and decreased postmenopausal bone loss.
	2. Endometrial proliferation, myometrial excitability	
	3. Genitalia development	
	4. Stromal development of breast	
	5. Fat deposition	
	6. Hepatic synthesis of transport proteins	
	7. Feedback inhibition of FSH	Unopposed estrogen therapy: increased risk of endometrial cancer; use of progesterone with estrogen decreases those risks.
	8. LH surge (estrogen feedback on LH secretion switches to positive from negative just before LH surge)	
	9. Increased myometrial excitability	

Progesterone

Source	Corpus luteum, placenta, adrenal cortex, testes.	Elevation of progesterone is indicative of ovulation.
Function	1. Stimulation of endometrial glandular secretions and spiral artery development	
	2. Maintenance of pregnancy	
	3. Decreased myometrial excitability	
	4. Production of thick cervical mucus, which inhibits sperm entry into the uterus	
	5. Increased body temperature (0.5 degree)	
	6. Inhibition of gonadotropins (LH, FSH)	
	7. Uterine smooth muscle relaxation	

Menstrual cycle

Follicular growth is fastest during second week of proliferative phase.

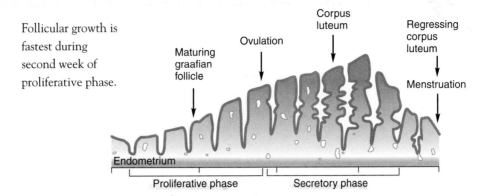

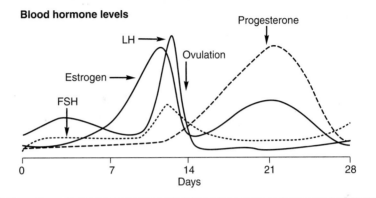

HCG

Source
: Trophoblast of placenta

Function
: 1. Maintains the corpus luteum for the first trimester because it acts like LH but is not susceptible to feedback regulation from estrogen and progesterone.
  In the second and third trimester, the placenta synthesizes its own estrogen and progesterone. As a result, the corpus luteum degenerates.
2. Used to detect pregnancy because it appears in the urine eight days after successful fertilization (blood and urine tests available).
3. Elevated HCG in women with hydatidiform moles or choriocarcinoma.

Nägele's rule:

due date = LMP + 7 days

– 3 months.

Prenatal care is critical to the delivery of a healthy baby. The due date can be estimated using Nägele's rule: LMP + 7 days – 3 months + 1 year. The pregnant patient's prenatal labs should be scheduled as described in Table 2.11–1.

Recommended weight gain is **25–35 lbs** for women of average pre-pregnancy weight (more for underweight women, less for heavier women), with only 1–2 lbs gained during the first trimester and 0.75–1 lb per week for the duration of the pregnancy. Average-weight women will require a **daily caloric intake of about 2500 kcal,** or an increase of about 300 kcal per day.

TABLE 2.11–1. Standard Prenatal Labs and Studies

Gestation	Labs to Be Obtained
Initial visit	CBC
	Type, Rh, and antibody screen
	Rubella antibody titer
	Cervical gonorrhea and chlamydia cultures
	VDRL/RPR for syphilis screening
	Hepatitis B surface antigen test
	Pap smear
	Urinalysis
If indicated	PPD
	Sickle prep in high-risk groups
	HIV testing (with consent), counseling in high-risk groups
	Glucose test if patient has risk factors for diabetes
15–20 weeks	**Maternal serum alpha-fetoprotein (MSAFP) level** should be measured to screen for any neural tube defect (very high level) and trisomy 21 (low level). Perform triple screen (AFP, HCG, estriol) at 16 weeks to screen for trisomy 18, trisomy 21, and neural tube defects. If abnormal or patient > 35 years of age, perform ultrasound or amniocentesis.
18–20 weeks	Ultrasound for dating if unknown or uncertain. This is the best time during fetal development to assess the age of the fetus if there is only one chance of obtaining an ultrasound.
26–28 weeks	**Glucose test** for everyone (risk factors or not). Repeat hematocrit. Repeat Rh antibody screen.
28–30 weeks	RhoGAM administered to patients determined to be Rh antibody negative in initial screen.
32–36 weeks	Cervical chlamydia and gonorrhea cultures in high-risk patients. Repeat hematocrit. Group B strep screening. If positive, penicillin is given at labor to prevent transmission to the infant.

- Increased demands for calcium and protein are best met through the diet with animal sources. Most requirements for vitamins and minerals during pregnancy can also be met through diet. Exceptions are folate and iron.
- **The administration of 1 mg of folate,** via diet or supplementation, is recommended for all women to decrease the risk of neural tube malformations.
- Iron must be supplemented owing to transfer to the growing fetus and placenta and increased volume of RBCs. Supplementation with **30–60 mg/day of elemental iron** is recommended in the latter half of pregnancy.
- Some practitioners also recommend a standard daily multivitamin.
- Strict vegetarians may require **vitamin B$_{12}$ supplementation.**

NORMAL PHYSIOLOGIC CHANGES DURING PREGNANCY

Maternal changes during pregnancy are summarized in Table 2.11–2.

TABLE 2.11–2. Normal Physiologic Changes in Pregnancy

Organ/ System	Physiologic Change
Vagina	Markedly increased blood flow lends a characteristic **violet color.** Thick, acidic secretions.
Cervix	Softens, becomes highly vascular. Thick mucus clot forms in the cervical os that is expelled at or near labor, causing the **"bloody show."** Cervical mucus changes in response to progesterone; a sample spread on a glass slide demonstrates *beading* crystallization (**ferning**). Tissue at the os is friable and bleeds easily upon contact.
Uterus	At **12 weeks,** the uterus contacts the anterior abdominal wall and begins to displace the intestines. By the third trimester, the uterus compresses the IVC when the mother is in the supine position, reducing venous return from the lower extremities. Irregular painless (**Braxton Hicks**) contractions occur throughout pregnancy and may become frequent and rhythmic late in the third trimester ("false labor").
Breasts	Colostrum can be expressed at 3–4 months. Prolactin from the pituitary stimulates lactose production. At birth, an abrupt drop in the level of progesterone allows prolactin to act unopposed. Suckling triggers the pituitary to release oxytocin, which stimulates contraction of the myoepithelium and ducts.

The lateral recumbent position allows maintenance of normal lower venous pressure and optimal perfusion to the fetus.

TABLE 2.11–2. (continued). Normal physiologic changes in pregnancy

Organ/ System	Physiologic Change
Fluids	Water retention occurs as a result of (1) a fall in plasma osmolality (see renal), (2) high water content of the placenta, fetus, and amniotic fluid, and (3) increases in maternal blood volume (see heme).
Renal	**GFR increases by 50%; RPF increases by 30%.** The threshold for thirst and for renal water absorption is altered, with decreased serum osmolality by 10 mOsm/L and an increase in blood volume.
Respiratory	**Progesterone stimulates the respiratory system.** Tidal volume increases by 40%, while total lung capacity, residual volume, and expiratory reserve volume are all reduced. Relative hyperventilation decreases pCO_2, facilitating diffusion of pCO_2 from the fetus to the mother. Patients may have a sensation of dyspnea, but respiratory rate is normal.
Cardiovascular	Cardiac output increases by 50%, with increased heart rate (by 10–15 bpm) and stroke volume. Systolic flow murmur and exaggerated S1 split heart sound occur due to the high-flow state. Estrogen, progesterone, and prostaglandins cause vasodilation with a drop in arterial blood pressure. The growing uterus displaces the heart upward and to the left. The apex is pushed laterally with enlargement of the cardiac silhouette on CXR.
Hematologic	Blood volume increases 40–45%, with increased plasma and RBCs. Increased RBC production. While hematocrit and hemoglobin concentrations decrease slightly with the hypervolemia of pregnancy, a **hemoglobin < 11.0 g/dL is abnormal and likely due to iron deficiency.** Pregnancy is a hypercoagulable state, with the greatest risk of DVT in the puerperium.
Endocrine	Increased demands of fetus, insulin resistance, and postprandial glucagon suppression cause: • **Mild fasting hypoglycemia** • **Postprandial hyperglycemia** • **Hyperinsulinemia** Can worsen existing diabetes or cause a gestational diabetes.
Musculoskeletal	Increased mobility of sacroiliac, sacrococcygeal, and pubic joints with hormonal changes of system pregnancy.
Skin	Increased estrogen may cause changes that resemble cirrhotic disease: • Striae over abdomen, breasts, and thighs • Pigmented linea nigra over the midline • Spider angiomas or palmar erythema Rectus muscles may separate in the midline (diastasis recti) so that a portion of the anterior uterus is covered only by skin, fascia, and peritoneum.

Dilation of the collecting system may be mistaken for hydronephrosis.

New diastolic murmurs in pregnancy are not normal.

Thromboembolic disease is the most common nonobstetric cause of postpartum death.

302

Alpha-Fetoprotein (AFP) in Prenatal Testing

AFP is produced by the fetus and is found primarily in amniotic fluid. Small amounts of AFP cross the placenta and enter the maternal circulation. **Maternal serum alpha-fetoprotein (MSAFP) should be measured at 16–18 weeks' gestation.** The results of AFP testing depend on accurate gestational dating. Causes of elevated MSAFP include open neural tube defects (anencephaly or spina bifida), abdominal wall defects, multiple gestation, incorrect gestational dating, fetal death, and placental abnormalities (e.g., placental abruption). An abnormally low MSAFP level warrants amniocentesis and karyotyping to rule out chromosomal abnormalities (such as trisomy 21).

A **triple screen** is AFP, estriol, and HCG. All three are low in trisomy 18; HCG is high and AFP and estriol are low in trisomy 21.

Amniocentesis

Transabdominal removal of amniotic fluid using an ultrasound-guided needle. Fetal cells in the fluid are evaluated for chromosomal abnormalities. There is ample amniotic fluid in weeks 15–17 to perform the test. Amniocentesis is used:

easly 11 – 14 wks

- In women > 35 years to detect Down's syndrome or other chromosomal abnormalities
- In combination with an abnormal triple-screen test to detect Down's syndrome or other chromosomal abnormalities
- In Rh-sensitized pregnancy to obtain fetal blood type or signs of fetal hemolysis

In combination with an abnormal triple screen, amniocentesis detects 65% of fetuses with Down's syndrome. Risks of the procedure are fetal–maternal hemorrhage (1–2%) and fetal loss (0.5%).

Chorionic Villus Sampling

Transvaginal or transabdominal aspiration of chorionic villus tissue. The advantage is that it can be used earlier, in weeks 9–12. However, it cannot be used to assess neural tube defects, and limb defects have been associated with chorionic villus sampling performed at or before nine weeks. The risk of fetal loss is 1%.

Percutaneous Umbilical Blood Sampling (PUBS)

Performed in the second and third trimesters. PUBS is used for:

- Fetal transfusions in Rh-isoimmunization/erythroblastosis fetalis
- Fetal karyotyping
- Fetal infection
- Evaluation of genetic diseases
- Evaluation of fetal acid–base status

HIGH-YIELD FACTS

Obstetrics

303

A disorder of late pregnancy, hyperglycemia in the first trimester usually suggests preexisting diabetes.

Gestational diabetes occurs in 3–5% of all pregnancies. Risk factors include past history of gestational diabetes, prior abortions, stillbirths, hypertension, obesity, a previous history of macrosomic baby, maternal age > 30, and a family history of diabetes. A prior history of polyuria, recurrent UTIs, and a fetus that is large for gestational age may indicate occult (preexisting) diabetes.

History/PE

Typically **asymptomatic.**

Differential

Preexisting diabetes mellitus, volume overload, sugar overload, urinary tract abnormalities.

Evaluation

A fetus that is large for gestational age may indicate occult diabetes.

UA reveals **glycosuria.** Other findings include **fasting hyperglycemia** (serum glucose > 105 mg/dL) and an **abnormal glucose tolerance test** (routinely performed between 24 and 28 weeks' gestation). One-hour (50 g) glucose tolerance testing with postprandial serum glucose > 140 mg/dL suggests the diagnosis for confirmation; this should be followed by a three-hour (100 g) glucose tolerance test (GTT). Diagnosis is made when any two of the following values are met or exceeded: fasting, 105; one hour, 190; two hours, 155; three hours, 145.

Management

Treatment consists of strict adherence to **ADA diet.** Administer **insulin** if the diabetes cannot be controlled by diet alone. **Avoid oral hypoglycemics** (can cause fetal hypoglycemia). Ultrasound to assess fetal growth.

Complications

Patients who can be managed with diet alone are at low risk for maternal or fetal complications or death. Patients with poor glycemic control requiring insulin therapy have increased mortality and are at risk for the same complications as are pregestational diabetics (see following entry). More than 50% of patients with gestational diabetes develop glucose intolerance and/or diabetes mellitus type II later on.

UCV OB.39

Poorly controlled diabetes mellitus ($HbA_{1C} > 10$) is associated with an increased risk of congenital malformations and greater morbidity to the mother during labor and delivery.

Management

Management consists of the following measures:

Mother:
- Routine prenatal screening and care.
- Nutritional counseling.
- Strict glucose control in order to minimize fetal defects. For patients with type I DM, insulin therapy with the goal of maintaining the following blood glucose levels:
  - Fasting morning: 60–90 mg/dL
  - Pre-lunch: 60–105 mg/dL
  - Two-hour postprandial: < 120 mg/dL
- Renal, ophthalmologic, and cardiac evaluation to assess the degree of end-organ damage.

Fetus:
- **16–20 weeks:** Ultrasound to determine fetal age and growth and to assess for macrosomia, polyhydramnios, and intrauterine growth retardation; AFP to screen for developmental anomalies.
- **20–22 weeks:** Echocardiogram to assess cardiac anomalies.
- **Third trimester:** Close fetal surveillance (including NSTs, biophysical profile). Admit at 32–36 weeks if maternal diabetes has been poorly controlled or if fetal parameters are a concern.

Delivery and postpartum:
- Maintain normoglycemia (80–100 mg/dL) during labor.
- Consider early delivery with the following conditions: poor maternal glycemic control, preeclampsia, macrosomia, evidence of fetal lung maturity.
- Cesarean delivery is indicated for fetal weight > 4000 g.
- Continue glucose monitoring postpartum; the need for insulin rapidly decreases at delivery.

Complications

See Table 2.11–3.

TABLE 2.11–3. Complications of Pregestational Diabetes Mellitus

Maternal Complications	Fetal Complications
DKA (type I) or HHNK (type II)	Macrosomia
Preeclampsia/eclampsia	Cardiac and neural tube defects
Cephalopelvic disproportion due to macrosomia and need for cesarean section	Hypoglycemia secondary to hyperinsulinemia
Preterm labor	Hypocalcemia
	Hyperbilirubinemia
	Polycythemia
	Respiratory distress syndrome
	IUGR
	Renal anomalies
	Perinatal mortality

HIGH-YIELD FACTS

Obstetrics

Pregnancy-induced hypertension (PIH) is defined by two BP measurements of 140/90 (without a history of hypertension) at least six hours apart at > 20 weeks' gestation. **Preeclampsia** is defined as **PIH, proteinuria** (> 300 mg/24 hours or 1–2+ protein on dipstick), and/or **nondependent (hand and face) edema**. **Eclampsia** is defined as **seizures** in a patient with preeclampsia. Risk factors include nulliparity, black race, extremes of age (< 15 or > 35), multiple gestations, molar pregnancy, vascular disease (secondary to SLE or diabetes), a family history of preeclampsia, and chronic hypertension. **HELLP syndrome** is a variant of preeclampsia that has a poor prognosis (see sidebar).

> **HELLP syndrome**
>
> **H**emolysis, **E**levated **L**FTs, **L**ow **P**latelets (thrombocytopenia)

History/PE

Mild and severe preeclampsia share a spectrum of signs and symptoms (Table 2.11–4). Mild preeclampsia is often asymptomatic, so routine prenatal screening is essential for early detection.

Differential

Molar pregnancy, essential hypertension, renal disease, renovascular hypertension, primary aldosteronism, Cushing's syndrome, pheochromocytoma, primary seizure disorder, TTP, and SLE.

Evaluation

UA, 24-hour urine protein, CBC, electrolytes, serum BUN/creatinine, uric acid, **amniocentesis** (to check for **fetal lung maturity**), LFTs, PT/PTT, fibrinogen, fibrin split products, urine tox screen, ultrasound, and nonstress tests/biophysical profiles (as indicated).

Treatment

Seizures require magnesium ± benzodiazepines.

The only cure for preeclampsia/eclampsia is delivery. Use IV **magnesium sulfate** for seizure prophylaxis in severe preeclampsia (continue 12–24 hours after delivery) and for seizure management. Management should also include precise measurement of fetal age, fetal monitoring until delivery, and control of hypertension (e.g., labetalol, nifedipine). Table 2.11–5 further details the management of preeclampsia and eclampsia.

Complications

Prematurity, fetal distress, intrauterine growth retardation (IUGR), placental abruption, seizure, DIC, cerebral hemorrhage, serous retinal detachment, acute renal failure, fetal/maternal death.

UCV *OB.51*

HIGH-YIELD FACTS

Obstetrics

TABLE 2.11–4. Signs and Symptoms of Preeclampsia and Eclampsia

Mild Preeclampsia	Severe Preeclampsia	Eclampsia
Rapid weight gain; edema Blood pressure greater than **140/90** measured two times six hours apart Proteinuria (> 300 mg/24 h or 1–2+ urine dipstick)	Signs and symptoms of mild preeclampsia plus: • **Cerebral changes** (headaches, somnolence) • **Visual changes** (blurred vision, scotomata) • **GI symptoms** (epigastric pain) • **Hyperactive reflexes,** clonus BP greater than **160/110** measured two times six hours apart Proteinuria (> 4 g over 24 hours, or > 2+ on urine dipstick) Oliguria Right upper quadrant/epigastric pain Pulmonary edema/cyanosis HELLP syndrome Oligohydramnios IUGR	The three most common symptoms preceding an eclamptic attack are **headache, visual changes, and right upper quadrant/ epigastric pain** **Seizures;** severe if not controlled with anticonvulsant therapy

TABLE 2.11–5. Management of Preeclampsia and Eclampsia

Preeclampsia	Eclampsia
If close to term or if fetal lungs are mature, induce delivery with IV oxytocin. **If mild** and far from term, modified bed rest, check BP q4h, reflexes, daily weight and urine protein output, fetal surveillance, patient education, 24-hour urine protein, weekly LFTs. **If severe, control BP** with antihypertensives with the goal of maintaining BP at < 160/110 but high enough to maintain fetal blood flow, keeping diastolic BP at 90–100 mmHg. (<u>ACE inhibitors are contraindicated in pregnancy.</u>) **Immediately hospitalize** and monitor for urine output and the presence of pulmonary edema. Give magnesium sulfate for seizure prophylaxis. Deliver as soon as possible by labor induction and/or cesarean section; delivery may be necessary before fetal lungs are mature. Postpartum: **continue magnesium sulfate** for the first 12–24 hours; check BP, pulmonary status, and fluid retention. Follow heme, renal, and liver labs. General course of disease: 30% of preeclampsia cases occur before 30 weeks' gestational age, with the highest number of cases occurring at 34 weeks' gestational age.	Supplemental oxygen. Place in left lateral decubitus position. Prevent maternal trauma. Control seizure with **magnesium sulfate** and consider benzodiazepines. **Control BP.** General measures: limit fluid intake, Foley catheter, monitor inputs and outputs, monitor blood magnesium level, carefully monitor fetal status, **initiate steps to delivery!** **Postpartum: same as preeclampsia.** General course of disease: 50% of seizures occur antepartum, 25% occur intrapartum, 25% occur within 24 hours postpartum.

Rh factor is an antigenic protein located on RBCs in Rh-positive individuals and is transmitted in an autosomal-dominant fashion. Thus, if the father is Rh-positive, an Rh-negative mother may have an Rh-positive fetus against which she can form antibodies. Since maternal anti-Rh IgG antibodies are able to cross the placenta, these maternal antibodies can react with the infant's RBCs, resulting in fetal RBC hemolysis **(erythroblastosis fetalis)** (see Figure 2.11–1). Hemolytic disease usually occurs during the second pregnancy as a result of the rapid production of anti-Rh IgG antibodies by memory plasma cells.

History/PE

Inquire after events that may have exposed the mother to Rh-positive blood, including ectopic pregnancy, abortion, prior blood transfusions, **previous delivery of an Rh-positive child,** amniocentesis, or other traumatic procedures during pregnancy.

Evaluation

- **Maternal:** Screen for anti-Rh IgG on initial visit. If negative, repeat Coombs' testing at 26–28 weeks. If positive, test serially for high titers of maternal anti-Rh IgG (> 1:16).
- **Paternal:** Test for Rh-positive blood.
- Perform fetal assessment during pregnancy using amniocentesis or ultrasound-guided umbilical blood sampling for fetal blood type, Coombs' titer, bilirubin levels, hematocrit, and reticulocytes; or determine Rh status and hematocrit postnatally using fetal cord blood.

Treatment

- **Prevention:** If the Coombs' test at 28 weeks is negative, **give RhoGAM** (anti-IgG Rh) if the father is Rh positive or unknown or if paternity is uncertain. RhoGAM should be given postpartum if the baby is Rh positive. RhoGAM should also be given to Rh-negative mothers who undergo spontaneous abortion, miscarriage, ectopic pregnancy, amniocentesis, vaginal bleeding, or placenta previa/placental abruption.

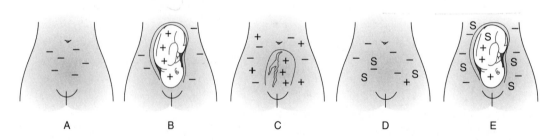

FIGURE 2.11–1. Rh disease. (A) Rh-negative woman before pregnancy. (B) Pregnancy occurs. The fetus is Rh-positive. (C) Separation of the placenta. (D) Following delivery, Rh-isoimmunization occurs in the mother, and she develops antibodies (S = antibodies). (E) The next pregnancy with an Rh-positive fetus. Maternal antibodies cross the placenta, enter the bloodstream, and attach to Rh-positive cells, causing hemolysis. RhoGAM (Rh IgG) is given to the Rh-negative mother to prevent sensitization. (Adapted, with permission, from DeCherney AH, *Current Obstetric & Gynecologic Diagnosis & Treatment,* 8th ed., Stamford, CT: Appleton & Lange, 1994: p. 339, Fig. 15–1.)

- Sensitized Rh-negative mothers with titers > 1:16 should be closely monitored (for evidence of fetal hemolysis) with serial ultrasound and amniocentesis.
- In severe cases, preterm delivery should be initiated when fetal lungs are mature (enhance pulmonary maturity with betamethasone). Prior to delivery, intrauterine blood transfusions may be given to correct a low fetal hematocrit.

Complications

Fetal hypoxia and acidosis, kernicterus, fetal prematurity, fetal death. **Hydrops fetalis** (decreased protein, decreased oncotic pressure, edema, high-output cardiac failure) occurs when hemoglobin decreases to > 7 g/dL below normal.

PLACENTAL ABRUPTION AND PLACENTA PREVIA

Placenta previa (Figure 2.11–2) and placental abruption are the two most common causes of **third-trimester bleeding.** Other causes include placenta accreta, bloody show, ruptured vasa previa, early labor, ruptured uterus, marginal placental separation, and genital tract lesions and trauma.

Table 2.11–6 compares the characteristics and management of the two conditions.

UCV OB.43, 44

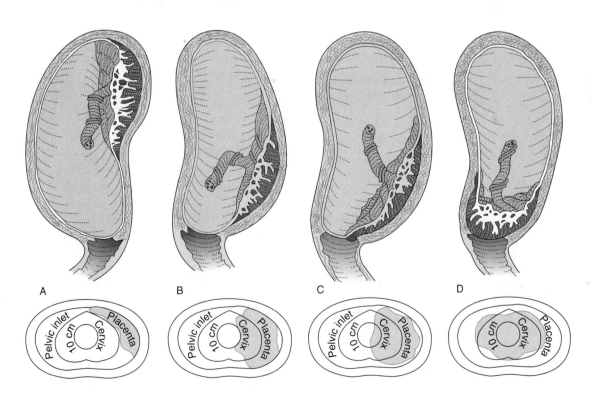

FIGURE 2.11–2. Placental implantation. (A) Normal placenta. (B) Low implantation. (C) Partial placenta previa. (D) Complete placenta previa. (Adapted, with permission, from DeCherney AH, *Current Obstetric & Gynecologic Diagnosis & Treatment*, 8th ed., Stamford, CT: Appleton & Lange, 1994: p. 404, Fig. 20–2.)

TABLE 2.11–6. Placental Abruption Versus Placenta Previa

	Placental Abruption	**Placenta Previa**
Pathophysiology	**Premature** (before the onset of labor) **separation** of normally implanted placenta.	**Abnormal implantation** of placenta **near or at the cervical os,** classified as: • Total: placenta covers cervical os • Partial: placenta partially covers os • Marginal: edge of placenta extends to margin of os • Low-lying: placenta in close proximity to os
Incidence	1/100	1/200
Risk factors	**Hypertension, abdominal/pelvic trauma, tobacco or cocaine use.**	**Prior cesarean sections, grand multiparous, advanced maternal age.**
Symptoms	**Painful** vaginal bleeding (although in 10% of cases there is no bleeding) that does not spontaneously cease. Abdominal pain, uterine hypertonicity. Fetal distress.	**Painless,** bright red bleeding (bleeding source is mom), with the first bleeding episode at 29–30 weeks' gestation. Bleeding often ceases in 1–2 hours with or without uterine contractions. Usually no fetal distress.
Diagnosis	Transabdominal/transvaginal ultrasound: look for retroplacental clot; can rule in diagnosis but cannot rule out.	**Transabdominal/transvaginal ultrasound:** look for abnormally positioned placenta; this test is very sensitive for the diagnosis.
Management	Stabilize patient with premature fetus; **expectant management** with continuous or frequent monitoring. **Moderate to severe abruption: immediate delivery** (vaginal delivery with amniotomy if fetal heart rate is stable; cesarean section if mom or fetus is in distress).	**NO vaginal exam!** **Stabilize patient with premature fetus;** bed rest. Tocolytics (magnesium sulfate). Serial ultrasound to assess fetal growth, resolution of partial previa. Amniocentesis to check fetal lung maturity; administer betamethasone to augment fetal lung maturity. Delivery by cesarean section. **Indications for delivery: persistent labor, blood loss of > 500 mL, unstable bleeding requiring multiple transfusion, coagulation defects, documented fetal lung maturity, 36 weeks' gestational age.**
Complications	Hemorrhagic shock. Coagulopathy: DIC in 10% of all abruptions. Recurrence risk is 5–16%; this risk increases to 25% after two previous abruptions. Fetal hypoxia.	↑ incidence of placenta accreta (abnormal adherence of placenta to uterine wall). Vasa previa (fetal vessels crossing the internal os). Twofold increase in congenital abnormalities, IUGR. Preterm delivery. Increased risk of postpartum hemorrhage.

HIGH-YIELD FACTS

Obstetrics

Gestational trophoblastic disease (GTD) includes a range of proliferative trophoblastic abnormalities and can be benign or malignant. **Benign GTD** (molar pregnancy, or hydatidiform mole) accounts for approximately 80% of cases of GTD. **Complete molar pregnancies,** which result from sperm fertilization of an empty ovum, most commonly have a chromosomal pattern of **46, XX** and are completely derived from the father. **Incomplete molar pregnancies,** which result when a normal ovum is fertilized by two sperm, most commonly have a chromosomal pattern of **69, XXY.** Fetal tissue is present.

Hydatidiform mole may progress to **malignant GTD,** which consists of invasive moles (10–15% of GTD) and choriocarcinoma (2–5% of GTD). Risk factors for GTD include extremes of age (< 20 or > 40), **inadequate folate** or beta-carotene in the diet, and low socioeconomic status. GTD may also follow normal pregnancy, ectopic pregnancy, or spontaneous abortion.

History/PE

First-trimester **uterine bleeding** (most common presenting sign), **uterine size > date discrepancy, preeclampsia** (may present at < 24 weeks), passage of molar vesicles, **hyperemesis gravidarum** (intractable nausea and vomiting), and hyperthyroidism. No fetal heartbeat is detected. Pelvic examination may reveal bilaterally enlarged ovaries with bilateral theca lutein cysts.

Differential

Normal pregnancy, spontaneous abortion, threatened abortion, ectopic pregnancy, preeclampsia, placenta previa, placental abruption, multiple-gestation pregnancy.

Evaluation

Findings include **markedly elevated serum β-HCG** (usually > 100,000 mIU/mL) and a **"snowstorm" appearance on pelvic ultrasound** with no gestational sac or fetus present. CXR may show lung metastases.

Treatment

Dilation and curettage revealing **"cluster-of-grapes"** tissue (Figure 2.11–3); continue to follow β-HCG closely. For malignant disease, treat with **chemotherapy (methotrexate** or dactinomycin) and **hysterectomy for residual disease** in the uterus. Chemotherapy and irradiation for metastases.

Complications

Development of malignant GTD from a benign mole; **pulmonary or CNS metastases,** trophoblastic pulmonary emboli, acute respiratory insufficiency.

Preeclampsia in the first trimester is pathognomonic for hydatidiform mole.

HIGH-YIELD FACTS

Obstetrics

311

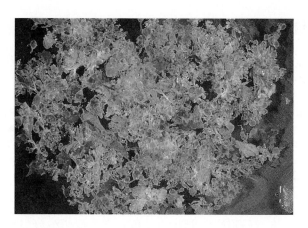

FIGURE 2.11–3. Hydatidiform mole. Note the characteristic "bunch of grapes" appearance on this gross specimen. (Reproduced, courtesy of Dr. Raoul Fresco, Loyola University.)

TESTS OF FETAL WELL-BEING

NONSTRESS TEST (NST)

Performed with the mother resting in the left lateral supine position. Fetal heart rate is monitored externally (by doppler) and correlated with spontaneous fetal movements as reported by the mother (Table 2.11–7). A normal response is acceleration of fetal heart rate of 15 beats or more per minute above baseline for at least 15 seconds. Two such accelerations within a 20-minute period are considered a normal "reactive" test. If the nonstress test is "nonreactive," further tests, such as the biophysical profile, may be performed to further evaluate fetal well-being.

TABLE 2.11–7. Fetal Heart Decelerations

Fetal Deceleration	Description	Most Common Cause
Early deceleration	Decelerations begin and end at approximately the same time as the maternal contraction.	Cephalic compression (**no fetal distress**).
Variable deceleration	Decelerations occur at any time during the maternal contraction.	Umbilical cord compression. Change mother's position (e.g., back to side).
Late deceleration	Decelerations begin at the peak of the contraction and persist until the contraction has finished.	Uteroplacental insufficiency and fetal hypoxemia, possibly due to abruption or hypotension. Further testing for fetal reassurance is necessary. If late decelerations are repetitious and severe, deliver the baby ASAP.

CONTRACTION STRESS TEST

Used in high-risk pregnancy (see IUGR) to assess uteroplacental dysfunction. During labor or induction of contractions using oxytocin, the fetal heart rate is monitored with an external fetal monitor, fetal scalp electrode, fetal scalp pH, and ultrasound. Long-term variability, beat-to-beat variability, and transient accelerations of heart rate are reassuring findings. See Figure 2.11–4.

BIOPHYSICAL PROFILE

Real-time ultrasonography is used to assess:

Test the Baby, MAN!

- Fetal **T**one
- Fetal **B**reathing
- Fetal **M**ovement
- **A**mniotic fluid volume
- **N**onstress test

A score of 2 (normal) or 0 (abnormal) is given to each. A score of 8–10 is "reassuring" of fetal well-being.

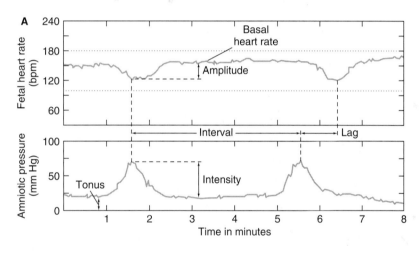

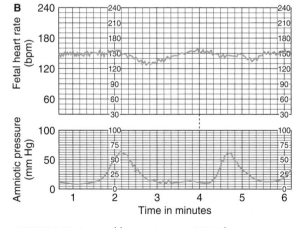

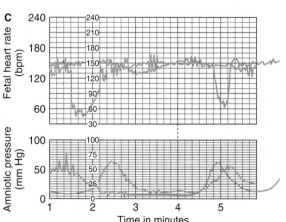

FIGURE 2.11–4. Fetal heart tracings. (A) Schematic tracing. (B) Late deceleration. (C) Variable deceleration. (Reproduced, with permission, from DeCherney AH, *Current Obstetrics & Gynecologic Diagnosis & Treatment*, 8th ed. Stamford, CT: Appleton & Lange, 1994: p. 301, Fig. 13–13A, C, and D.)

Intrauterine fetal growth less than expected. Occurs in 3–7% of all pregnancies. There are two types:

Symmetric IUGR is generally a FETAL problem.

1. **Symmetric:** Twenty percent of cases of IUGR are symmetric, with an overall decrease in size that affects both the head and the body. Common causes are congenital infections, chromosomal abnormalities, congenital abnormalities, or maternal drug use (alcohol, smoking, cocaine). The insult usually occurs **early in pregnancy.**

Asymmetric IUGR is considered a MATERNAL problem.

2. **Asymmetric:** Eighty percent of IUGR cases are asymmetric, with a decrease in subcutaneous fat and abdominal girth with relative sparing of head circumference and femur length. Causes include placental defects, multiple gestations, and chronic maternal disease, particularly vascular disease (hypertension, diabetes, renal disease), which leads to decreased uteroplacental blood flow and oxygenation. The etiologic insult occurs **late in pregnancy.**

Evaluation

- **Fundal height:** A discrepancy of > 4 between fundal height (in centimeters) and gestational age (in weeks) is cause for concern.
- **Ultrasound:** Assess amniotic fluid volume, placental function, estimated fetal weight, fetal gestational age, congenital anomalies, and head-to-abdominal circumference (HC/AC) +/– femur length to abdominal circumference (FL/AC) ratios.
  - HC/AC and FL/AC are increased in **asymmetric** IUGR.
  - Ratios are normal in **symmetric** IUGR.
  - **Increased HC/AC with decreased amniotic fluid volume and estimated fetal weight below the tenth percentile indicates the presence of IUGR.**

Treatment

- Serial exams.
- Ultrasound evaluation every 3–4 weeks.
- Fetal monitoring. Nonstress test, contraction stress test, or biophysical profile or doppler flow studies to evaluate uterine/umbilical artery flow.
- Steroids to accelerate fetal lung maturity.
- Consider early delivery, particularly with asymmetric IUGR, in which the uterine environment later in pregnancy is critical.
- Continuous fetal heart rate monitoring during labor with cesarean section if decelerations persist.

Table 2.11–8 summarizes the effects of some common teratogens.

TABLE 2.11–8. Birth Defects

Teratogen	Effect
DES	Clear cell adenocarcinoma of the vagina/cervix; genital tract abnormalities
Thalidomide	Limb abnormalities (**phocomelia**) as well as auricle, eye, and visceral malformations
Amphetamines	Transposition of the great vessels, cleft palate
Ethanol	Fetal alcohol syndrome (microcephaly, mental retardation, facial abnormalities, limb dislocation, heart/lung fistulas)
Iodide	Congenital goiter, hypothyroidism, mental retardation
Tetracycline	Inhibition of bone growth, small limbs, syndactyly, discoloration of teeth
Fluoroquinolones	Cartilage damage
Aminoglycosides	Eighth-nerve damage, macromelia, multiple skeletal abnormalities
Sulfonamides	Kernicterus
Griseofulvin	Multiple anomalies
Isotretinoin	Multiple anomalies
Warfarin	Skeletal and facial abnormalities, mental retardation, stillbirth, IUGR
Phenytoin, carbamazepine	Multiple anomalies, including cleft lip/palate, hypoplasia of distal phalanges, and sacral teratomas (fetal anticonvulsive syndrome)
Valproic acid	Fetal anticonvulsive syndrome, neural tube defects
ACE inhibitors	Fetal renal damage

FETAL PRESENTATIONS

The fetus may have a **cephalic** presentation, with the head closest to the birth canal.

- Ninety-five percent of cephalic presentations are vertex with chin to chest, occiput presenting.
- The face may present with a fully extended neck.
- The brow may present with the neck only partially extended.

Three percent of all deliveries are **breech** (see Figure 2.11–5).

- **Frank breech (50–75%):** Thighs are flexed and knees are extended.
- **Footling (incomplete) breech (20%):** One or both legs are extended below the buttocks.
- **Complete breech (5–10%):** Thighs and knees are flexed.

Any presentation other than vertex is considered abnormal. The increased fetal mortality associated with breech presentation is due to congenital abnormalities, hypoxia, birth injury, and prematurity.

Evaluation

Leopold maneuvers are used to identify the location of the fetal head, back, and breech to determine the orientation of the fetus.

Treatment

- Follow. Seventy-five percent will spontaneously change to vertex presentation by the 38th week.
- External version. If the fetus has not reverted spontaneously, pressure may be applied to the maternal abdominal wall to turn the infant to a vertex position. The success rate is about 75%; risks are placental abruption and cord compression, so the clinician must be prepared to perform an emergency cesarean.

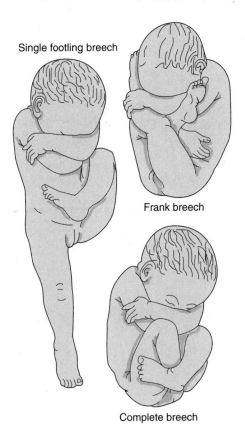

FIGURE 2.11–5. Types of breech presentations. (Reproduced, with permission, from DeCherney AH, *Current Obstetrics & Gynecologic Diagnosis & Treatment*, 8th ed., Stamford, CT: Appleton & Lange, 1994: p. 411, Fig. 21–1.)

- Cesarean section is the standard of care in many hospitals for breech presentations; however, it has NOT been shown to improve outcome.
- Criteria for a trial of labor:
  - Frank breech presentation.
  - Gestational age of ≥ 36 weeks; fetal weight 2500–3800 g.
  - Adequate maternal pelvic dimensions (by x-ray or history of delivery of large baby).
  - Ultrasound evaluation does not show fetal anomalies, placental anomalies, or extension of the fetal head.
  - No other indication for cesarean section.

LABOR STAGES

Table 2.11–9 and Figure 2.11–6 depict the normal stages of labor.

			Duration (hours)	
TABLE 2.11–9. Stages of Labor				
Stage	**Starts/End**	**Events**	**Duration (hours)**	
First			Nulli*	Multi**
Latent	Regular uterine contractions/cervix dilated to 4 cm	Highly variable duration; cervix **effaces** (cervical canal shortens) and slowly dilates.	6–11	4–8
Active	4-cm cervical dilation/ complete cervical dilation (10 cm) or progressing at ~1 cm/hr	Regular and intense uterine contractions; cervix effaces and dilates more quickly; fetal head progressively descends into pelvis.	4–6	2–3
Second	Complete cervical dilation/delivery of the baby	Baby undergoes all stages of cardinal movements.	1–2	0.5–1
Third	Delivery of baby/ delivery of placenta	Placenta separates and uterus contracts to establish hemostasis.	0–0.5	0–0.5

*Nulli = nulliparous (first-time mother).

**Multi = multiparous (pregnant and delivered before).

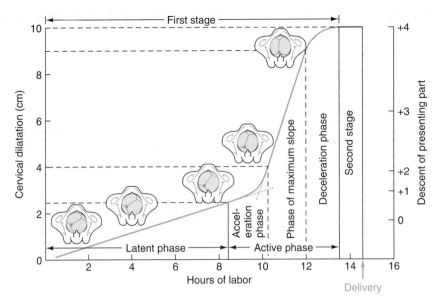

FIGURE 2.11–6. Stages of labor. Cervical dilatation, level of descent, and orientation of occipitoanterior presentation during various stages of labor. (Reproduced, with permission, from DeCherney AH, *Current Obstetrics & Gynecologic Diagnosis & Treatment*, 8th ed., Stamford, CT: Appleton & Lange, 1994: p. 211, Fig. 10–5.)

INDICATIONS FOR CESAREAN SECTION

Indications for performing cesarean section are as follows:

- Previous cesarean section due to risk of uterine rupture (the most common indication, but many women elect a trial of labor even if they have had a previous C-section)
- Cephalopelvic disproportion
- Placenta previa
- Placental abruption
- Fetal malposition (e.g., posterior chin position, transverse lie, brow presentation, shoulder presentation, footling or complete breech)
- Fetal distress
- Erythroblastosis fetalis (Rh incompatibility)
- Cord prolapse
- Carcinoma of the cervix
- Post-term pregnancy (relative indication)
- Failed operative vaginal delivery
- Active genital herpes infection
- Maternal trauma/demise

Defined as a loss of > 500 mL of blood within the first 24 hours of delivery. Table 2.11–10 summarizes the common causes of postpartum hemorrhage. Complications include excessive blood loss and transfusion-related risks.

TABLE 2.11–10. Common Causes of Postpartum Hemorrhage

	Uterine Atony	Genital Tract Trauma	Retained Placental Tissue
Risk factors	Overdistention of the uterus (multiple gestations, macrosomia) Abnormal labor (prolonged labor, precipitous labor) Conditions interfering with uterine contractions (uterine myomas, magnesium sulfate, general anesthesia) Uterine infection	Precipitous labor Operative vaginal delivery (forceps, vacuum extraction) Large infant Inadequate episiotomy repair	Placenta accreta/increta/percreta Preterm delivery Placenta previa Previous cesarean section/ curettage Uterine leiomyomas
Diagnosis	Palpation of a softer, flaccid, "boggy" uterus without a firm fundus **Most common cause of postpartum hemorrhage** (90%)	Careful visualization of the lower genital tract looking for any laceration > 2 cm in length	Careful inspection of the placenta for missing cotyledons. Ultrasound may also be used to examine the uterus.
Treatment	Bimanual **uterine massage,** which is usually successful **Oxytocin** infusion Methylergonovine maleate (Methergine) if not hypertensive and/or prostaglandin F2-alpha if patient is not asthmatic or hypertensive	Surgical repair of the physical defect	Manual removal of the remaining placental tissue. Curettage with suctioning may also be used with care taken to avoid perforating the uterine fundus. In cases of true placenta accreta/increta/percreta where the placental villi invade into the uterine tissue, hysterectomy is often required as a life-preserving therapy.

HIGH-YIELD FACTS

Obstetrics

319

Effect of progesterone on the respiratory system.	Stimulant; increases tidal volume, creating a relative hyperventilation in pregnancy
Most common cause of postpartum death.	Thromboembolic disease
Pregnant woman has hematocrit of 10 g/dL; is this the normal anemia of pregnancy?	No; below 11 g/dL should raise the suspicion of iron deficiency
Tests to assess neural tube defects.	AFP or amniocentesis
Test that can be used in the tenth week of gestation to screen for chromosomal abnormalities.	Chorionic villus sampling
Fetal complications with poorly controlled maternal diabetes.	Include macrosomia, cardiac and renal defects, RDS, IUGR
Abnormal heart rate pattern in contraction stress test.	Late decelerations, indicating fetal hypoxia
Indicated by increased fetal head-to-abdominal circumference and decreased amniotic fluid.	Intrauterine growth retardation
When to administer prenatal glucose testing.	26–28 weeks
Seizure prophylaxis in severe preeclampsia.	IV magnesium sulfate
HELLP syndrome.	Hemolysis, elevated LFTs, and low platelets; a variant of preeclampsia with a poor prognosis
Cure for preeclampsia/eclampsia.	Delivery
Erythroblastosis fetalis.	Fetal RBC hemolysis due to maternal antibodies against infant's Rh-positive RBCs
Hydrops fetalis.	Decreased production of protein by fetal liver, with resulting drop in oncotic pressure, edema, and high-output cardiac failure
Preeclampsia in the first trimester is pathognomonic for what condition?	Hydatidiform mole
Classic ultrasound and gross appearance in hydatidiform mole.	Snowstorm on ultrasound; cluster-of-grapes gross appearance
Symptoms of placental abruption.	Painful vaginal bleeding, continuous
Symptoms of placenta previa.	Painless vaginal bleeding, self-limited
When should vaginal exam be performed with suspected placenta previa?	Never
Antibiotics with teratogenic effects.	Tetracycline, fluoroquinolones, aminoglycosides, sulfonamides

The following clinical questions and accompanying answers are reproduced, with permission, from Evans MI, *PreTest: Obstetrics & Gynecology*, 9th ed., New York: McGraw-Hill, 2001.

Questions

1. In terms of birth defect potential, the safest of the following drugs is
   a. Alcohol
   b. Isotretinoin (Accutane)
   c. Tetracyclines
   d. Progesterones
   e. Phenytoin (Dilantin)

2. A 19-year-old woman comes to the emergency room and reports that she fainted at work earlier in the day. She has mild vaginal bleeding. Her abdomen is diffusely tender and distended. In addition, she complains of shoulder and abdominal pain. Her temperature is 36.4°C (97.6°F), pulse rate is 120 beats/min, and blood pressure is 96/50 mmHg. To confirm the diagnosis suggested by the available clinical data, the best diagnostic procedure would be
   a. Pregnancy test
   b. Posterior colpotomy
   c. Dilation and curettage
   d. Culdocentesis
   e. Laparoscopy

3. A 24-year-old woman appears at eight weeks of pregnancy and reveals a history of pulmonary embolism seven years ago during her first pregnancy. She was treated with intravenous heparin followed by several months of oral warfarin (Coumadin) and has had no further evidence of thromboembolic disease for over six years. Which of the following statements about her current condition is true?
   a. Having no evidence of disease for over five years means that the risk of thromboembolism is not greater than normal
   b. Impedance plethysmography is not a useful study to evaluate her for deep venous thrombosis in pregnancy
   c. Doppler ultrasonography is not a useful technique to evaluate her for deep venous thrombosis in pregnancy
   d. The patient should be placed on low-dose heparin therapy throughout pregnancy and puerperium
   e. The patient is at highest risk for recurrent thromboembolism during the second trimester of pregnancy

4. A 29-year-old, gravida 3, para 2 black woman in the 33rd week of gestation is admitted to the emergency room because of acute abdominal pain that developed and is increasing during the past 24 hours. The pain is severe and is radiating from the epigastrium to the back. The patient has vomited a few times and has not eaten or had a bowel movement since the pain started. On examination you observe an acutely ill patient lying on the bed with her knees drawn up. Her blood pressure is 150/100 mmHg, her pulse is 110 beats/min, and her temperature is 38.18°C (100.68°F). On palpation the abdomen is somewhat distended and tender, mainly in the epigastric area, and the uterine fundus reaches 31 cm above the symphysis. Hypotonic bowel sounds are noted. Fetal monitoring reveals a normal pat-

321

tern of fetal heart rate (FHR) without uterine contractions. On ultrasonography the fetus is in vertex presentation and appropriate in size for gestational age; fetal breathing and trunk movements are noted and the volume of amniotic fluid is normal. The placenta is located on the anterior uterine wall and of grade 2 to 3. Laboratory values show mild leukocytosis (12,000 cells/μL); a hematocrit of 43; mildly elevated serum glutamic-oxaloacetic transaminase (SGOT), serum glutamic-pyruvic transaminase (SGPT), and bilirubin; and serum amylase of 180 U/dL. Urinalysis is normal.

The most probable diagnosis in this patient is
    a. Acute degeneration of uterine leiomyoma
    b. Acute cholecystitis
    c. Acute pancreatitis
    d. Acute appendicitis
    e. Severe preeclamptic toxemia

5. When treating urinary tract infection (UTI) in the third trimester, the antibiotic of choice should be
    a. Cephalosporin
    b. Tetracycline
    c. Sulfonamide
    d. Nitrofurantoin

Answers

1. **The answer is d.** Alcohol is an enormous contributor to otherwise preventable birth defects. Sequelae include retardation of intrauterine growth, craniofacial abnormalities, and mental retardation. The occasional drink in pregnancy has not been proved to be deleterious. Isotretinoin (Accutane) is a powerful drug for acne that has enormous potential for producing congenital anomalies when ingested in early pregnancy; it should never be used in pregnancy. Tetracyclines interfere with development of bone and can lead to stained teeth in children. Progesterones have been implicated in multiple birth defects but controlled studies have failed to demonstrate a significant association with increased risk. Patients who have inadvertently become pregnant while on birth control pills should be reassured that the incidence of birth defects is no higher for them than for the general population. Phenytoin (Dilantin) is used for epilepsy and can be associated with a spectrum of abnormalities, including digital hypoplasia and facial abnormalities.

2. **The answer is d.** The clinical history presented in this question is a classic one for a ruptured tubal pregnancy accompanied by hemoperitoneum. Because pregnancy tests are negative in almost 50% of cases, they are of little practical value in an emergency. Dilation and curettage would not permit rapid enough diagnosis, and the results obtained by this procedure are variable. Posterior colpotomy requires an operating room, surgical anesthesia, and an experienced operator with a scrubbed and gowned associate. Refined optic and electronic systems have improved the accuracy of laparoscopy, but this new equipment is not always available, and the procedure requires an operating room and, usually, surgical anesthesia. Culdocentesis is a rapid, nonsurgical method to confirm the presence of unclotted intraabdominal blood from a ruptured tubal pregnancy. Culdocentesis, however, is also not perfect, and a negative culdocentesis should not be used as the sole criterion for whether or not to operate on a patient.

3. **The answer is d.** Patients with a history of thromboembolic disease in pregnancy are at high risk to develop it in subsequent pregnancies. Impedance plethysmography and doppler ultrasonography are useful techniques even in pregnancy and should be done as baseline studies. Patients should be treated prophylactically with low-dose heparin therapy through the postpartum period as this is the time of highest risk of this disease. Coumadin is contraindicated in pregnancy.

4. **The answer is c.** The most probable diagnosis in this case is acute pancreatitis. The pain caused by a myoma in degeneration is more localized to the uterine wall. Low-grade fever and mild leukocytosis may appear with a degenerating myoma, but liver function tests are usually normal. The other obstetric cause of epigastric pain, severe preeclamptic toxemia (PET), may exhibit disturbed liver function (sometimes associated with the HELLP syndrome [hemolysis, elevated liver enzymes, low platelets]), but this patient has only mild elevation of blood pressure and no proteinuria. Acute appendicitis in pregnancy is one of the more common nonobstetric causes of abdominal pain. In pregnancy, symptoms of acute appendicitis are similar to those in nonpregnant patients, but the pain is more vague and poorly localized and the point of maximal tenderness moves with advancing gestation to the right upper quadrant. Liver function tests are normal with acute appendicitis. Acute cholecystitis may cause fever, leukocytosis, and pain of the right upper quadrant with abnormal liver function tests, but amylase levels would be elevated only mildly, if at all,

and pain would be less severe than described in this patient. The diagnosis that fits the clinical description and the laboratory findings is acute pancreatitis. This disorder may be more common during pregnancy, with an incidence of 1:100 to 1:10,000 pregnancies. Cholelithiasis, chronic alcoholism, infection, abdominal trauma, some medications, and pregnancy-induced hypertension are known predisposing factors. Patients with pancreatitis are usually in acute distress—the classic finding is a person who is rocking with knees drawn up and trunk flexed in agony. Fever, tachypnea, hypotension, ascites, and pleural effusion may be observed. Hypotonic bowel sounds, epigastric tenderness, and signs of peritonitis may be demonstrated on examination.

Leukocytosis, hemoconcentration, and abnormal liver function tests are common laboratory findings in acute pancreatitis. The most important laboratory finding is, however, an elevation of serum amylase levels, which appears 12–24 hours after onset of clinical disease. Values may exceed 200 U/dL (normal values are 50 to 160 U/dL). A useful diagnostic tool in the pregnant patient with only modest elevation of amylase values is the amylase/creatinine ratio. In patients with acute pancreatitis, the ratio of amylase clearance to creatinine clearance is always greater than 5–6%.

Treatment considerations for the pregnant patient with acute pancreatitis are similar to those in nonpregnant patients. Intravenous hydration, nasogastric suction, enteric rest, and correction of electrolyte imbalance and of hyperglycemia are the mainstays of therapy. Careful attention to tissue perfusion, volume expansion, and transfusions to maintain a stable cardiovascular performance are critical. Gradual recovery occurs over 5–6 days.

5. **The answer is a.** Although quite effective, sulfonamides should be avoided during the last few weeks of pregnancy because they competitively inhibit the binding of bilirubin to albumin, which increases the risk of neonatal hyperbilirubinemia. Nitrofurantoin may not be tolerated in pregnancy because of the effect of nausea. It should also be avoided in late pregnancy because of the risk of hemolysis due to the deficiency of erythrocyte phosphate dehydrogenase in the newborn. Tetracyclines are contraindicated during pregnancy because of dental staining in the fetus. Thus, the drugs of choice for treatment of UTI in pregnancy are ampicillin and the cephalosporins.

Gynecology

Amenorrhea is defined as the absence of menstruation. **Primary amenorrhea** is the absence of menses and the lack of secondary sexual characteristics by age 14 or the absence of menses by age 16 with or without secondary sexual characteristics. **Secondary amenorrhea** is the absence of menses for three cycles or for six months with prior normal menses.

Differential

The causes of primary amenorrhea include gonadal failure/agenesis (e.g., Turner's syndrome), müllerian duct abnormality, androgen insensitivity syndrome, hypopituitary failure, and constitutional developmental delay. The causes of secondary amenorrhea include **pregnancy** (most common), hyper- or hypothyroidism, polycystic ovarian syndrome, premature menopause, hypothalamic/pituitary failure (e.g., Sheehan's syndrome, Kallmann's syndrome), hyperprolactinemia (galactorrhea), and anorexia nervosa.

Evaluation

Consider the disorder at three levels:

- Outflow tract
- Uterus/ovaries
- Pituitary/hypothalamus/CNS

Evaluation may include the following (see Figures 2.12–1 and 2.12–2):

- β-HCG (the most common cause of amenorrhea is pregnancy).
- Physical exam may reveal an obvious outflow tract abnormality (absent uterus, vaginal agenesis).

Always rule out pregnancy in a patient with amenorrhea.

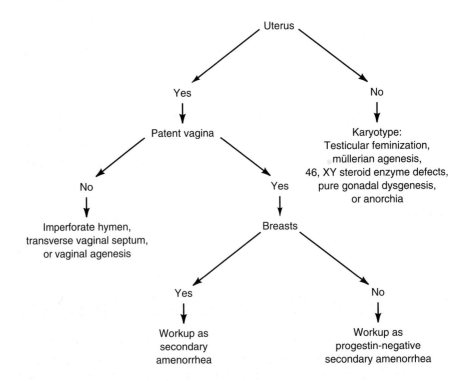

FIGURE 2.12–1. Workup for patients with primary amenorrhea. (Reproduced, with permission, from DeCherney AH, *Current Obstetric & Gynecologic Diagnosis & Treatment*, 8th ed., Stamford, CT: Appleton & Lange, 1994: p. 1010, Fig. 54–2.)

HIGH-YIELD FACTS

Gynecology

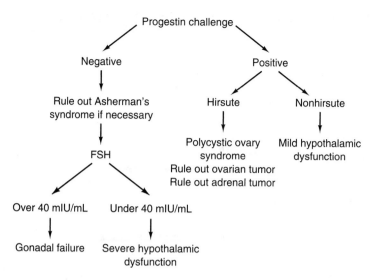

FIGURE 2.12–2. Workup for patients with secondary amenorrhea without hyperprolactinemia. (Reproduced, with permission, from DeCherney AH, *Current Obstetric & Gynecologic Diagnosis & Treatment,* 8th ed., Stamford, CT: Appleton & Lange, 1994: p. 1012, Fig. 54–4.)

- **Prolactin:** Elevated prolactin levels cause decreased release of FSH and LH. Causes of hyperprolactinemia are pituitary tumor, hypothyroidism, and dopamine-antagonizing drugs (such as phenothiazines). Test TSH; obtain CT or MRI to visualize the pituitary. If negative, perform a progestin test.
- **Progestin challenge:** If withdrawal bleeding occurs after a five-day course of progesterone (positive test), the patient has a patent outflow tract and is producing estrogen; the problem is anovulation. Causes of anovulation include hypothalamic dysfunction due to weight loss, obesity, exercise, or emotional stress; polycystic ovarian syndrome; ovarian or adrenal tumor; or Cushing's syndrome. If there is no bleeding, estrogen–progesterone challenge is performed.
- **Estrogen–progesterone challenge:** If bleeding occurs, the problem is at the follicle or the hypothalamic–pituitary axis. The absence of bleeding indicates **Asherman's syndrome** (endometrial fibrosis due to IUD or D&C).
- **Gonadotropins (FSH/LH):** If gonadotropins are low (hypogonadotropism), hypothalamic/pituitary dysfunction (Sheehan's syndrome, pituitary tumor) exists. If high (hypergonadotropism), gonadal failure (Turner's syndrome, 17-hydroxylase deficiency, gonadal agenesis) is the problem.

Treatment

Treat the underlying cause.

UCV OB.22, 23, 26

ABNORMAL UTERINE BLEEDING

Abnormal uterine bleeding can be of many types, including menorrhagia (excessive or prolonged menses), metrorrhagia (irregularity), menometrorrhagia (irregular, prolonged, heavy menstrual bleeding), polymenorrhea (increased frequency of menstruation), or oligomenorrhea (scanty menstruation).

Uterine bleeding is considered abnormal if any of the following are present:

- Menstrual flow lasting > 8 days.
- A menstrual interval of < 21 days.
- Total blood loss/menstrual cycle > 80 mL.

Common causes include threatened abortion, ectopic pregnancy, uterine fibroids/polyps, adenomyosis, endometriosis, and cervical or **endometrial cancer.** If other pathologic causes are ruled out, the abnormal bleeding is termed "dysfunctional uterine bleeding," which is usually associated with disturbance of the hypothalamic–gonadal axis and anovulation.

Evaluation

Laboratory tests include β-HCG (to rule out pregnancy), CBC, coagulation studies, and endocrine tests (serum TSH/prolactin/FSH/LH). Rule out uterine lesions by D&C and transvaginal ultrasound. Obtain a Pap smear and an endometrial biopsy on postmenopausal women to rule out cancer.

Treatment

Treat the underlying cause. Anovulatory bleeding can be treated with hormone replacement therapy. Dysfunctional uterine bleeding can be treated with **OCPs.** Patients with severe, uncontrollable uterine bleeding may require D & C with **endometrial ablation.** Vaginal packing and uterine artery ligation may be necessary. **Hysterectomy** may be performed as a last resort.

UCV OB.8

ECTOPIC PREGNANCY

Any pregnancy outside the uterine cavity (Figure 2.12–3). It most commonly occurs in the ampulla of the oviduct (95%). Risk factors include a history of **PID** (most common), prior ectopic pregnancy, tubal/pelvic surgery, DES exposure in utero, and IUD use. It occurs in 1 in 200 pregnancies.

History/PE

Suspect ectopic pregnancy whenever a pregnant patient presents with bleeding and/or unilateral abdominal/pelvic pain. **Vaginal bleeding** usually occurs 7–14 days after the last menstrual period. A **pelvic mass** may be palpated. Ruptured ectopic pregnancy may present with orthostatic hypotension, tachycardia, generalized abdominal and adnexal tenderness with rebound, shoulder pain, and shock.

Evaluation

Measure β-HCG and follow the rate of rise. Quantitative β-HCG levels are lower than expected for normal pregnancies of the same duration with **prolonged doubling times** (normal doubling time is two days). Serum progesterone is also below normal (usually < 15 ng/mL). An **elevated β-HCG in the absence of an intrauterine pregnancy on ultrasound** is highly suspicious.

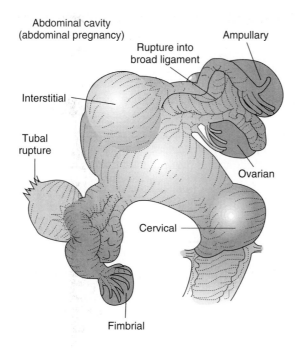

Abdominal cavity
(abdominal pregnancy)

Rupture into
broad ligament

Ampullary

Interstitial

Tubal
rupture

Ovarian

Cervical

Fimbrial

FIGURE 2.12–3. Sites of ectopic pregnancy. (Adapted from Benson RC, *Handbook of Obstetrics & Gynecology*, 8th ed., Stamford, CT: Appleton & Lange, 1983.)

Evidence of an intrauterine pregnancy (to rule out an ectopic) can be found by transabdominal ultrasound (when β-HCG levels reach 5000 mIU/mL) or by transvaginal ultrasound (when β-HCG is 1500 mIU/mL). The return of > 5 cc of nonclotting blood on culdocentesis identifies hemoperitoneum but is not sensitive or specific. Definitive diagnosis is made by laparoscopy or laparotomy.

Treatment

Patients with an ectopic pregnancy or suspicion of having one should be closely followed with serial β-HCG and ultrasound studies. Management is as follows:

- Patients with falling β-HCG levels, fallopian tube pregnancy, no evidence of intra-abdominal bleeding by ultrasound, and a < 3.5-cm ectopic mass can be managed expectantly for spontaneous resolution.
- Medical treatment for stable unruptured ectopic pregnancies < 3.5 cm of < 6-week gestation is with **methotrexate.**
- All other ectopic pregnancies require surgery.
- Surgical options include salpingostomy, salpingectomy, and salpingo-oophorectomy.
- Give a **RhoGAM** shot if appropriate.

Complications

Inevitable loss of fetus, hemorrhagic shock, **future ectopic pregnancy,** infertility, maternal death, Rh sensitization.

UCV *OB.41*

Spontaneous abortion is defined as a nonelective termination of a pregnancy at < **20 weeks' gestational age** or at an estimated fetal weight of < 500 g. It is a common cause of first-trimester bleeding. Types of spontaneous abortion and their management are summarized in Table 2.12–1. Causes of recurrent spontaneous abortion include cervical incompetence, infections, uterine abnormalities, hormonal dysfunction, hypercoagulable states, and **chromosomal abnormalities** (most often a trisomy). It occurs in 15% of recognized pregnancies. Risk factors include increasing maternal/paternal age, increased gravidity, minority status, and a history of previous losses.

History/PE

Obtaining a medical history of prior abortions, infections, and genetic abnormalities in the family is important. Examination shows vaginal bleeding and may reveal passage of tissue. Note closed versus open cervical os on pelvic examination.

Evaluation

Evaluation includes qualitative/quantitative β-HCG to confirm pregnancy, establish gestational age, or ensure that there is no remaining tissue after completed abortion; transvaginal ultrasound to assess fetal viability; and possibly culdocentesis.

Treatment

Ensure hemodynamic stability if there has been significant bleeding. Management generally consists of **uterine evacuation,** prevention of infection, and **RhoGAM if appropriate.**

Complications

Sepsis, hemorrhage.

TABLE 2.12–1. Types of Spontaneous Abortion

Abortion	Definition	Treatment
Threatened abortion EM.38	Less than 20 weeks' gestation **No products of conception expelled** Membranes remain intact Internal **cervical os closed** Uterine bleeding Abdominal pain may be present Fetus is still viable	Avoid heavy activity Pelvic rest Bed rest RhoGAM if appropriate
Inevitable abortion	Less than 20 weeks' gestation **No products of conception expelled** Membranes ruptured Internal **cervical os open** Uterine bleeding and cramps	Emergent D&C RhoGAM if appropriate
Complete abortion OB.33	Less than 20 weeks' gestation **All products of conception expelled** Internal **cervical os closed** Uterine bleeding	RhoGAM if appropriate
Incomplete abortion	Less than 20 weeks' gestation **Some products of conception expelled** Internal **cervical os open** Uterine bleeding	D&C RhoGAM if appropriate
Missed abortion	Fetal demise (no cardiac activity) No products of conception expelled Retained fetal tissue Uterus not growing Internal cervical os closed No uterine bleeding	Evacuate uterus D&C RhoGAM if appropriate
Septic abortion	Infection associated with abortion Endometritis leading to septicemia Maternal mortality 10–50%	Complete uterine evacuation D&C Intravenous antibiotics RhoGAM if appropriate
Intrauterine fetal death	No cardiac activity (fetal heart tones) Greater than eight weeks' gestation, with 15 mm or larger crown–rump length	Evacuate uterus D&C RhoGAM if appropriate

The permanent cessation of menstruation secondary to end-organ ovarian resistance to gonadotropins. The median age of onset of menopause in U.S. women is 50–52 years. Premature menopause is the cessation of menstruation before **age 40** and is often secondary to idiopathic premature ovarian failure. Early menopause is frequently associated with **cigarette smoking.** Postmenopausal women lose the protective effects of estrogen and are thus at increased risk of developing **osteoporosis** and **heart disease.**

History/PE

Menstrual irregularities (e.g., menorrhagia, polymenorrhea, oligomenorrhea, amenorrhea), **hot flashes** (secondary to vasomotor instability), **sweats,** sleep disturbances, **mood changes,** decreased libido, depression, dyspareunia (secondary to vaginal wall atrophy), cystocele, urinary frequency/incontinence, and **dysuria.** Examination reveals vaginal dryness and genital tract atrophy.

Evaluation

Elevated serum FSH is suggestive. Diagnosis requires one year without menses.

Treatment

- **Hormone replacement therapy** (HRT) gives some patients symptomatic relief and is useful in the prevention of osteoporosis and cardiovascular disease.
- Use a regimen of opposed progesterone/estrogen if the patient still has her uterus.
- Use unopposed estrogen if the patient has undergone TAH/BSO.
- Alternatives to HRT include calcium, vitamin D, and bisphosphonates.

Complications

Osteoporosis, atrophic vaginitis, **cardiovascular disease (MI, stroke).**

UCV *OB.14*

Endometriosis is the most common cause of female infertility, followed by PID.

Failure on the part of a couple to achieve pregnancy after **repeated attempts over a 12-month period.** Infertility can be classified into four etiologies: male dysfunction (30–40%), ovulatory problems (15–20%), pelvic factors (30%), and cervical factors (5%). In approximately 5–20% of cases, the cause of infertility is unknown.

Differential

Ovulatory dysfunction (e.g., ovarian failure, prolactinoma), genital tract damage/scarring (endometriosis, PID, Asherman's syndrome), defects in spermatogenesis, varicoceles (interfere with normal sperm development).

Evaluation

Evaluation includes semen analysis, postcoital test (to assess cervical mucus), daily basal body temperature measurements (to verify ovulation), endometrial biopsy, serum FSH/LH/midcycle progesterone/prolactin (to rule out endocrine dysfunction), and hysterosalpingogram (to rule out tubal disease and uterine cavity abnormalities). Assess cervical mucus for antisperm antibodies.

UCV *OB.13*

CONTRACEPTIVES

Table 2.12–2 describes various methods of contraception.

TABLE 2.12–2. Contraceptive Methods

Method	Description	Side Effects
Rhythm	Uses body temperature and cervical mucus consistency to predict the time of fertility.	Not very effective.
OCPs	Suppress ovulation by inhibiting FSH/LH; changing the consistency of cervical mucus makes the endometrium unsuitable for implantation.	Nausea, breast tenderness, headache, acne, mood changes, hypertension, hepatic adenoma, post-pill amenorrhea, and **increased incidence of DVT** (but protective effects against PID and ovarian and endometrial cancer).
Levonorgestrel (Norplant)	Progestin-only subdermal implant that inhibits ovulation by suppressing LH peak. Contraceptive effects last for five years.	Irregular vaginal bleeding, weight gain, galactorrhea, acne, breast tenderness. Difficult to remove.
Postcoital "morning-after" pill	Estrogen or estrogen/progesterone taken within 72 hours of unprotected sex to suppress ovulation or discourage implantation of fertilized ovum.	Clear-cell vaginal carcinoma associated with unopposed estrogen use; congenital malformation if pregnancy does occur.
Medroxyprogesterone (Depo-Provera)	Intramuscular injection of medroxyprogesterone acetate given every three months, which suppresses ovulation by suppressing LH.	Irregular vaginal bleeding, weight gain, galactorrhea, acne, breast tenderness, mood changes, hair loss.
IUD	Causes local sterile inflammatory reaction within the wall of the uterus that prevents implantation.	Increased vaginal bleeding, uterine perforation, infection, increased risk of PID and ectopic pregnancy, IUD migration.
Barrier methods (e.g., condoms, diaphragms, sponges)	Physically block entrance of sperm into the uterine cavity. Protective effects against PID, STDs, and cervical cancer. When used with spermicides, condoms are as effective as OCPs.	Very few (possible allergic reactions to latex or spermicides).
Surgical sterilization (e.g., tubal ligation, vasectomy) *OB.50*	Tubes are ligated, cauterized, or mechanically occluded.	Essentially irreversible; bleeding, infection, failure, ectopic pregnancy.

The vagina normally contains mixed bacterial flora in an acidic environment (pH 3.5–4.5) maintained by lactic acid–producing lactobacilli. A change in this acidic environment (e.g., due to medications, illness, or frequent sexual intercourse) can lead to overgrowth of other bacterial species and hence to clinical infection. Vaginal infections are either bacterial (most commonly *Gardnerella vaginalis*), fungal (*Candida*), or protozoan (*Trichomonas*).

History/PE

Increased vaginal discharge is the most common symptom of **vulvovaginal pruritus** with or without a burning sensation or odor.

Differential

UTIs, STDs, normal physiologic secretions, malignancy.

Workup

Obtain vaginal discharge slide smears with saline and KOH (see Figure 2.12–4). A Gram stain of the vaginal discharge and chlamydia antigen tests should also be performed to rule out STDs. Also obtain a clean-catch urine culture and a UA to rule out UTI. Findings are noted in Table 2.12–3.

Treatment

See Table 2.12–3.

Complications

Increased risk of PID (with bacterial vaginosis). Increased risk of preterm labor or rupture of membranes if occurring during pregnancy.

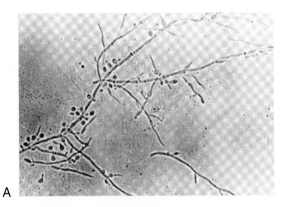
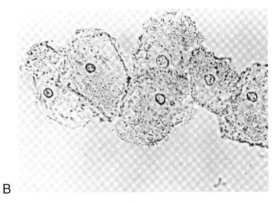

A   B

FIGURE 2.12–4. Causes of vaginitis. (A) Candidal vaginitis. Branched and budding *Candida albicans* are evident on KOH preparation of vaginal discharge. (B) *Gardnerella vaginalis.* Saline wet mount of vaginal fluid reveals granulations on vaginal epithelial cells ("clue cells") due to adherence of *G. vaginalis* organisms to the cell surface. (Reproduced, with permission, from DeCherney AH, *Current Obstetric & Gynecologic Diagnosis & Treatment,* 8th ed., Stamford, CT: Appleton & Lange, 1994: p. 692, Figs. 34–2 and 34–4.)

HIGH-YIELD FACTS

Gynecology

TABLE 2.12–3. Causes of Vaginitis

Variable	Bacterial Vaginosis (usually *Gardnerella*)	*Trichomonas*	Yeast (usually *Candida*)
Relative frequency	50%	25% (may coexist with bacterial vaginosis)	25%
Exam	Mild vaginal irritation	Strawberry petechiae in upper vagina/cervix	Erythematous, excoriated vulva/vagina
Discharge	Homogenous, grayish-white, watery, fishy and stale odor	Profuse, malodorous, yellow-green, frothy	Thick, white, cottage-cheese texture
Vaginal pH	> 4.5	> 4.5	Normal vaginal pH
Saline smear*	**Clue cells** (epithelial cells coated with bacteria; see Figure 2.12–4B)	**Motile trichomonads** (flagellated organisms just larger than WBCs)	Nothing
KOH prep	Positive whiff test (**fishy smell**)	Whiff test may be positive	**Pseudohyphae** (see Figure 2.12–4A)
Treatment	Metronidazole (oral or intravaginal cream)**	Oral metronidazole.** **Treat partner;** this is considered an STD. Test for coexisting STDs.	Topical antifungals (miconazole, nystatin)

*On saline smear, if you see lots of WBCs and no organism, suspect chlamydia.
**Patients taking metronidazole should not drink alcohol, which would lead to an Antabuse-like effect. Not recommended during pregnancy owing to teratogenic effects.

UCV *OB.1, 30, 31*

CERVICITIS

Neisseria gonorrhoeae and *Chlamydia trachomatis* can infect the glandular epithelium of the cervix. Both organisms cause a yellowish-green, mucopurulent cervical discharge.

History/PE

Patients may complain of discharge, dyspareunia (painful intercourse), or postcoital bleeding, or they may be asymptomatic. Examination reveals a purulent endocervical discharge along with erythema and edema of the endocervix.

Evaluation

Intracellular gram-negative diplococci on smear yields a diagnosis of gonorrhea; if negative, a presumptive diagnosis of chlamydial cervicitis is made, which can be confirmed in several days by culture. Culture for *N. gonorrhoeae* on Thayer–Martin agar; immunoassays for chlamydia should also be obtained.

Treatment

Ceftriaxone for gonorrhea; doxycycline or azithromycin for chlamydia (erythromycin if pregnant). Sexual partners should also be treated.

(See the Infectious Disease section, p. 207, for further discussion of STDs.)

Ascending genital tract infection secondary to cervical and/or vaginal infection. Causes of PID include *Neisseria gonorrhoeae*, *Chlamydia trachomatis*, and aerobic/anaerobic bacteria. Risk factors include multiple sexual partners, unprotected sexual intercourse, high frequency of intercourse, high-risk behavior, young age at first intercourse, and IUD use. Use of OCPs and barrier contraception decreases the incidence of PID.

Use of OCPs and barrier contraception decreases the incidence of PID.

History

One- to three-day history of **lower abdominal pain** with or without fever, **vaginal discharge, recent menses,** history of sexual exposure, or a past history of PID. Patients often believe they have appendicitis (especially if pain is right-sided).

PE

Diffuse lower **abdominal tenderness, cervical motion tenderness (CMT), adnexal tenderness,** and/or purulent cervical discharge.

Differential

Ectopic pregnancy, endometriosis, ovarian tumors, hemorrhagic ovarian cyst, appendicitis, UTI, diverticulitis.

Evaluation

"Chandelier sign": severe CMT on exam that makes the patient "jump for the chandelier."

The diagnosis of PID is made in the presence of clinical findings along with **leukocytosis** (WBC > 10,000) and **fever** (> 38°C), plus a swab for chlamydia or gonorrhea, pus in the cul de sac, or abscess on examination or ultrasound. Obtain β-HCG (to check pregnancy status) and Gram stain/cultures of the cervical discharge. Consider RPR/VDRL, HIV serology, and hepatitis serology. For definitive diagnosis, consider ultrasound, culdocentesis, and/or laparoscopy.

Treatment

Antibiotic treatment should address the most common pathogens (e.g., *N. gonorrhoeae*, *C. trachomatis*, and anaerobes).

- **Inpatient IV antibiotic regimen:** Cefoxitin and doxycycline.
- **Outpatient antibiotic regimen:** Ceftriaxone and doxycycline for 2–4 weeks.

Hospitalize for pelvic or tubo-ovarian abscess, pregnancy, peritonitis, nausea/vomiting (preventing PO intake of meds), failure of the outpatient regimen to improve symptoms in 48 hours, or high fever or WBC.

Complications

Tubo-ovarian abscess (TOA) should be suspected in patients with severe pain, high fever, nausea/vomiting, signs of sepsis, peritoneal signs, or adnexal mass (if examination is even possible). TOA requires hospitalization for IV antibiotics and hydration and possible surgical intervention (drainage or TAH/BSO). Other complications include **ectopic pregnancy,** chronic pelvic pain, **infertility,** and Fitz-Hugh–Curtis syndrome (perihepatitis with RUQ pain; occurs in 5–10% of PID patients).

UCV OB.18

ENDOMETRIOSIS

Defined as the presence of endometrial glands and stroma outside the uterus. The most common sites of endometriosis are the ovaries, broad ligament, and cul de sac. Proposed etiologies include direct implantation of endometrial cells by retrograde menstruation, vascular and lymphatic dissemination of endometrial cells, and metaplasia within the peritoneal cavity. Risk factors include positive family history, nulliparity, and infertility.

History/PE

Dysmenorrhea, **dyschezia** (painful defecation), **chronic pelvic pain, dyspareunia,** abnormal bleeding, and/or **infertility.** Pelvic examination may reveal nodular thickening along the uterosacral ligament, a fixed, retroverted uterus, and/or tender, fixed adnexal masses.

Endometriosis is the most common cause of infertility.

Differential

PID, pelvic adhesions, ectopic pregnancy, appendicitis, adnexal torsion, ruptured corpus luteal cyst, primary/secondary amenorrhea, endometrioma.

Evaluation

Definitive diagnosis can be made by **laparoscopic examination**/biopsy, which will reveal functioning endometrial glands, **"chocolate cysts,"** or dark, spotted "powder-burn" lesions. Laboratory tests include β-HCG, UA, and ultrasound (may reveal endometriomas).

Treatment

Medical options include suppressing ovulation and menstruation with OCPs or progestin and suppressing estrogen production with danazol or GnRH agonists. Surgical options include **laparoscopic ablation** of visible endometriosis or **total abdominal hysterectomy** with lysis of adhesions in patients with severe, recurrent disease.

UCV OB.10

UTERINE LEIOMYOMA

The most **common** benign gynecologic lesion, also known as uterine fibroids. More common in black women and those > 35 years of age. Leiomyomas can change in size with the menstrual cycle but usually regress after menopause.

History

Asymptomatic or may present with dysmenorrhea, abdominal pain, menorrhagia (excessive uterine bleeding), metrorrhagia (irregular uterine bleeding), anemia, infertility, or urinary frequency.

PE

Firm, irregular, palpable uterine mass on pelvic examination.

Differential

Cervical or endometrial carcinoma, leiomyosarcoma, pregnancy, ovarian carcinoma, endometriosis, adenomyosis.

Evaluation

The condition can usually be diagnosed by **ultrasound.**

Treatment

- Can be followed with **ultrasound.**
- If symptoms worsen, the lesion can be **resected.** Myomectomy is performed if fertility is to be preserved; hysterectomy if not.
- Rarely, a myoma resected for symptomatic relief turns out to be a leiomyosarcoma, an aggressive tumor that is usually not responsive to therapy.

UCV OB.28

POLYCYSTIC OVARIAN SYNDROME

Also known as Stein–Leventhal syndrome, polycystic ovarian syndrome affects **women aged 15–30,** resulting in chronic amenorrhea and infertility. It is thought to involve a disorder of the hypothalamic–pituitary axis in which excess LH and androgen production causes virilization and anovulation with cyst formation in the ovary (see Figure 2.12–5).

History

Hirsutism, amenorrhea/oligomenorrhea, **obesity,** and **infertility.**

PE

Bilaterally enlarged ovaries are found on bimanual exam. Patients also present with acne.

If a uterine mass continues to grow after menopause, it is not a leiomyoma.

HIGH-YIELD FACTS

Gynecology

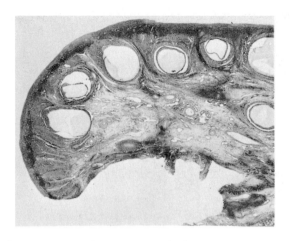

FIGURE 2.12–5. Polycystic ovary with prominent multiple cysts. (Reproduced, with permission, from DeCherney AH, *Current Obstetric & Gynecologic Diagnosis & Treatment*, 8th ed., Stamford, CT: Appleton & Lange, 1994: p. 747, Fig. 37–3.)

Differential

Androgen-secreting ovarian tumor, endometriosis, adrenal tumor, Cushing's syndrome, congenital adrenal hyperplasia.

Evaluation

Findings include a **serum LH:FSH ratio > 3** and **increased serum androstenedione and DHEA.** Ultrasound shows bilaterally enlarged ovaries with numerous large subcapsular cysts.

Treatment

Weight reduction alone may resolve symptoms; **clomiphene citrate** (induces ovulation and may result in multiple pregnancies) and **OCPs** (which suppress pituitary LH secretion) may also be given.

Complications

Infertility, increased risk of ovarian torsion, increased risk of diabetes and endometrial cancer (secondary to unopposed estrogen stimulation).

UCV *OB.20*

GYNECOLOGIC MALIGNANCIES

BREAST CANCER

Risk factors include breast cancer in first-degree relatives, personal history of breast cancer, history of benign breast disease with atypia, nulliparity, early menarche, and late menopause. Women who have their first child at age 35 or older are also at greater risk. Risk is decreased by late menarche. Breast cancer is rarely seen in males. BRCA1 and BRCA2 mutations are associated with multiple/early-onset breast and ovarian cancer.

Increased exposure to estrogen (early menarche, late menopause, nulliparity) increases the risk of breast cancer.

History

Patients can present with a **breast lump,** breast infection, or **nipple discharge.** Many are asymptomatic and present with a nonpalpable **mammographic abnormality.** Breast cancer most often presents in the **upper outer quadrant** of the breast.

PE

Firm, immobile, painless lump in the breast; **skin changes** (redness, ulceration, edema, nodularity) and axillary adenopathy indicate more advanced disease.

Differential

Mammary dysplasia, fibroadenoma, papilloma *(OB.14)*, mastitis, fat necrosis.

Evaluation

Diagnosis is suggested by a palpable mass or by **mammographic abnormalities** (microcalcifications, hyperdense regions). **Ultrasound** may be used to examine a lump (if cystic, follow or biopsy; if solid, proceed to biopsy). **Biopsy** may be performed by multiple modalities: direct needle/core biopsy (of a palpable lump), stereotactic core biopsy (of a mammographic lesion), or open surgical biopsy (with needle localization if there is no palpable mass). Special variants include:

- **Inflammatory breast cancer:** Highly malignant, rapidly growing, invades lymphatics; poor prognosis.
- **Paget's disease:** Ductal carcinoma in situ of the nipple with itching, burning, and erosion of the nipple (may be mistaken for infection).
- **Bilateral breast cancer** (more commonly seen with lobular carcinoma).

Treatment

Treatment depends on the type and stage:

- **Carcinoma in situ** (CIS) is classified as lobular (LCIS) or ductal (DCIS). LCIS carries a risk of subsequent invasive carcinoma in both breasts, so patients should elect either close follow-up or bilateral mastectomy (especially if there is a positive family history). DCIS can be treated with surgical excision plus radiation (no node dissection is necessary) and follow-up.
- **Invasive cancer** can also be either lobular or ductal. The tumor must be staged based on size, node status, and metastases (bone scan, CBC, serum calcium, and CXR). Localized disease can be treated either with lumpectomy + axillary node dissection + radiation or with mastectomy + axillary node dissection. The decision to use chemotherapy is based on the **number of positive nodes** or the presence of **metastases.**
- Positive **estrogen receptor status** makes tamoxifen therapy an option.
- Metastatic or recurrent disease is treated with chemotherapy +/– BMT.
- Metastatic sites include **bone marrow, chest wall, brain,** and **liver.**

Positive estrogen receptor status of the tumor is a good prognostic factor.

Prevention

- **Monthly breast self-exam** for women ≥ 20 years old.

- **Clinical breast exam** every 2–3 years until age 40, then annually.
- **Screening mammography** should be performed yearly in all women > 40–50 years old and earlier in patients with a positive family history.
- Data suggest that prophylactic **tamoxifen** therapy decreases the incidence of breast cancer in high-risk women (those with a positive family history). Tamoxifen increases the risk of uterine cancer, so this is an individual decision.
- Consider genetic testing in high-risk families.
- Do not use estrogen replacement therapy in postmenopausal women with estrogen receptor–positive breast cancer.

UCV *OB.2, 3*

CERVICAL CANCER

Risk factors include intercourse early in life, multiple sexual partners, **tobacco use,** and HPV infection.

History

Cervical cancer is usually diagnosed in asymptomatic patients by Pap smear, colposcopy, and biopsy, but patients may present with dysfunctional uterine bleeding, **postcoital bleeding,** pelvic pain, and vaginal discharge.

PE

Cervical discharge/ulceration, pelvic mass, or fistulas.

Differential

Cervicitis, vaginitis, STDs, actinomycosis.

Evaluation

A positive Pap smear/colposcopy must be followed with cone biopsy. The diagnosis may be invasive cervical carcinoma or cervical intraepithelial neoplasia (CIN), which is divided into low-grade squamous intraepithelial lesion (LSIL) and high-grade squamous intraepithelial lesion (HSIL).

Treatment

- CIN is usually treated with **cryosurgery** or **loop resection** (LSIL) or with **conization** of the cervix (HSIL/carcinoma in situ).
- Invasive carcinoma is treated with **surgical resection**—simple **hysterectomy** for early disease, and radical hysterectomy +/– radiation for advanced/extracervical disease.

Prevention

- **Annual Pap smears** should be obtained beginning with the onset of sexual activity or at 18 years of age. Indeterminate (atypical squamous cells of undetermined significance—ASCUS) or low-grade lesions are followed up in 3–6 months. After three consecutive normal Pap smears, regular screening may resume.

UCV *OB.4*

Screening with annual Pap smears has dramatically reduced the incidence of invasive cervical cancer.

ENDOMETRIAL CANCER

Usually adenocarcinoma (70–80%), endometrial cancer is more common than vaginal or ovarian cancers and carries a better prognosis. Its incidence is strongly linked to exposure to high levels of estrogen, as with exogenous estrogens, polycystic ovarian syndrome, ovarian granulosa cell tumors, obesity, and tamoxifen. Other risk factors are diabetes, hypertension, nulliparity, and positive family history. Peak incidence is between 50 and 70 years of age.

Metastasis of endometrial cancer occurs by direct extension (to the cervix), by intraperitoneal seeding, lymphatically (to the aortic and pelvic nodes), or hematogenously (to the lungs and vagina). Lymph node metastases have a high incidence of recurrence.

History/PE

Postmenopausal bleeding should never be attributed to atrophic vaginitis until endometrial sampling has ruled out carcinoma.

Abnormally heavy menstrual bleeding, bleeding midcycle, or postmenopausal bleeding. With cancer that has spread to the adnexa and peritoneum, the uterus may be fixed and immobile on exam. Patients may complain of lower abdominal pain and cramping.

Evaluation

- Endometrial biopsy shows hyperplasia and anaplasia of glandular cells with invasion of stroma, myometrium, or blood vessels. If the sample is inadequate, curettage is used. Although the Pap smear may incidentally detect disease in asymptomatic patients, it is *not* a very sensitive test for confirming a diagnosis.
- CA-125 levels are elevated.
- Chest x-ray may show metastases in patients with advanced disease.
- Staging is done surgically.

Treatment

- Total abdominal hysterectomy and bilateral salpingo-oophorectomy (TAH-BSO).
- Adjuvant radiation therapy in patients with cervical involvement.
- **Hormone therapy:** Progesterone and/or tamoxifen when surgery and irradiation fail (best response rate with well-differentiated tumors).
- **Chemotherapy:** Doxorubicin and cisplatin are also used for advanced or recurrent endometrial cancer.

UCV *OB.9*

EVALUATION OF AN ADNEXAL MASS

- Note risk factors for malignancy (family history, nulliparity, infertility), previous malignancy, and previous ovarian cysts (e.g., polycystic ovarian syndrome). Feel for a palpable mass. Check for ascites, cervical motion tenderness, and abdominal tenderness.
- Perform a transvaginal ultrasound.
- CT/MRI may help delineate the lesion.

- Check CA-125 level.
- The mass should be **resected** if imaging suggests possible malignancy, if the patient has risk factors for ovarian cancer, and if CA-125 is elevated.

OVARIAN CANCER

Risk factors for ovarian cancer include a family history of **breast or ovarian cancer, infertility,** and **nulliparity.** BRCA1 and BRCA2 syndromes are associated with an increased risk of breast and ovarian cancer.

History

Ovarian cancer is **usually asymptomatic until late in the course of the disease.** Patients may present with abdominal pain and bloating, early satiety, constipation, vaginal bleeding, and systemic symptoms (fatigue, malaise, weight loss).

PE

Physical findings can include a palpable abdominal/adnexal mass and ascites **(increasing abdominal girth).**

Differential

Uterine leiomyomas (should not increase in size after menopause), ectopic pregnancy, pelvic kidney, retroperitoneal fibrosis/tumor, colorectal cancer, PID, ovarian cyst, metastasis.

Evaluation

Elevated CA-125; transvaginal ultrasound and possibly CT/MRI; biopsy with **diagnostic laparoscopy or open resection.** Epithelial tumors are the most common histologic variant; other types include germ cell/functional tumors.

CA-125 levels may be elevated in ovarian cancer.

Treatment

- Primary therapy consists of **resection** as part of a **TAH/BSO.**
- Postsurgical **chemotherapy** (cisplatin, paclitaxel) is warranted for almost all patients.
- Ovarian cancer has a **poor prognosis;** most recur despite treatment.
- Germ cell tumors may be treated with radiation therapy.

Prevention

- Women with a strong family history (two or more affected first-degree relatives) can be screened annually with **CA-125** and **transvaginal ultrasound. Prophylactic oophorectomy** is sometimes recommended after childbearing is complete.
- **Oral contraceptive** use decreases the risk of ovarian cancer.

HIGH-YIELD FACTS

Gynecology

First test to perform when a woman presents with amenorrhea.	β-HCG; the most common cause of amenorrhea is pregnancy
Cause of amenorrhea with normal prolactin, no response to estrogen–progesterone challenge, and history of D&C.	Asherman's syndrome
First-line conservative therapy for polycystic ovarian syndrome.	Weight loss
Diagnostic step required in a postmenopausal woman who presents with vaginal bleeding.	Endometrial biopsy
Indications for medical treatment of ectopic pregnancy.	Stable unruptured ectopic pregnancy < 3.5 cm and < 6 weeks' gestation
Medical options for endometriosis.	OCPs, danazol, GnRH agonists
Uterine bleeding at 18 weeks' gestation; no products expelled; cervical os closed.	Threatened abortion
Uterine bleeding at 18 weeks' gestation; no products expelled; membranes ruptured; cervical os open.	Inevitable abortion
Laparoscopic findings in endometriosis.	Chocolate cysts, powder burns
How to diagnose and follow leiomyoma.	Ultrasound
Natural history of leiomyoma.	Regress after menopause
Patient complains of increased vaginal discharge; on exam, petechial patches seen in upper vagina and cervix.	*Trichomonas* vaginitis
Treatment for bacterial vaginosis.	Oral or topical metronidazole
Contraceptive methods that protect against PID.	OCP and barrier contraception
Causes of secondary amenorrhea with elevated prolactin levels.	Pituitary tumor, hypothyroidism, or dopamine antagonists
Unopposed estrogen contraindicated in which cancers?	Endometrial or estrogen receptor-positive breast cancer
Patient with recent PID complains of right upper quadrant pain.	Consider Fitz-Hugh–Curtis syndrome, perihepatic inflammation following PID
Breast malignancy presenting as itching, burning, and erosion of the nipple.	Paget's disease
Annual screening for women with family history of ovarian cancer.	CA-125 and transvaginal ultrasound

The following clinical questions and accompanying answers are reproduced, with permission, from Evans MI, *PreTest: Ob/Gyn*, 9th ed., New York: McGraw-Hill, 2001.

Questions

1. A 62-year-old woman presents for annual examination. Her last spontaneous menstrual period was nine years ago, and she has been reluctant to use postmenopausal hormone replacement because of a strong family history of breast cancer. She now complains of diminished interest in sexual activity. Which of the following is the most likely cause of her complaint?
   a. Decreased vaginal length
   b. Decreased ovarian function
   c. Alienation from her partner
   d. Untreatable sexual dysfunction
   e. Physiologic anorgasmia

2. Which of the following contraceptives appear to increase the risk for development of pelvic inflammatory disease?
   a. Condoms without spermicide
   b. Oral contraceptives
   c. Intrauterine device
   d. Diaphragm
   e. Vasectomy

3. A patient is diagnosed with carcinoma of the breast. The most important prognostic factor in the treatment of this disease is
   a. Age at diagnosis
   b. Size of tumor
   c. Axillary metastases
   d. Estrogen receptors on the tumor
   e. Progesterone receptors on the tumor

4. Women who have ovarian carcinoma most commonly present with which of the following symptoms?
   a. Vaginal bleeding and anorexia
   b. Weight loss and dyspareunia
   c. Nausea and vaginal discharge
   d. Constipation and frequent urination
   e. Abdominal distention and pain

5. Women who have endometrial carcinoma most frequently present with which of the following symptoms?
   a. Bloating
   b. Weight loss
   c. Postmenopausal bleeding
   d. Vaginal discharge
   e. Hemoptysis

1. **The answer is b.** Sexuality continues despite aging. However, there are physiologic changes that must be recognized. Diminished ovarian function may lower libido, but estrogen replacement therapy (ERT) may help. Sexual dysfunction can be physiologic, e.g., from lowered libido. As with younger patients, however, lowered libido is in most cases treatable. Because aging does not alter the capacity for orgasm or produce vaginismus, a further evaluation should be initiated if these symptoms persist after a postmenopausal woman is placed on ERT.

2. **The answer is c.** Acute salpingitis, or pelvic inflammatory disease (PID), is a disease predominantly of nulliparous young women. The intrauterine device (IUD) increases the risk of developing salpingitis three- to fivefold; the number of sexual partners and the incidence of sexually transmitted disease in a population also influence the development of PID in IUD users. Oral contraceptives are felt to have a protective effect on developing infections; the risk is 30–90% that of nonusers. Condoms, diaphragms, and chemical barriers also provide protection from disease. Vasectomy does not appear to influence the risk for development of PID.

3. **The answer is c.** Recognition of the high risk associated with axillary metastases for early death and poor five-year survival have led to the use of postsurgical adjuvant chemotherapy in these patients. Patients who have estrogen- or progesterone-receptive tumors (i.e., receptor present or receptor positive) are particular candidates for this adjuvant therapy, as 60% of estrogen-positive tumors will respond to hormonal therapy. Age and size of the tumor are certainly factors of importance, but they are secondary in importance to the presence or absence of axillary metastases.

4. **The answer is e.** Approximately 50% of women who have ovarian cancer present with abdominal distention, and 50% present with abdominal pain. Gastrointestinal symptoms, which occur in about 20% of affected women, are often secondary to the development of ascites or partial bowel obstruction from the tumor. Urinary tract symptoms, caused by the pressure exerted by a rapidly growing mass, and abnormal vaginal bleeding are the initial symptoms of ovarian cancer in only 15% of affected women.

5. **The answer is c.** Postmenopausal bleeding is the most common presenting symptom of women who have endometrial carcinoma. Because this warning signal is present even in the earliest stages of disease, early diagnosis and treatment are possible and likely.

Pediatrics

Autosomal trisomies

Down's syndrome (trisomy 21), 1:700	**Most common chromosomal disorder** and cause of congenital mental retardation. **Findings:** mental retardation, flat facial profile, prominent epicanthal folds, simian crease, duodenal atresia, congenital heart disease (most common malformation is endocardial cushion defect), Alzheimer's disease in affected individuals > 35 years old, increased risk of ALL. Ninety-five percent of cases are due to meiotic nondisjunction of homologous chromosomes; **meiotic nondisjunction** is associated with **advanced maternal age** (from 1:1500 in women < 20 to 1:25 in women > 45). Four percent of cases are due to Robertsonian translocation, and 1% of cases are due to Down mosaicism (no maternal association).	Drinking age (21) "**ALL** or **ALL**zheimer's go **DOWN** together."
Edwards' syndrome (trisomy 18), 1:8000	Findings: severe mental retardation, rocker bottom feet, low-set ears, micrognathia, congenital heart disease, clenched hands (flexion of fingers), prominent occiput. Death usually occurs within one year of birth.	Election age (18)
Patau's syndrome (trisomy 13), 1:6000	Findings: severe mental retardation, microphthalmia, microcephaly, cleft lip/palate, abnormal forebrain structures, polydactyly, congenital heart disease. Death usually occurs within one year of birth.	Puberty (13)

Genetic gender disorders

Klinefelter's syndrome [male] (XXY), 1:850 *Path2.4, Bio.23*	Testicular atrophy, eunuchoid body shape, tall, long extremities, gynecomastia, female hair distribution. Presence of inactivated X chromosome (Barr body).	One of the most common causes of hypogonadism in males.
Turner's syndrome [female] (XO), 1:3000 *Path2.6*	Short stature, ovarian dysgenesis, webbing of neck, coarctation of the aorta, most common cause of primary amenorrhea. No Barr body.	"Hugs & kisses" (XO) from Tina **Turner** (female).
Double Y males [male] (XYY), 1:1000	Phenotypically normal, very tall, severe acne, antisocial behavior (seen in 1–2% of XYY males).	Observed with increased frequency among inmates of penal institutions.

Common congenital malformations

1. Heart defects (congenital rubella)
2. Hypospadias
3. Cleft lip with or without cleft palate
4. Congenital hip dislocation
5. Spina bifida
6. Anencephaly
7. Pyloric stenosis (associated with polyhydramnios); projectile vomiting

Neural tube defects (spina bifida and anencephaly) are associated with increased levels of A-FP (in the amniotic fluid and maternal serum). Their incidence is decreased with maternal folate ingestion during pregnancy.

Congenital heart disease

R-to-L shunts (early cyanosis) "blue babies"	1. Tetralogy of Fallot (most common cause of early cyanosis)
	2. Transposition of great vessels
	3. Truncus arteriosus
		The 3 T's:
		  Tetralogy
		  Transposition
		  Truncus
		Children may squat to increase venous return.

L-to-R shunts (late cyanosis) "blue kids"	1. VSD (most common congenital cardiac anomaly) 2. ASD 3. PDA (close with indomethacin)	Frequency: VSD > ASD > PDA Increased pulmonary resistance due to arteriolar thickening. → progressive pulmonary hypertension; R → L shunt (Eisenmenger's).

Table 2.13–1 highlights major developmental milestones in the first three years of a child's life.

TABLE 2.13–1. Developmental Milestones

Age (months)	Motor	Social/Cognitive
2	Holds head up	Social smile
4–5	Rolls over; grasps object	Laughs
7	Sits without support	Stranger anxiety
9	Crawls	Says "Mama/Dada" (nonspecific)
12	Walks; pincer grasp	Says "Mama/Dada" (specific)
18	Runs	Names common objects
24	Walks up and down stairs	Uses 2-word combinations (**2 years = 2 words**) Understands 2-step commands
36	Pedals a tricycle; copies a circle	Uses plurals and 3-word combinations (**3 years = 3 words**)

CHILDHOOD VACCINATIONS

Table 2.13–2 summarizes the recommended timetable for childhood immunizations.

- Avoid live vaccines in immune-compromised patients (oral polio, varicella, MMR). However, MMR and varicella may be administered to HIV-positive patients without immune compromise.
- For previously unvaccinated patients, Hib is not necessary for patients > 5 years of age and pertussis is not necessary for patients > 6 years of age.

TABLE 2.13–2. Timetable for Childhood Vaccinations

Vaccine	Age
Diphtheria–tetanus–pertussis (DTP or DTaP)	2, 4, 6, 15–18 months/4–6 years; tetanus booster at 15 years and 10 years thereafter
Polio	2, 4, 6–18 months/4–6 years
MMR	> 12 months/4–6 years
H. influenzae type B (HIB)	2, 4, 6, 12 months
Varicella	> 12 months
Hepatitis B	Birth/1–4, 6–18 months

- HIB is not indicated in patients > 5 years of age.
- Avoid DTP in children with progressive neurologic disorders.
- Avoid influenza vaccine and MMR in patients with egg allergies.
- Asplenic patients should receive pneumococcal, meningococcal, and HIB vaccines.

FAILURE TO THRIVE (FTT)

Failure to thrive, or growth deficiency, refers to an infant or child whose weight or weight gain is significantly below that of children of similar age (Table 2.13–3). Cases are traditionally divided into two categories: **organic,** in which an underlying medical condition is responsible, and **inorganic** or psychosocial, in which no underlying medical condition can be found. Risk factors include chronic illness, low socioeconomic status, low maternal age, chaotic family situation, CF and other genetic diseases, and inborn errors of metabolism. Infants born with HIV comprise an increasing number of cases of FTT.

History

Patients are of **low weight for their age and height** and exhibit little or no weight gain or even weight loss. Note caloric intake and parent–child interaction.

PE

Plot height, weight, and head circumference on a standardized chart and compare the values to the population norms; look for signs of systemic disease.

Differential

The differential is vast **(often no organic cause is identified)** and includes poverty, inadequate breast feeding, improper feeding, mechanical GI dysfunction, structural abnormalities (e.g., pyloric stenosis, intestinal atresia), infection, endocrine disease, congenital heart disease, lung disease, and neurologic disorders.

TABLE 2.13–3. Definitions of Failure to Thrive

Attained growth

    Weight < 3rd percentile on NCHS* growth chart

    Weight for height < 5th percentile on NCHS growth chart

    Weight 20% or more below ideal weight for height

    Triceps skin-fold thickness ≤ 5 mm

Rate of growth

    Depressed rate of weight gain

        < 20 g/day from 0–3 months of age

        < 15 g/day from 3–6 months of age

    Falloff from previously established growth curve:

        downward crossing of ≥ 2 major percentiles on NCHS growth charts

    Documented weight loss

*NCHS = National Center for Health Statistics.

Evaluation

Evaluation should include CBC, electrolytes, creatinine, albumin, total protein, sweat test, UA/culture, stool ova and parasites, and assessment of bone age. Take a careful diet history, including calorie count.

Treatment

Hospitalize children if there is evidence of neglect or severe malnourishment.

Treatment depends on cause.

- Start a calorie count.
- Encourage **nutritional supplementation** if breast feeding is inadequate (a common cause of early FTT is poorly managed mammary engorgement).
- **Hospitalize** the patient if there is evidence of neglect or severe malnourishment.

IMMUNODEFICIENCY DISORDERS

Congenital immunodeficiencies are rare, with an overall frequency of about 1 in 10,000. **B-cell deficiencies** are the most common (50%) and generally present with recurrent URIs and bacteremia with encapsulated organisms (pneumococcus, *Staphylococcus*, *H. influenzae*); they are likely to present **after 6 months of age,** when transplacentally acquired maternal antibodies decline. **T-cell deficiencies** tend to present earlier (1–3 months) and with a broader range of infections, including fungal, viral, and intracellular bacteria (e.g., mycobacteria), and may also secondarily cause B-cell dysfunction. **Phagocyte defects** characteristically result in mucous membrane infections and poor wound healing; catalase-positive (*S. aureus*) and enteric gram-negative organisms are typical. Distinguishing features of specific immunodeficiencies are listed in Table 2.13–4.

Treatment

Treatment is as follows:

- **B-cell disorders:** Generally, prophylactic antibiotic treatment, but IVIG may be used in X-linked agammaglobulinemia and common variable disease.
- **T-cell disorders:** If severe, bone marrow transplantation; IVIG if humoral immunity is affected as well.
- **Phagocytic disorders:** Antibiotics; surgical debridement of wounds.

TABLE 2.13–4. Pediatric Immunodeficiency Disorders

Disorder	Description
B-cell	
X-linked (Bruton's) agammaglobulinemia	Males only. Profound B-cell deficiency; may present < 6 months. *Pseudomonas* infections.
Ped.36	Initially normal, immunoglobulin levels drop severely in the second
Common variable immunodeficiency	or third decade of life. Recurrent URIs; **chronic diarrhea** and **autoimmune disease.**
T-cell	
DiGeorge syndrome	Agenesis of the third and fourth pharyngeal pouch. **CATCH 22** = **C**ardiac anomalies, **A**bnormal facies, **T**hymic hypoplasia, **C**left palate, **H**ypocalcemia, defect on chromosome **22.** May result in severe combined immunodeficiency.
Ataxia–telangectasia	Cutaneous and conjunctival telangectasias and cerebellar ataxia with decreased T-cell function and antibody levels.
Combined	
Severe combined immunodeficiency (SCID) *Ped.37*	Profound lack of T and B cells. Severe bacterial infections, chronic candidiasis, opportunistic organisms. Skin manifestations (eczema) due to graft-versus-host disease.
Phagocytic	
Chronic granulomatous disease	X-linked; affects males only. Deficient **superoxide** production by neutrophils and macrophages. Lymphadenopathy, hypergammaglobu-linemia, anemia; many sites affected: chronic bronchitis, GI infec-tions, UTIs, osteomyelitis, hepatitis.
Chédiak–Higashi syndrome	Autosomal recessive; defect of neutrophil **chemotaxis.** Oculocutaneous albinism, neuropathy, **neutropenia.**

CHILD ABUSE

Includes physical abuse, sexual abuse, emotional abuse, neglect, and, rarely, Munchausen's syndrome by proxy. The diagnosis of physical abuse is based on a **history discordant with the physical findings.**

Red flags should rise if the caretaker's story does not match the child's injury.

History

Pain, swelling, and multiple ecchymoses. Infants may present with irritability and failure to thrive. Evidence of neglect (poor hygiene) may be noted.

PE

Physical findings may include the following:

- **Cutaneous findings:** Oddly situated (e.g., head/face, back, thighs) **bruises of varying ages** (note: bruises on the shins, elbows, and knees occur with normal childhood activity) as well as **pattern injuries** such as wire-loop marks (electrical cords), burns (cigarettes, immersion, etc.), and belt marks. Ophthalmologic examination may reveal **retinal hemorrhages** (shaken baby syndrome; see Clinical Images, plate. 7).

- **Skeletal trauma: Spiral fractures** of the humerus and femur in patients < 3 years of age indicate abuse until proven otherwise; **epiphyseal/metaphyseal injuries** in infants are suggestive as well (they result from pulling, twisting, or shaking of the limbs). Look for **rib injuries** in infants < 2 years (ribs are extremely pliant).
- **Sexual abuse:** Symptoms of **STDs, genital trauma,** or behavioral abnormalities.

Spiral fractures suggest child abuse.

Evaluation

Skeletal survey shows multiple fractures in various stages of healing. Perform coagulation studies if there are multiple bruises. Obtain gonorrhea and chlamydia cultures and HIV testing if sexual abuse is suspected. Ophthalmic exam may reveal retinal hemorrhages. In a shaken baby, CT may reveal bilateral subdural hemorrhages, and MRI will show white matter changes.

Treatment

Notify child protective services (CPS) for appropriate evaluation and possible removal from the home environment. If the child is in immediate danger, consider hospitalizing to ensure safety pending CPS evaluation.

UCV *Ped.53, Psych.13*

CEREBRAL PALSY (CP)

A broad term used to describe a range of **nonprogressive,** nonhereditary disorders of impaired motor function and posture. CP most commonly results from a perinatal neurologic insult. Risk factors include prematurity, mental retardation, low birth weight, fetal malformation, neonatal seizures, neonatal cerebral hemorrhage, and perinatal asphyxia. Categories of CP include:

- **Pyramidal (spastic):** About 75% of cases are pyramidal; such cases involve spastic paresis of any or all limbs. Approximately 90% of patients are mentally retarded.
- **Extrapyramidal (nonspastic):** Extrapyramidal CP results from damage to extrapyramidal tracts. This category includes choreoathetoid, ataxic, rigid, hypotonic, and dystonic types. Movements worsen with stress and disappear during sleep.
- **Mixed:** Marked by spasticity and extrapyramidal symptoms.

History/PE

Patients may have an associated **seizure** disorder, **mental retardation,** or sensory and speech deficits. **Contractures** of the upper and lower extremities are common. Hip dysplasia/dislocation and scoliosis may develop.

Differential

Metabolic disorders, cerebellar dysgenesis, spinocerebellar degeneration.

Evaluation

EEG may be useful in patients with seizures; otherwise CP is largely a **clinical diagnosis.**

Treatment

Administer diazepam, dantrolene, or baclofen for spasticity. Special education, physical therapy, bracing, and surgical release/lengthening of contractures are often helpful. Baclofen pumps and posterior rhizotomy may alleviate contractures in severe cases.

UCV *Neuro.5*

FEBRILE SEIZURES

Fever-associated seizures that occur in children 6 months to 6 years of age.

History/PE

Febrile seizures may be classified as simple or complex.

- **Simple:** High fever (> 39°C), short duration (< 15 minutes), **generalized,** one per 24-hour period, fever onset within hours of the seizure.
- **Complex:** Low-grade fever, duration > 15 minutes, **focal** seizure, > 1 seizure per 24-hour period, fever for several days before seizure onset.

Etiologies

Meningitis, sepsis, dehydration, electrolyte imbalance, CNS malformations, tumors, intoxication.

Evaluation

None indicated if the presentation is consistent with febrile seizures. Obtain electrolytes, serum glucose, blood cultures, UA, and CBC with differential if presentation is atypical. Perform an LP if CNS infection is suspected. Obtain an **EEG and MRI** of the brain for **complex febrile seizures.**

Perform LP if CNS infection is suspected in a patient with a febrile seizure.

Treatment

Administer **antipyretics** (acetaminophen; avoid aspirin in children owing to the risk of Reye's syndrome) and treat underlying illness. Children with febrile seizures should receive aggressive antipyretic therapy even with low-grade fevers. Children with complex febrile seizures should have a thorough neurologic evaluation and may require chronic anticonvulsant therapy.

Complications

For simple febrile seizures there is **no increased risk** of epilepsy or of developmental, intellectual, or growth abnormalities. With complex seizures, the risk of epilepsy is 10%.

Patients with complex febrile seizures may require chronic anticonvulsant therapy.

UCV *Neuro.42*

An acute inflammatory disease of the larynx, primarily within the subglottic space; also known as **laryngotracheobronchitis**. Croup affects children from 3 months to 5 years of age. **Parainfluenza type 1** is the most common pathogen; others include parainfluenza type 2 and 3, RSV, influenza, rubeola, adenovirus, and Mycoplasma pneumoniae.

History/PE

There is usually a prodrome of URI symptoms followed by low-grade fever, mild dyspnea, inspiratory stridor that worsens with agitation, and the characteristic **barking cough** (usually at night).

Differential

Epiglottitis, foreign body aspiration, bacterial tracheitis, angioedema, retropharyngeal abscess.

Evaluation

Diagnosis is primarily **clinical.** Lateral neck film may show subglottic narrowing (**"steeple sign"**; see Figure 2.13–1).

Treatment

- Manage mild cases **supportively** on an outpatient basis.
- **Mist therapy,** oxygen, **aerosolized racemic epinephrine,** and **corticosteroids** may be useful.
- Hospitalize patients with severe symptoms (such as stridor at rest).

UCV *Ped.28*

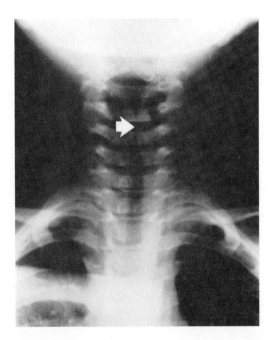

FIGURE 2.13–1. Croup. The x-ray shows marked subglottic narrowing of the airway (arrow). (Reproduced, with permission, from Saunders C, *Current Emergency Diagnosis & Treatment,* 4th ed., Stamford, CT: Appleton & Lange, 1992: p. 448, Fig. 26–9.)

A serious and rapidly progressive infection of the epiglottis and contiguous structures that can cause life-threatening airway obstruction. Epiglottitis affects **children aged 2–7** and is most commonly caused by ***Haemophilus influenzae* type B** infection. Other common pathogenic organisms include *Streptococcus* species and nontypeable *H. flu.* The incidence of epiglottitis has decreased with the widespread use of the *H. flu* vaccine.

Epiglottitis may cause life-threatening airway obstruction.

History/PE

Sudden-onset high **fever** (39–40°C), **dysphagia, drooling, muffled voice,** inspiratory retractions, cyanosis, and **soft stridor.** Patients sit with the neck hyperextended and the chin protruding (**"sniffing dog"** position). If untreated, it may progress to total airway obstruction and respiratory arrest.

Differential

Croup, tracheitis, foreign body aspiration, angioedema, retropharyngeal abscess (see Table 2.13–5).

Evaluation

Diagnosis is primarily clinical. **Do not examine the patient's throat** unless an anesthesiologist is present. Definitive diagnosis is made by direct fiberoptic vi-

Throat examination may precipitate laryngospasm and airway obstruction.

TABLE 2.13–5. Characteristics of Croup, Epiglottitis, and Tracheitis

Croup	Epiglottitis	Tracheitis
Age: 3 months to 5 years	Age: 2–7 years	Age: older child, but may affect any age
Usually viral etiology, commonly parainfluenza	*Haemophilus influenzae* type B, Group A *Streptococcus*	Often *Staphylococcus aureus*
Develops over **2–3 days**	**Rapid onset** over hours	**Gradual onset** over 2–3 days followed by acute decompensation
Low-grade fever	High fever	High fever
Usually only mild to moderate respiratory distress	Commonly severe respiratory distress	Commonly severe respiratory distress
Prefers sitting up, leaning against parent's chest	Prefers perched position with neck extended	May have position preference
Stridor improves with aerosolized racemic epinephrine	No response to racemic epinephrine	No response to racemic epinephrine
"Steeple sign" on AP neck films	"Thumbprint sign" on lateral neck films	Subglottic narrowing

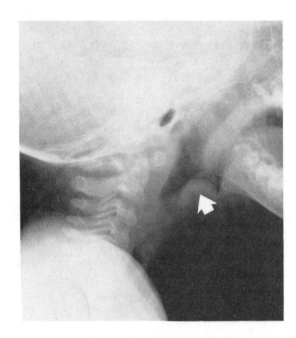

FIGURE 2.13–2. Epiglottitis. The classic swollen epiglottis ("thumbprint sign"; arrow) and obstructed airway are seen on lateral neck x-ray. (Reproduced, with permission, from Saunders C, *Current Emergency Diagnosis & Treatment,* 4th ed., Stamford, CT: Appleton & Lange, 1992: p. 447, Fig. 26–8B.)

sualization of cherry-red and swollen epiglottis and arytenoids. Lateral x-ray demonstrates a swollen epiglottis obliterating the valleculae (the classic **"thumbprint sign";** see Figure 2.13–2).

Treatment

This disease is a true emergency.

- Keep the patient (and his or her parents) calm, call anesthesia immediately, and **transfer the patient to the OR.**
- Treat with **endotracheal intubation** and **IV antibiotics** (ceftriaxone, chloramphenicol, ampicillin).

UCV *EM.25*

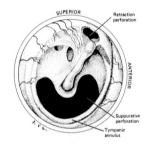

FIGURE 2.13–3. Perforated TM. Common sites of TM perforation. (Reproduced, with permission, from Saunders C, *Current Emergency Diagnosis & Treatment,* 4th ed., Stamford, CT: Appleton & Lange, 1992: p. 433, Fig. 26–2.)

OTITIS MEDIA

Middle ear infection most commonly caused by **S. pneumoniae, H. flu,** or **Moraxella catarrhalis.** Children are predisposed to otitis media because the middle ear canal is shorter and more horizontal in children than it is in adults. Other predisposing conditions include URIs, trisomy 21, CF, immune deficiencies, passive smoke exposure, day care, and previous ear infections.

History/PE

Parents may report **fever, ear tugging,** crying, **hearing loss, irritability,** feeding difficulties, and vomiting. Otoscopic examination may reveal a **bulging or hyperemic tympanic membrane (TM), decreased movement of the TM with insufflation, loss of the TM light reflex,** or TM perforation (Figure 2.13–3).

Differential

Otitis externa, toothache, foreign body in the ear, ear canal furuncle, ear canal trauma, hard cerumen.

Evaluation

Diagnosis is clinical.

Treatment

Treat with **amoxicillin for ten days;** amoxicillin–clavulanic acid or trimetho-prim–sulfamethoxazole may be required in recurrent otitis media to cover *H. flu.*

Complications

Mastoiditis, sigmoid sinus thrombosis, meningitis, brain abscess, hearing loss.

UCV *EM.12*

RESPIRATORY DISTRESS SYNDROME

The most common form of respiratory failure in **preterm infants;** results from **surfactant deficiency,** causing poor lung compliance and atelectasis. Respiratory distress syndrome is seen in 65% of infants born at 29–30 weeks' gestation.

History/PE

Patients present in the **first 48–72 hours of life** with a **respiratory rate > 60/min,** progressive **hypoxemia,** cyanosis, **nasal flaring, intercostal retractions,** and **expiratory grunting.**

Differential

Transient tachypnea of the newborn (TTN), meconium aspiration syndrome, congenital pneumonia, spontaneous pneumothorax, diaphragmatic hernia, cyanotic heart disease.

Evaluation

Evaluation depends primarily on characteristic CXR. Check ABGs, CBC, and blood cultures to rule out infection. Classic CXR findings include:

- **Respiratory distress syndrome:** Bilateral atelectasis causes a **"ground-glass"** appearance.
- **TTN:** Retained amniotic fluid causes prominent perihilar streaking in the interlobular fissures.
- **Meconium aspiration:** Coarse, irregular infiltrates and hyperexpansion.
- **Congenital pneumonia:** CXR is not helpful; neutropenia, tracheal aspirate, and Gram stain suggest the diagnosis.

Treatment

- **Intubation** is often required to maintain adequate oxygenation.
- **Surfactant replacement therapy** decreases mortality.
- Supportive care in a neonatal ICU is required.

- Prevent by administering **corticosteroids** to mothers at high risk for premature delivery and monitor fetal lung maturity with amniotic-fluid **lecithin-to-sphingomyelin ratio.**

UCV *Ped.41*

CARDIAC ANOMALIES

ATRIAL SEPTAL DEFECT (ASD)

An opening in the atrial septum that allows the flow of blood between the atria. It usually begins as a left-to-right shunt but may reverse if pulmonary hypertension develops **(Eisenmenger's syndrome).**

History

May present at any age, but usually not until late childhood or early adulthood. Presentation varies from asymptomatic to severe cyanosis and symptoms of CHF, depending on the size of the defect. Other symptoms include dyspnea, easy fatigability, and failure to thrive.

PE

Heaving cardiac impulse at the lower left sternal border, wide and often **fixed split S2,** and systolic ejection murmur (SEM) at the upper left sternal border; there may be a mid-diastolic rumble at the lower left sternal border, suggesting high flow.

Differential

Patent ductus arteriosus, VSD, aortopulmonary window.

Evaluation

Echo with color flow doppler is diagnostic, showing blood flow between the atria as well as paradoxic ventricular wall motion and a dilated right ventricle. EKG shows right-axis deviation; CXR shows cardiac enlargement and increased pulmonary vasculature markings.

Treatment

Small defects do not require treatment but should undergo preventive measures such as prophylactic antibiotics before dental procedures. Surgical closure is recommended for infants presenting with CHF and for patients with > 2:1 ratio of pulmonary to systemic blood flow. Early identification and correction of a defect improves the prognosis by preventing late complications such as **arrhythmias** and right ventricular dysfunction.

UCV *Surg.1*

VENTRICULAR SEPTAL DEFECT (VSD)

A congenital "hole" in the ventricular septum that causes symptoms which depend on the degree of **left-to-right** shunting. VSD can be membranous, perimembranous, or muscular (the last two often close spontaneously). VSDs are more common in patients with Apert's syndrome, Down's syndrome, cri-du-chat syndrome, and trisomies 13 and 18. VSD is the most common congenital heart defect.

VSD is the most common congenital heart defect.

History

Usually **asymptomatic** at birth if the defect is small. Frequent respiratory infections, failure to thrive, dyspnea, exercise intolerance, shortness of breath from pulmonary edema, and other symptoms of cardiac failure may be seen in severe cases.

PE

Pansystolic murmur at the lower left sternal border; loud pulmonic S2. If severe, systolic thrill, cardiomegaly, and crackles may be present.

Distinguish VSD from ASD by ASD's fixed, split S2.

Differential

Mitral regurgitation, aortic stenosis, cardiomyopathy, other congenital heart defects (including VSD as part of tetralogy of Fallot).

Evaluation

Diagnosis is made by clinical presentation and **echocardiogram.** EKG may show RVH or LVH. EKG is normal in patients with small VSDs.

Treatment

- Treat cardiac failure (with diuretics and inotropes) and respiratory infections.
- Follow small VSDs, since most will close spontaneously.
- Surgically repair large VSDs (or VSDs in patients with Down's syndrome) as soon as possible to prevent pulmonary vascular disease and heart failure.
- If a VSD remains open, Eisenmenger's syndrome may develop. Eisenmenger's syndrome is characterized by pulmonary vascular hyperplasia and consequent pulmonary hypertension that leads to RVH (cor pulmonale) and reversal to a right-to-left shunt. Eisenmenger's syndrome presents as cyanosis, is often **irreversible,** and may render the patient inoperable.
- Patients with patent VSDs are at increased risk for **endocarditis** and septic emboli.

Eisenmenger's syndrome: L → R shunt causes pulmonary hypertension and shunt reversal.

UCV Ped.3

PATENT DUCTUS ARTERIOSUS (PDA)

Failure of the ductus arteriosus to close within the first few days of life, resulting in a left-to-right shunt as blood flows from the aorta to the pulmonary artery. Risk factors include prematurity, high altitude (low O_2 tension), and maternal first-trimester rubella infection. It is more common in females and preterm infants.

History

Asymptomatic or may present with symptoms of heart failure, lower extremity clubbing, and dyspnea.

PE

Wide pulse pressure, a continuous **"machinery" murmur** at the second intercostal space on the left upper sternal border, loud S2, and bounding peripheral pulses.

Differential

Aortopulmonary window, truncus arteriosus, mitral regurgitation, VSD, aortic stenosis, Eisenmenger's syndrome.

Evaluation

Echocardiography shows left atrial and ventricular enlargement; angiography with increased O_2 in the pulmonary artery confirms the diagnosis. EKG may show LVH. CXR may show cardiomegaly.

Treatment

- Treat with **indomethacin** unless the PDA is necessary for survival (transposition of the great vessels).
- If indomethacin fails or if a child is > 6–8 months old, surgical closure is preferred.

UCV *Ped.1*

TRANSPOSITION OF THE GREAT VESSELS

A condition in which the pulmonary and systemic circulations exist in **parallel:** the aorta is connected to the right ventricle and the pulmonary artery to the left ventricle. Risk factors include Apert's syndrome, Down's syndrome, cri-du-chat syndrome, and trisomy 13/18.

In transposition of the great vessels, a PDA or VSD is required for mixing of pulmonary and systemic blood flow.

History

Patients usually present immediately after birth with **cyanosis** and are **critically ill.** The condition is fatal without correction unless the patient has a PDA or VSD.

PE

Cyanosis, tachypnea, and progressive respiratory failure. Some may present with signs of CHF.

Differential

Large VSD, aortic coarctation, tetralogy of Fallot, hypoplastic left ventricle.

Evaluation

Echocardiography. CXR may show narrow heart base and absence of main pulmonary artery segment.

Treatment

- Keep the ductus open with **prostaglandin E$_1$(PGE$_1$).**
- **Balloon atrial septostomy** if immediate surgery is not feasible.
- **Surgical correction** (arterial or atrial switch).

PERSISTENT TRUNCUS ARTERIOSUS

A congenital heart defect in which a failure of separation leads to a single great vessel supplying both the systemic and pulmonary arterial beds with a mixture of oxygenated and deoxygenated blood.

History

Usually presents shortly after birth with cyanosis. Further symptoms develop in the first weeks to months of life and include dyspnea, easy fatigability, failure to thrive, and symptoms of CHF.

PE

Presents with a harsh systolic murmur at the lower left sternal border with a loud systolic ejection click, loud S1/S2, cardiomegaly, and bounding pulses.

Differential

Tetralogy of Fallot, VSD, large ASD.

Evaluation

Angiocardiography is diagnostic, showing the single great vessel, which may also be seen on echo. EKG usually shows normal axis, often with evidence of RVH and LVH. CXR may show boot-shaped heart, absence of the main pulmonary artery, and a large aorta arching to the right.

Treatment

Surgical repair is necessary.

TETRALOGY OF FALLOT

Tetralogy consists of VSD, right ventricular outflow obstruction, RVH, and overriding aorta. Early cyanosis results from right-to-left shunting across the VSD. Risk factors include Down's syndrome, cri-du-chat syndrome, and trisomy 13/18.

History

Patients present during infancy with **cyanosis, dyspnea,** and easy fatigability. Children often **squat for relief ("tet spells")** during hypoxemic episodes. They may have failure to thrive or mental status changes secondary to hypoxemia.

PE

Systolic ejection murmur at the left sternal border, **RV lift,** and single second heart sound. May present with signs of CHF.

Differential

Tricuspid or pulmonary atresia, transposition of the great vessels, hypoplastic left heart syndrome, PDA.

Evaluation

Echocardiography and catheterization. CXR shows a **"boot-shaped" heart.** EKG shows right-axis deviation and RVH.

Treatment

- Administer **PGE$_1$** to keep the ductus arteriosus open.
- Treat cyanotic spells with oxygen, propranolol, knee–chest position, fluids, and morphine.
- **Surgical correction.** Temporary palliation can be achieved through the creation of an artificial shunt (e.g., balloon atrial septostomy).
- There is an increased risk of arrhythmia even after correction.
- Prognosis depends on the degree of pulmonary stenosis.

UCV *Ped.2, Surg.3*

COARCTATION OF THE AORTA

Constriction of the aorta leading to decreased flow below the coarctation and increased flow above it (to the upper extremities). **Turner's syndrome** is a risk factor, and males are affected more frequently than females. One-fourth of patients have a bicuspid aortic valve.

History

Coarctation of the aorta is a cause of secondary hypertension.

Patients often present during childhood with asymptomatic hypertension. Dyspnea on exertion, syncope, claudication, epistaxis, and headache may be present.

PE

Higher systolic BP in the upper extremities than in the lower extremities, decreased femoral and distal pulses, a late systolic murmur (heard in the left axilla), and forceful apical impulses. BP in the right arm may be greater than that in the left arm depending on the location of the coarctation.

Differential

Primary hypertension, pheochromocytoma, aortic stenosis, renal artery stenosis, renal disease, Cushing's syndrome, hyperaldosteronism.

Evaluation

Perform EKG (LVH), echocardiography, and possibly MRI. Diagnosis can be made by cardiac catheterization (aortography). CXR may reveal a **"reverse 3 sign"** due to pre- and postdilatation of the coarct segment as well as **"rib notching"** due to collateral circulation through the intercostal arteries.

Treatment

- **Surgical correction** is often only partially successful and does not correct the intercostal aneurysms that result from long-standing coarctation.
- **Balloon angioplasty** is an alternative to surgical repair.
- Continue **endocarditis prophylaxis** even after treatment.
- **Initiate repair** as **early** as possible given the risks of heart failure, premature CAD, and intracerebral hemorrhage.
- Twenty-five percent of patients continue to have hypertension after repair.

UCV *Surg.2*

In advanced cases of coarctation, patients may have a well-developed upper body and lower-extremity wasting.

PYLORIC STENOSIS

Hypertrophy of the pyloric sphincter causing gastric outlet obstruction. Males are most often affected. Incidence is 1 in 500 births.

History

Nonbilious emesis progressing to **projectile emesis** in the **first two weeks to four months of life.** Babies feed well initially but eventually suffer from malnutrition and dehydration.

PE

Palpable **epigastric olive-shaped mass** or visible gastric peristaltic waves.

Differential

Hiatal hernia, duodenal atresia ("double bubble" sign), malrotation/volvulus, meconium ileus, GERD, gastroenteritis.

Evaluation

Obtain plain abdominal films and electrolytes (look for hypokalemia and metabolic alkalosis secondary to emesis). Barium studies may reveal a narrow pyloric channel (**"string sign"**) or a **pyloric beak.** Abdominal ultrasound may reveal the hypertrophic pylorus.

Treatment

- Correct dehydration and electrolyte abnormalities.
- **Surgical correction** (pyloromyotomy).

UCV *Ped.42*

NEONATAL JAUNDICE

Direct hyperbilirubinemia is never physiologic.

Jaundice in the first day of life is not physiologic. "Physiologic" jaundice occurs after the first day of life and within 3–5 days of birth; bilirubin commonly rises to 9 mg/dL and then slowly falls. If bilirubin levels rise more quickly or to a higher level, infants need treatment and a search for a cause. **Kernicterus** results from the irreversible deposition of bilirubin in the basal ganglia, pons, and cerebellum; it occurs with bilirubin levels of > 20 mg/dL and is potentially fatal.

History/PE

Neonates may be jaundiced with bilirubin levels > 5 mg/dL. Search for signs of infection, congenital malformations, cephalohematomas, and hepatomegaly. Note a history of maternal–fetal ABO or Rh incompatibilities. Kernicterus presents with lethargy, poor feeding, a high-pitched cry, hypertonicity, and seizures.

Differential

Physiologic jaundice, breast milk jaundice, breast-feeding jaundice, Crigler–Najjar syndrome, Gilbert's syndrome, hemolysis, neonatal hepatitis, biliary atresia, alpha-1-antitrypsin deficiency, infections, metabolic disorders, and hypothyroidism.

Evaluation

A jaundiced neonate with abnormal vital signs requires a full septic workup.

Assess direct (conjugated) and indirect (unconjugated) bilirubin levels. If indirect (but not direct) bilirubin is elevated, check blood smear **(hemolysis)**. Coombs' test distinguishes between immune-mediated disorders (ABO incompatibility) and non-immune-mediated hemolytic disorders (G6PD deficiency, hereditary spherocytosis). If direct bilirubin is elevated, check liver enzymes, alkaline phosphatase, bile acids, sweat test, and tests for aminoacidopathies and alpha-1-antitrypsin deficiency. Blood cultures are warranted, and a jaundiced neonate who is febrile, hypotensive, and/or tachypneic needs a full septic workup and ICU monitoring.

Treatment

- Treat infectious causes (e.g., TORCHeS) with appropriate therapy.
- If bilirubin rises above 15–20 mg/dL (regardless of cause), initiate **phototherapy.**
- Diarrhea is a common side effect of this procedure and can be managed by a lactose-free formula.
- In more severe cases, **exchange transfusion** may be used. Hypocalcemia and hypoglycemia are common complications of this procedure.

UCV *Ped.45*

The telescoping of a segment of bowel into itself, usually proximal to the ileo-cecal valve (Figure 2.13–4). Intussusception is the **most common cause of bowel obstruction in the first two years of life** and affects males more than females. In most cases the cause is not apparent, but risk factors include Meckel's diverticulum, intestinal lymphoma, **Henoch–Schönlein purpura,** parasites, adenovirus or rotavirus infection, celiac disease, and cystic fibrosis.

Intussusception is the most common cause of bowel obstruction in the first two years of life.

History

Abrupt-onset abdominal pain in apparently healthy children. The pain is often **colicky** in nature and is accompanied by emesis and bloody mucus in the stool **("currant jelly" stool).**

PE

Abdominal tenderness, positive stool guaiac, and pallor/diaphoresis. A **"sausage-shaped" abdominal mass** may be palpated.

Differential

Meckel's diverticulum, constipation, lymphoma (children > 6 years), GI infection, and meconium ileus (neonates).

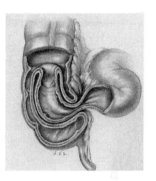

FIGURE 2.13–4. Intussusception. A segment of bowel telescopes into an adjacent segment, causing obstruction. (Reproduced, with permission, from Way L, *Current Surgical Diagnosis & Treatment,* 10th ed., Stamford, CT: Appleton & Lange, 1994: p. 1222, Fig. 46–13.)

Evaluation

CBC (leukocytosis), air contrast enema (if clinically stable), abdominal plain films, and ultrasound.

Treatment

- Correct volume/electrolyte abnormalities.
- **Air contrast enema** is diagnostic and often curative. If the child is not stable or if enema reduction is unsuccessful, proceed to **surgical reduction** and resection of gangrenous bowel.
- The appendix is usually removed during surgery as a preventive measure.

UCV *EM.17*

Air contrast enema is both diagnostic and curative for intussusception.

A remnant of the omphalomesenteric duct that persists as an outpouching of the distal ileum and can contain ectopic (usually gastric or pancreatic) mucosa. Meckel's diverticulum affects 1–3% of the population and conforms to the **"rule of 2's"** (see sidebar).

History

Often asymptomatic and noted incidentally during surgery. Patients may present with **painless rectal bleeding,** intussusception, intestinal ulceration, peptic perforation, diverticulitis, fistula, obstruction, or abscess.

HIGH-YIELD FACTS

Pediatrics

Meckel's diverticulum is rarely seen on barium studies.

PE

Usually **unremarkable.** Possible physical findings include rectal bleeding, abdominal pain secondary to obstruction from intussusception, purulent or other discharge from the umbilicus, and umbilical cellulitis.

Differential

Omphalomesenteric fistula, enterocystoma, appendicitis, umbilical sinus, other GI structural abnormalities.

Evaluation

Evaluation should include a **technetium radionuclide scan** (detects ectopic gastric mucosa). The condition is rarely seen on barium studies.

Treatment

- Hydrate/transfuse as needed.
- Perform **surgical exploration if symptomatic. Resection** of bowel may be required depending on the location and complexity of the lesion.

UCV *Ped.10*

WILMS' TUMOR

An **embryonal tumor of renal origin** that is the most common renal tumor in children (usually seen in 1- to 4-year-olds). Risk factors include a positive family history, Beckwith–Wiedemann syndrome, neurofibromatosis, aniridia, hemihypertrophy, congenital GU anomalies, and WAGR syndrome (Wilms', aniridia, ambiguous genitalia, and mental retardation).

History

Painless abdominal/flank mass, hematuria (usually microscopic), weight loss, nausea, emesis, bone pain, dysuria, and polyuria.

PE

Physical examination may reveal an **abdominal/flank mass,** abdominal tenderness, **fever,** and **hypertension.**

Differential

Neuroblastoma, abdominal neoplasms.

Evaluation

Abdominal CT/ultrasound will show an **intrarenal mass.** Assess the extent of disease with CXR, chest CT, CBC, LFTs, and BUN/creatinine.

Treatment

- **Transabdominal nephrectomy.**
- Administer chemotherapy after surgery **(vincristine/dactinomycin).**
- Flank irradiation is used in some cases.
- Prognosis is good in most cases, but depends on staging and tumor histology.

UCV *Ped.48*

NEUROBLASTOMA

A tumor of **neural crest cell origin.** Risk factors include neurofibromatosis, tuberous sclerosis, Klippel–Feil syndrome, Waardenburg syndrome, pheochromocytoma, and Hirschsprung's disease. Children < 5 years of age are most commonly affected.

History

Lesions can appear anywhere in the body, so symptoms vary. May present as an **abdominal mass,** abdominal distention, anorexia, weight loss, malaise, fever, diarrhea, bone pain, irritability, or **neuromuscular symptoms** (if paraspinal).

PE

Abdominal mass, tenderness, distention, hepatomegaly, skull mass, leg edema, hypertension, fever, pallor, and periorbital bruising.

Differential

Wilms' tumor, Ewing's sarcoma, rhabdomyosarcoma, peripheral neuroepithelioma, lymphoma.

Evaluation

Diagnose with abdominal CT plus 24-hour urinary catecholamines (look for **elevated VMA** and **HVA**). Assess the extent of disease with CXR, bone scan, CBC, LFTs, BUN/creatinine, and coagulation screen.

Treatment

- Localized tumors are usually cured with **excision.**
- Localized but unresectable tumors also have a favorable prognosis.
- Chemotherapy includes **cyclophosphamide and doxorubicin.**
- Radiation is a useful adjunct.
- Prognosis is improved if diagnosis is made at < 1 year of age.

UCV *Neuro.47*

Child has just begun to sit on his own, cries when separated from his parents, and laughs often. How old is he?	Six months
Vaccines to avoid in immune-compromised patients.	Live vaccines: oral polio, varicella, MMR
A 15-year-old patient has stepped on a nail. Last tetanus shot was at 5 years of age. What does she receive?	Tetanus booster
Patients with allergy to egg should avoid which vaccines?	MMR and influenza
Wide, fixed split S2 is pathognomonic for . . .	Atrial septal defect
A continuous machine-like murmur in the upper left sternal border.	PDA
Close PDA with . . .	Indomethacin
A condition in which PDA is necessary for survival.	Transposition of the great vessels
Classic CXR finding in tetralogy of Fallot.	Boot-shaped heart
Rib notching on CXR.	Coarctation of the aorta
Abrupt onset of colicky abdominal pain in 2-year-old boy, with bloody mucus in stool.	Intussusception
Jaundice, lethargy, and seizures in an infant with bilirubin level of 25 mg/dL.	Kernicterus
Finding on barium swallow study in patient with pyloric stenosis.	"String sign" or "beak sign"
Flank mass, hematuria, weight loss, and bony pain in a 3-year-old child.	Wilms' tumor
Tumor associated with Hirschsprung's disease.	Neuroblastoma
After what age, in general, is a well-appearing, febrile child treated as an outpatient rather than admitted for a sepsis workup?	One month
Most common pathogen of croup.	Parainfluenza type 1
Classic finding on lateral x-ray in epiglottitis.	"Thumbprint" sign from swollen epiglottis obstructing the airway
First-line treatment for otitis media.	Amoxicillin
Most common cause of respiratory failure in preterm infants.	RDS

Questions 1, 2, and 3: Reproduced, with permission, from Yetmar KJ, *PreTest: Pediatrics*, 9th ed., New York: McGraw-Hill, 2001.

Question 4: Reproduced, with permission, from Ratelle S, *PreTest: Preventive Medicine and Public Health*, 9th ed., New York: McGraw-Hill, 2001.

Questions

1. You are called to the nursery to see a baby who was noted to be jaundiced and has a serum bilirubin concentration of 13 mg/dL at 18 hours of age. The baby is a 3500-g boy who was born at term to a 27-year-old primigravida 16 hours after membranes ruptured. There were no prenatal complications. Breast-feeding has been well tolerated. Of the following, which is LEAST likely to be responsible for the jaundice in this baby?
   a. Rh or ABO hemolytic disease
   b. physiologic jaundice
   c. sepsis
   d. congenital spherocytic anemia
   e. glucose-6-phosphate dehydrogenase (G6PD) deficiency

2. During a regular checkup on an 8-year-old child, you note a loud first heart sound with a fixed and widely split second heart sound at the upper left sternal border that does not change with respirations. The patient is otherwise active and healthy. The most likely heart lesion to explain these findings is
   a. atrial septal defect
   b. ventricular septal defect
   c. isolated tricuspid regurgitation
   d. tetralogy of Fallot
   e. mitral valve prolapse

3. A 4-year-old boy presents with a history of constipation since the age of 6 months. His stools, produced every 3–4 days, are described as large and hard. Physical examination is normal; rectal examination reveals a large ampulla, poor sphincter tone, and stool in the rectal vault. The next step in the management of this infant would be
   a. lower GI barium study
   b. parental reassurance and counseling
   c. serum electrolyte measurement
   d. upper GI barium study
   e. initiation of synthroid

4. A 20-month-old child presents to your office with a mild viral infection. The results of examination are normal except for a temperature of 37.2°C (99°F) and clear nasal discharge. Review of her vaccination records reveals that she received only two doses of polio vaccine and diphtheria–tetanus–pertussis (DTaP) vaccine, and that she did not receive the measles–mumps–rubella (MMR) vaccine. The mother is 20 weeks pregnant. Her brother is undergoing chemotherapy for leukemia. Which of the following is the most appropriate intervention?
   a. Schedule a visit in two weeks for DTaP
   b. Administer inactivated polio vaccine (IPV) and DTaP
   c. Administer DTaP, oral polio vaccine (OPV), and MMR
   d. Administer DTaP, IPV, and MMR
   e. Administer DTaP and OPV and schedule a visit in three months for MMR

Answers

1. **The answer is b.** The development of jaundice in a healthy full-term baby may be considered the result of a normal physiologic process if the time of onset and duration of the jaundice and the pattern of serially determined serum concentrations of bilirubin are in conformity with currently accepted safe criteria. Physiologic jaundice becomes apparent on the second or third day of life, peaks to levels no higher than about 12 mg/dL on the fourth or fifth day, and disappears by the end of the week. The rate of rise is less than 5 mg/dL per 24 h and levels of conjugated bilirubin do not exceed about 1 mg/dL. Concern about neonatal jaundice relates to the risk of the neurotoxic effects of unconjugated bilirubin. The precise level and duration of exposure necessary to produce toxic effects are not known, but bilirubin encephalopathy, or kernicterus, is rare in term infants whose bilirubin level is kept below 18 to 20 mg/dL. Certain risk factors affecting premature or sick newborns increase their susceptibility to kernicterus at much lower levels of bilirubin. The diagnosis of physiologic jaundice is made by excluding other causes of hyperbilirubinemia by means of history, physical examination, and laboratory determinations. Jaundice appearing in the first 24 hours is usually a feature of hemolytic states and is accompanied by an indirect hyperbilirubinemia, reticulocytosis, and evidence of red-cell destruction on smear. In the absence of blood group or Rh incompatibility, congenital hemolytic states (e.g., spherocytic anemia) or G6PD deficiency should be considered. With infection, hemolytic and hepatotoxic factors are reflected in the increased levels of both direct and indirect bilirubin.

    Studies should include maternal and infant Rh types and blood groups and Coombs' tests to detect blood group or Rh incompatibility and sensitization. Measurements of total and direct bilirubin concentrations help to determine the level of production of bilirubin and the presence of conjugated hyperbilirubinemia. Hematocrit and reticulocyte count provide information as to the degree of hemolysis and anemia, and a complete blood count screens for the possibility of sepsis and the need for cultures. Examination of the blood smear is useful in differentiating common hemolytic disorders. Except for determinations of total and direct bilirubin, tests of liver function are not particularly helpful in establishing the cause of early-onset jaundice. Transient elevations of transaminases (AST and ALT) related to the trauma of delivery and to hypoxia have been noted. Biliary atresia and neonatal hepatitis can be accompanied by elevated levels of transaminase but characteristically present as chronic cholestatic jaundice with mixed hyperbilirubinemia after the first week of life.

2. **The answer is a.** Most commonly, children with an atrial septal defect (ASD) are asymptomatic with the lesion found during a routine examination. In older children, exercise intolerance can be noted if the lesion is of significant size. On examination, the pulses are normal, a right ventricular systolic lift at the left sternal border is palpable, and a fixed splitting of the second heart sound is audible. For lesser degrees of ASD, surgical treatment is more controversial. Ventricular septal defects commonly present as a harsh or blowing holosystolic murmur best heard along the left lower sternum, often with radiation throughout the precordium. Tricuspid regurgitation is a mid-diastolic rumble at the lower left sternal border. Often, a history of birth asphyxia or findings of other cardiac lesions are present. Tetralogy of Fallot is a very common form of congenital heart disease. The four abnormalities include right ventricular outflow obstruction, ventricular septal defect, dextroposition of the aorta, and right ventricular hyper-

trophy. The cyanosis presents in infants and in young children. Mitral valve prolapse occurs with the billowing into the atria of one or both mitral valve leaflets at the end of systole. It is a congenital abnormality that frequently only manifests during adolescence or later. It is more common in girls than in boys and seems to be inherited in an autosomal dominant fashion. On clinical examination, an apical murmur is noted late in systole, which can be preceded by a mid systolic click. The diagnosis is confirmed with an echocardiogram that shows prolapse of the mitral leaflets during mid to late systole. Antibiotic prophylaxis is recommended for dental work (especially if a murmur is present) as the incidence of endocarditis can be higher in these patients.

3. **The answer is b.** Hirschsprung's disease is usually suspected in the chronically constipated child despite the fact that 98% of such children have functional constipation. Finding a dilated, stool-filled anal canal with poor tone on the physical examination of a well-grown child supports the diagnosis of functional constipation. The difficulty in treating functional constipation once it has been established emphasizes the need for prompt identification and treatment of problems with defecation and for counseling of parents regarding proper toileting behavior. The extensive workup of this patient would likely be negative and expensive and is not indicated.

4. **The answer is d.** Children who are late in their immunization schedule should be vaccinated when the opportunity arises. Mild acute illness or antibiotic use is not a contraindication to immunization. MMR is not contraindicated in children of pregnant women. OPV, but not MMR, is contraindicated in any household contact of a severely immunocompromised person. In fact, in an effort to reduce vaccine-associated paralytic polio (VAPP), OPV is no longer recommended for the first two doses of polio immunizations in infants since 1997, and effective January 2000, the CDC recommendations are to give four doses of IPV at 2 months, 4 months, 6–18 months, and then at 6–8 years. OPV can be considered only under a few specific circumstances. If the parents refuse the schedule, OPV could be given only for the third or fourth dose and parents should be counseled about the possible occurrence of VAPP. In this case scenario, however, OPV would not be acceptable given the sibling situation. Live and inactivated vaccines can be given at the same time.

HIGH-YIELD FACTS

Pediatrics

Antipsychotics (neuroleptics)
Thioridazine, haloperidol, fluphenazine, chlorpromazine

Mechanism	Most antipsychotics block dopamine D_2 receptors (excess dopamine effects connected with schizophrenia).
Clinical use	Schizophrenia, psychosis.

Toxicity — Extrapyramidal system side effects, sedation, endocrine side effects, and side effects arising from blocking muscarinic, alpha, and histamine receptors.
Neuroleptic malignant syndrome: rigidity, autonomic instability, hyperpyrexia (treat with dantrolene and dopamine agonists). *Pharm.57,58*
Tardive dyskinesia: stereotypic oral–facial movements probably due to dopamine receptor sensitization; results of long-term antipsychotic use. *Pharm.59*

Evolution of EPS side effects:
4 h acute dystonia
4 d akinesia
4 wk akathisia
4 mo tardive dyskinesia (often irreversible).

Atypical antipsychotics
Clozapine, olanzapine, risperidone

Mechanism	Block $5HT_2$ and dopamine receptors.
Clinical use	Treatment of schizophrenia; useful for positive and negative symptoms. **Olanzapine** is also used for OCD, anxiety disorder, and depression.
Toxicity	Fewer extrapyramidal and anticholinergic side effects than other antipsychotics. **Clozapine** may cause agranulocytosis (requires weekly WBC monitoring).

Lithium

Mechanism	Not established; possibly related to inhibition of phosphoinositol cascade.
Clinical use	Mood stabilizer for bipolar affective disorder, blocks relapse and acute manic events.
Toxicity	Tremor, hypothyroidism, polyuria (ADH antagonist causing nephrogenic DI), teratogenesis. Narrow therapeutic window requiring close monitoring of serum levels.

Tricyclic antidepressants
Imipramine, amitriptyline, desipramine, nortriptyline, clomipramine, doxepin

Mechanism	Block reuptake of norepinephrine and serotonin.
Clinical use	Endogenous depression, bedwetting (imipramine), obsessive–compulsive disorder (clomipramine).
Side effects	Sedation, alpha-blocking effects, atropine-like (anticholinergic) side effects (tachycardia, urinary retention). Tertiary TCAs (amitriptyline) have more anticholinergic effects than secondary TCAs (nortriptyline). Desipramine is the least sedating.
Toxicity	"Tri-C"s: convulsions, coma, cardiotoxicity (arrhythmias); also respiratory depression, hyperpyrexia. Confusion and hallucinations in elderly.

SSRIs
Fluoxetine, sertraline, paroxetine, citalopram.

Mechanism	Serotonin-specific reuptake inhibitors.
Clinical use	Endogenous depression.
Toxicity	Fewer than TCAs. CNS stimulation: anxiety, insomnia, tremor, anorexia, nausea, and vomiting; "serotonin syndrome" with MAOIs: hyperthermia, muscle rigidity, CV collapse.

It normally takes 2–3 weeks for antidepressants to have an effect.

Heterocyclics	Second- and third-generation antidepressants with varied and mixed mechanisms of action. Used in major depressive disorders.
Trazodone	Primarily inhibits serotonin reuptake. Toxicity: sedation, nausea, priapism, postural hypotension.
Bupropion	Also used for smoking cessation. Mechanism not well known. Toxicity: stimulant effects (tachycardia, agitation), dry mouth, aggravation of psychosis.
Venlafaxine	Also used in generalized anxiety disorder. Inhibits serotonin and dopamine reuptake. Toxicity: stimulant effects (anxiety, agitation, headache, insomnia).
Mirtazapine	Alpha-2-antagonist (increases release of norepinephrine and serotonin) and potent $5HT_2$ receptor antagonist. Toxicity: sedation, increased serum cholesterol, increased appetite.

Monoamine oxidase (MAO) inhibitors	Phenelzine, isocarboxazid, tranylcypromine
Mechanism	Nonselective MAO inhibition.
Clinical use	Atypical depressions (i.e., with psychotic or phobic features), anxiety, hypochondriasis.
Toxicity	Hypertensive crisis with tyramine ingestion (in many foods) and meperidine; CNS stimulation. Contraindicated with SSRIs or beta-agonists.

Major depression has a lifetime prevalence of 15%. **Females** are affected twice as often as males. While socioeconomic status does not correlate with the likelihood of developing depression, **chronic illness** does. Incidence of depression is high in both inpatient (15%) and outpatient (10%) populations.

History/PE

Symptoms include depressed mood and symptoms described by the mnemonic **SIG E CAPS** (see sidebar).

Differential

Medical illness, bipolar disorder, substance-induced mood disorder, dysthymia, dementia, schizophrenia, schizoaffective disorder.

Evaluation

In order to be diagnosed with depression, a patient must have five or more of the above symptoms for a two-week period with impairment in daily living. At least one of the symptoms must be either depressed mood or loss of interest/pleasure. A depressed patient should always be assessed for suicide risk.

Treatment

- **Pharmacotherapy** (may require 3–4 weeks for effect):

  - **Selective serotonin reuptake inhibitors (SSRIs):** Relatively well tolerated and considered first-line therapy for depression. There is relatively little toxicity in overdose. Drawbacks include cost and high incidence of sexual dysfunction. Other potential side effects include restlessness, anxiety, insomnia, GI distress, anorexia, and drug interactions.
  - **Tricyclic antidepressants (TCAs):** Cheap and well studied but have significant side effects, including **anticholinergic effects, cardiac arrhythmias,** orthostatic hypotension, sexual dysfunction, and seizures. TCAs can be lethal in overdose and should be used with caution in suicidal patients. Check EKG before initiating therapy.
  - **Monoamine oxidase inhibitors (MAOIs):** **Inexpensive** and the best drugs for atypical depression (hypersomnolence, hyperphagia), but have **dietary restrictions** and serious side effects, including **hypertensive crises** (tyramine or "cheese reaction"), headache, dizziness, and sleep abnormalities.

- **Electroconvulsive therapy (ECT):** Possibly the most effective therapy, but reserved for refractory or catatonic depression (6–12 treatments are often needed). Adverse effects include postictal confusion, arrhythmias, and retrograde amnesia. Relative contraindications include intracranial mass, seizure disorder, and high anesthetic risk.

- **Psychotherapy:** May be effective alone, although a combination of psychotherapy and pharmacotherapy is thought to be most effective. Many techniques have been described. Cognitive therapy, behavioral therapy, and interpersonal therapy are among those with proven efficacy.

UCV *Psych.39, 41, 42, 43*

Symptoms of depression— SIG E CAPS

Sleep, (↓ or ↑)
Interest
Guilt

Energy

Concentration
Appetite (↓ or ↑)
Psychomotor retardation
Suicidal ideations

TCAs are lethal in overdose.

Avoid cheese and red wine when taking an MAOI.

HIGH-YIELD FACTS

Psychiatry

Bipolar disorder has a prevalence of approximately 1% and affects males and females equally. It is divided into two types. **Bipolar I disorder** is characterized by the occurrence of manic episodes that often (though not always) alternate with depressive episodes. **Bipolar II disorder** is characterized by a history of depressive episodes and at least one hypomanic episode.

History/PE

The mnemonic **DIG FAST** describes the clinical presentation of mania (see sidebar). Patients may have a history of excessive spending, speeding tickets, or excessive sexual activity. Episodes may be accompanied by psychotic features. Antidepressants may trigger manic episodes in patients with bipolar disorder.

Differential

Major depression, cyclothymic disorder, substance-induced mood disorder, schizophrenia, schizoaffective disorder, borderline personality disorder, and ADHD. Medical conditions such as metabolic derangements, CNS infections, or tumors may mimic bipolar disorder.

Evaluation

A manic episode must include **three of the above symptoms and must last at least one week** (less if hospitalization is necessary). Symptoms cannot be substance-related or due to a preexisting medical condition. Hypomanic episodes are similar but do not cause marked impairment in social or occupational functioning.

Treatment

- **Acute mania:** Control mood (lithium, valproic acid); resolve psychosis (antipsychotics) and manage agitation (benzodiazepines).
- **Bipolar depression:** Mood stabilizers (lithium, valproic acid) +/– antidepressant. ECT may be used in cases that fail to respond to pharmacologic intervention.

Lithium levels should be monitored to prevent acute side effects (CNS findings, including seizures) as well as chronic side effects (renal insufficiency). **Valproic acid** may be associated with GI distress, sedation, hepatotoxicity, and thrombocytopenia. Monitor platelets and LFTs. **Carbamazepine,** a second-line agent, has been associated with aplastic anemia and Stevens–Johnson syndrome (monitor CBC).

UCV *Psych.40*

> **Bipolar disorder—**
>
> **DIG FAST**
> **D**istractibility
> **I**nsomnia
> **G**randiosity
>
> **F**light of ideas
> Increase in goal-
>   directed **A**ctivities/
>   psychomotor
>   **A**gitation
> Pressured **S**peech
> **T**houghtlessness

Suicide is the **eighth-leading cause of death** in the United States and is the second-leading cause of death (after accidents) among 15- to 24-year-olds. Risk factors include depression, other major psychiatric disorders, a past history of suicide attempts, alcohol/substance abuse, a recent severe stressor, and a family history of suicide. Also at risk are unmarried individuals with poor so-

Women are more likely to attempt suicide, whereas men are more likely to commit suicide.

cial support; patients recovering from suicidal depression or from a first schizo-phrenic episode; and patients with a chronic medical condition (e.g., AIDS). Police officers and doctors are at increased risk compared to the general population, and whites commit suicide more frequently than blacks.

Evaluation

Look for an expressed desire to kill oneself, a **plan,** a positive family history, a previous suicide attempt, ambivalence toward death, and feelings of hopelessness. **Ask directly about suicidal ideation, intent, and plan.** Look for available means of committing suicide; perform a mental status exam.

Treatment

A patient who expresses a desire to kill himself, or who you believe may do so, requires **emergent inpatient hospitalization** even if it is against his wishes. ECT may be used for actively suicidal patients who are refractory to medication and psychotherapy. Note that there may be greater risk for suicide in the first few weeks after antidepressant medication is started because a patient's energy often returns before the depressed mood lifts.

UCV *EM.44*

ANXIETY DISORDERS

PANIC DISORDER

Panic disorder is characterized by the spontaneous occurrence of panic attacks along with persistent fear or worry about these attacks. It is often associated with agoraphobia, the fear of being in public places. An increased incidence of panic disorder has been found in patients with mitral valve prolapse.

History/PE

Recurrent panic attacks characterized by feelings of marked anxiety accompanied by chest pain, palpitations, diaphoresis, nausea, tachypnea, trembling, and/or dizziness. Attacks reach a peak after 10 minutes and usually last 20–30 minutes. In order to be diagnosed with panic disorder, a patient must also have persistent concern about having additional attacks or about the implications of the attacks (e.g., fear of "going crazy" or having a heart attack).

Differential

Angina, hyperthyroidism, substance-induced anxiety disorder, social phobia, posttraumatic stress disorder, generalized anxiety disorder.

Treatment

Cognitive-behavioral therapy, respiratory training, and pharmacotherapy have all been shown to be effective. Antidepressants, including tricyclics and SSRIs, are effective but require 3–4 weeks to take effect. Benzodiazepines may be started for more immediate relief but should be avoided for long-term use owing to their addictive potential.

UCV *Psych.8*

SPECIFIC PHOBIA

Specific phobia is the most common mental disorder among women and the second most common in men (after substance-related disorders), affecting 10–25% of the population. There is a 2:1 female-to-male ratio.

History/PE

Patients exhibit irrational fear and avoidance of an object, activity, or situation (e.g., animals, storms, heights). Phobias most often begin in childhood, and there may be a related history of traumatic events or panic attacks.

Differential

Appropriate fear, normal shyness, obsessive–compulsive disorder, generalized anxiety disorder, avoidant personality disorder, panic disorder, social phobia.

Treatment

Exposure therapy is the most common treatment. It involves gradually desensitizing the patient with incremental exposures to the feared object or situation. Relaxation and breathing techniques are helpful in conjunction with this method. Other approaches include hypnosis, supportive and family therapy, insight-oriented psychotherapy, and cognitive-behavioral therapy.

OBSESSIVE–COMPULSIVE DISORDER (OCD)

Obsessive–compulsive disorder has a lifetime prevalence of 2–3%. An obsession is a recurrent, intrusive, and usually unpleasant thought. A compulsion is a conscious, repeated thought or behavior performed to reduce the anxiety created by the obsession. It may occur in childhood or adulthood.

History/PE

In order to be diagnosed with OCD, patients must have obsessions or compulsions that cause them significant distress or lead to functional impairment. Common obsessions include cleanliness or contamination and fear of harm coming to oneself or to loved ones. Compulsions may take the form of excessive cleaning (e.g., hands may be chafed owing to frequent or caustic washing), elaborate rituals for conducting ordinary tasks (e.g., walking through a doorway), or excessive checking (e.g., multiple trips back home to check that the door is locked). When the disorder occurs in adulthood, patients realize that their thoughts or behaviors are excessive or unreasonable but are nonetheless unable to control them.

Differential

Tourette's syndrome, specific phobia, major depression, obsessive–compulsive personality disorder (patients do not see anything wrong with behaviors), psychosis, generalized anxiety disorder.

Treatment

Cognitive-behavioral therapy and pharmacotherapy with SSRIs or clomipramine.

UCV *Psych.7*

POSTTRAUMATIC STRESS DISORDER (PTSD)

Occurs after an individual is exposed to a traumatic event outside the realm of normal human experience (e.g., combat, natural disasters, physical/sexual assault, accidents). PTSD has a lifetime prevalence of 1–3%. Its prevalence in individuals exposed to traumatic events is as high as 60%.

History/PE

Patients reexperience traumatic events by having **intrusive thoughts** or **nightmares** and often have feelings of detachment, anhedonia, and amnesia. PTSD is associated with an increased state of arousal **(hypervigilance)** and leads to social and occupational impairment. Also watch for survivor guilt, avoidance behavior, personality change, substance abuse, depression, and suicidality.

Differential

Acute stress disorder (lasts < 1 month), adjustment disorder, depression, obsessive–compulsive disorder, anxiety disorder, borderline personality disorder.

Treatment

First-line agents include **antidepressants (SSRIs)** and **mood stabilizers** (lithium, valproic acid, carbamazepine). Adjunctive agents to **target anxiety** include beta-blockers, benzodiazepines, and alpha-2-agonists (clonidine). **Cognitive-behavior therapy** and **support groups** are also effective.

UCV *Psych.9*

GENERALIZED ANXIETY DISORDER

Generalized anxiety disorder affects 3–8% of the population and commonly coexists with other mental disorders. Women are affected twice as often as men.

History/PE

Patients usually come to clinical attention in their 20s. The disorder is characterized by excessive anxiety or worry occurring more days than not for > 6 months about a variety of activities or events, causing significant impairment or distress. The anxiety may be accompanied by restlessness, fatigue, difficulty concentrating, irritability, muscle tension, or sleep disturbance.

Differential

Medical disorders (e.g., hyperthyroidism), substance abuse, obsessive–compulsive disorder, specific phobia, panic disorder, major depression, dysthymic disorder, hypochondriasis.

Treatment

Treatment is with psychotherapy and/or pharmacotherapy (tricyclic antidepressants, benzodiazepines, or SSRIs). Buspirone has also been shown to be effective and may be preferable to benzodiazepines owing to a decreased risk of addiction and the absence of withdrawal effects.

UCV *Psych.6*

SCHIZOPHRENIA

Schizophrenia is characterized by psychotic symptoms that significantly impair social/occupational functioning. Schizophrenia has a prevalence of 1%, with males and females affected equally. Risk is increased in first-degree relatives of schizophrenic patients. Schizophrenia most commonly manifests itself in males 15–25 years of age and in females 25–35 years of age. Schizophrenics are at high risk for **suicide.**

Schizophrenic patients are at high risk for suicide.

History/PE

Positive symptoms include **delusions, auditory hallucinations,** thought alienation (thought broadcasting, withdrawal and insertion), and disorganized thought and behavior. **Negative symptoms** include **social withdrawal,** apathy, and **flattened affect.**

Differential

Schizoaffective disorder, brief psychotic disorder (symptoms last < 1 month), major depression, bipolar disorder, substance-induced psychotic disorder, drug withdrawal, and psychotic disorder due to a general medical condition (e.g., seizure disorder, CNS tumor, Cushing's syndrome, SLE).

Evaluation

In order to be diagnosed, patients must exhibit two or more of the above signs and symptoms with **an impaired level of social/occupational functioning for at least six months' duration.**

Treatment

Treat with **antipsychotics** and with hospitalization during psychotic episodes. Supportive psychotherapy and social skills training may also be useful. Negative symptoms are often more difficult to treat than positive symptoms. Paranoid schizophrenia has the best overall prognosis.

UCV *Psych.49*

Traditional Antipsychotics

Lower-potency drugs have more anticholinergic side effects, whereas higher-potency drugs have more extrapyramidal side effects.

Antipsychotics block dopamine receptors (mostly D_2 and D_4 subtypes). High-potency drugs include haloperidol, droperidol, fluphenazine, and thiothixene. Medium-potency drugs include trifluoperazine and perphenazine. Low-potency drugs include thioridazine and chlorpromazine.

Side effects include the following:

- **Extrapyramidal symptoms:** Acute dystonia, akathisia (treat with propranolol or benzodiazepine), parkinsonism (tremor, rigidity, bradykinesia), and tardive dyskinesia (lip smacking, etc.).
- **Anticholinergic effects:** Dry mouth, urinary retention, constipation, sedation, orthostatic hypotension, etc.
- **Neuroleptic malignant syndrome:** Fever, rigidity, autonomic instability, clouding of consciousness. Withdraw neuroleptic; treat with dantrolene/bromocriptine and IV fluids *(EM.39)*.
- **Hyperprolactinemia:** Amenorrhea, gynecomastia, galactorrhea.
- **Other:** Seizures, EKG changes.

Atypical Antipsychotics

Atypical antipsychotics have fewer anticholinergic and extrapyramidal side effects.

Atypical antipsychotics have fewer anticholinergic and extrapyramidal side effects. **Clozapine,** a first-generation drug, has a 1–2% incidence of **agranulocytosis** and requires weekly CBCs. Although clozapine is the most effective antipsychotic, its use is reserved for treatment-resistant psychosis owing to the high incidence of agranulocytosis. Side effects of atypical agents include sedation, anticholinergic effects, drooling, weight gain, seizures, and arrhythmias. Newer agents (risperidone, olanzapine, sertindole, and quetiapine) do not cause agranulocytosis and may have fewer side effects. The favorable side effect profile of atypical antipsychotics has resulted in their use as first-line agents in the treatment of chronic psychotic disorders.

UCV *Psych.26*

SOMATOFORM AND RELATED DISORDERS

Consider malingering in any case involving litigation or potential for secondary gain.

In all somatoform disorders, patients have no conscious control over their symptoms. These patients should never be told that they are imagining their symptoms (Table 2.14–1).

Table 2.14-1. Somatoform and Related Disorders

Disorder	Characteristics
Somatization *Psych.53*	Multiple, seemingly unrelated physical complaints with excessive seeking of medical help and significant impairment in functioning. Incidence is 5:1 female to male.
Conversion *Psych.51*	One or more neurologic complaints (e.g., paralysis, paresthesia, blindness) that cannot be explained by a medical disorder. Psychological factors must be associated with symptom onset in order to make the diagnosis. Most common in women, usually adolescents and young adults.
Hypochondriasis *Psych.52*	Preoccupation with and fear of having a serious disease that results in significant psychological distress and/or impaired social or occupational functioning. Men and women are equally affected. Onset most commonly occurs between the ages of 20 and 30.
Body dysmorphic *Psych.50*	Preoccupation with an imagined physical defect or abnormality that causes significant distress or impaired social or occupational functioning. Patients often present to dermatologists or plastic surgeons. Women are affected slightly more often than men. May be associated with depression, and SSRIs are helpful in some cases.
Factitious (Munchausen) *Psych.36*	NOT a somatoform disorder, since the patient consciously simulates physical or psychiatric illness in order to receive attention from medical personnel. Munchausen by proxy involves simulation of illness in another person, usually a child by a parent.
Malingering *Psych.37*	Also not a somatoform disorder. Patients simulate illness for personal gain. Differs from factitious disorder in that some concrete, usually material gain is sought, such as financial compensation, avoiding work, or gaining food and shelter.

ANOREXIA NERVOSA

An eating disorder in which patients refuse to maintain a normal body weight and are **> 15% below ideal body weight.** Patients either restrict themselves (fast, diet, and **exercise excessively**) or engage in binge-eating/purging behavior. Patients have a distorted body image (they **perceive themselves as fat**) and deny the potential medical consequences of their behavior. Ninety percent of cases of anorexia nervosa occur in females (1% prevalence in adolescent females).

Anorexic patients deny any health risks associated with their behavior, making them resistant to treatment.

History/PE

Amenorrhea, lanugo, cold intolerance, lethargy, excess energy, emaciation, bradycardia, hypotension, hypothermia, dry skin, electrolyte abnormalities, and hypercarotenemia. Patients are often preoccupied with food rituals, **intensely fear becoming fat,** and judge themselves by their weight.

Evaluation

Evaluation should include height and weight measurements, CBC, electrolytes, endocrine tests, EKG, and psychiatric evaluation.

Treatment

Early treatment centers on monitoring caloric intake to stabilize weight and then focuses on **weight gain.** In severe cases, hospitalization may be required to restore nutritional status and/or correct electrolyte imbalances. Later treatment includes individual, family, and group **psychotherapy.** SSRIs may help treat comorbid depression. Mortality is as high as 5–10%.

UCV *Psych.27*

BULIMIA

Bulimic patients tend to be more disturbed by their behavior and consequently are more easily engaged in therapy.

An eating disorder in which patients are usually **ashamed of their eating behaviors,** tend to keep them secret, and often maintain **normal body weight.** Bulimia has a 3–5% prevalence rate among late adolescent girls and can be classified into purging and nonpurging types.

History/PE

Dental enamel erosion (from vomiting), **enlarged parotid glands, scars on the dorsal surfaces of the hands** (from inducing vomiting), menstrual irregularities, electrolyte abnormalities, and laxative dependence. Patients' self-esteem is overly dependent on body weight.

Evaluation

Diagnosis is based on recurrent episodes of **binge eating** and **recurrent compensatory behaviors** to prevent weight gain (**induced vomiting, laxative abuse,** diuretic use, enemas, fasting, and excessive exercise), occurring at least twice weekly for three months.

Treatment

Psychotherapy focuses on behavior modification and body self-image. **Antidepressants** are effective in both depressed and nondepressed patients.

UCV *Psych.28*

SUBSTANCE ABUSE/DEPENDENCE

Substance abuse/dependence has a 13% lifetime prevalence. Abuse is diagnosed if the patient's life has been disrupted by substance use. Dependence can be diagnosed if three of the following are observed over a one-year period: tolerance; withdrawal; desire to cut back; a significant amount of time involved in substance use; withdrawal from former activities; and persistent use despite awareness of these problems.

Differential

Differentiate from other axis I psychiatric disorders and delirium. The signs and symptoms of intoxication and withdrawal for some drugs are summarized in Table 2.14–2.

Evaluation

Toxicology screen, LFTs, Breathalyzer or serum ethanol level. Offer HIV testing (especially to IV drug users).

Treatment

Management of substance intoxication is described in Table 2.14–3.

TABLE 2.14–2. Signs and Symptoms of Substance Abuse

Drug	Intoxication	Withdrawal
Alcohol *Psych.17*	Disinhibition, emotional lability, incoordination, slurred speech, ataxia, coma, blackouts (retrograde amnesia).	Tremor, tachycardia, hypertension, malaise, nausea, seizures, delirium tremens (DTs), tremulousness, agitation, hallucinations.
Opioids *EM.40, Psych.24*	CNS depression, nausea and vomiting, constipation, **pupillary constriction,** seizures, respiratory depression (overdose is life-threatening).	Anxiety, insomnia, anorexia, sweating, fever, rhinorrhea, piloerection, nausea, stomach cramps, diarrhea.
Amphetamines *EM.39*	Psychomotor agitation, impaired judgment, **pupillary dilation,** hypertension, tachycardia, euphoria, prolonged wakefulness and attention, cardiac arrhythmias, delusions, hallucinations, fever.	Post-use "crash," including anxiety, lethargy, headache, stomach cramps, hunger, severe depression, dysphoric mood, fatigue, insomnia/hypersomnia.
Cocaine *Psych.19*	Euphoria, psychomotor agitation, impaired judgment, tachycardia, **pupillary dilation,** hypertension, hallucinations (including tactile), paranoid ideations, angina, and sudden cardiac death.	Hypersomnolence, fatigue, depression, malaise, severe craving, suicidality.
PCP *Psych.25*	Belligerence, impulsiveness, fever, psychomotor agitation, **vertical and horizontal nystagmus,** tachycardia, ataxia, homicidality, psychosis, delirium.	Recurrence of symptoms due to reabsorption from lipid stores; sudden onset of severe, random, violence.
LSD *Psych.22*	Marked anxiety or depression, delusions, visual hallucinations, flashbacks.	
Marijuana *Psych.18*	Euphoria, anxiety, paranoid delusions, slowed time sense, impaired judgment, social withdrawal, increased appetite, dry mouth, conjunctival injection, persecutory delusions, hallucinations, amotivational syndrome.	
Barbiturates	Low safety margin, respiratory depression.	Anxiety, seizures, delirium, life-threatening cardiovascular collapse.
Benzodiazepines	Alcohol interactions, amnesia, ataxia, sleep, minor respiratory depression.	Rebound anxiety, seizures, tremor, insomnia, hypertension, tachycardia.
Caffeine	Restlessness, insomnia, diuresis, muscle twitching, cardiac arrhythmias.	Headache, lethargy, depression, weight gain.
Nicotine	Restlessness, insomnia, anxiety, arrhythmias.	Irritability, headache, anxiety, weight gain, craving, tachycardia.

TABLE 2.14–3. Management of Substance Intoxication

Drug	Management
Hallucinogens (e.g., LSD)	If severe, benzodiazepines or traditional antipsychotics; otherwise provide reassurance.
Cocaine/crack	Severe agitation is treated with haloperidol, benzodiazepines, antiemetics, anti-diarrheals, and NSAIDs (for muscle cramps).
PCP	If severe, benzodiazepines; otherwise provide reassurance.
Amphetamines EM.39	Same as with cocaine/crack.
Opioids	Naloxone/naltrexone block opioid receptors, reversing their effects. Beware of antagonist being cleared before opioid, particularly with longer-acting opioids such as methadone.

HIGH-YIELD FACTS

Psychiatry

ALCOHOLISM

DTs are a medical emergency with a mortality rate of 15–20%.

Alcohol is the most commonly abused substance (not counting tobacco and caffeine), and alcoholism has a lifetime prevalence of 6%. Males are affected almost four times as often as females, but the incidence of alcoholism among females is increasing. The highest prevalence is in males aged 21–34. Abuse and dependence criteria are similar to those of other substances.

History/PE

Alcohol intoxication results in **euphoria, disinhibition, hypoglycemia, ataxia, impaired judgment and reflexes,** and CNS depression. Acute overdose can result in respiratory depression, coma, or death. See Selected Topics in Emergency Medicine (p. 445) for symptoms and signs of alcohol withdrawal.

Evaluation

Evaluation is similar to that of substance abuse. Screen with the CAGE questionnaire (see sidebar). Monitor vital signs in hospitalized patients to assess for signs of withdrawal.

Treatment

- Rule out medical complications.
- Start benzodiazepine taper for withdrawal symptoms.
- Give **multivitamins with thiamine and folate;** correct electrolyte abnormalities.
- For patients with alcohol seizure history, give anticonvulsants and avoid neuroleptics, which decrease seizure threshold.
- Alcohol dependence can be treated with group therapy (Alcoholics Anonymous), disulfiram, or naltrexone.

CAGE questions:

1. Have you ever felt the need to **C**ut down on your drinking?

2. Have you ever felt **A**nnoyed by criticism of your drinking?

3. Have you ever felt **G**uilty about drinking?

4. Have you ever had to take a morning **E**ye opener?

More than one "yes" answer makes alcoholism likely.

Complications

GI bleeding (gastritis, ulcers, varices, or Mallory–Weiss tears), pancreatitis, liver disease, susceptibility to infections, electrolyte disturbances, delirium tremens.

UCV *Psych.17*

DELIRIUM

Delirium is a transient global disorder of consciousness. Etiologies include infectious disease, hypoxia, ICU psychosis, "sundowning," CVA, endocrine causes, autoimmune disease, uremia, hepatic encephalopathy, Wilson's disease, electrolyte abnormalities, and drugs (alcohol withdrawal, corticosteroids, psychedelic drugs, amphotericin B, antihistamines, anticholinergics, TCAs, phenytoin, heavy metal poisoning, beta-blockers, digitalis, lithium, barbiturates, and benzodiazepines).

History/PE

Waxing and waning levels of consciousness and perceptual disturbances (hallucinations or illusions). Patients may be anxious, restless, paranoid, or combative and may have a short attention span, decreased short-term memory, and autonomic disturbances (tachycardia, diaphoresis).

Differential

Must be distinguished from dementia, schizophrenia, mania, psychotic depression, and substance abuse.

Evaluation

Check vitals, pulse oximetry, and glucose; conduct a thorough physical and neurologic exam. Note recently started meds, overdose, alcohol use, previous history, concurrent medical problems, signs of organ failure, and signs of infection (occult UTI is common in the elderly). Laboratory studies include CBC, electrolytes, toxicology screen, UA, ABG, CXR, ECG, LP, and head CT.

Always check the medication list of delirious patients.

Treatment

Treat the underlying cause; normalize fluid and electrolyte status. Use antipsychotics for agitation. Benzodiazepines may also be used. Physical restraints may be necessary to prevent patients from harming themselves or others.

UCV *Psych.1*

DEMENTIA

Dementia is a chronic and progressive syndrome of global intellectual impairment. Dementia has its highest prevalence among those > 85 years old. The most common etiologies are Alzheimer's disease (70–80%), vascular dementia (10%), alcohol use, and Huntington's and Parkinson's diseases. Fewer than 10% of dementias are reversible (e.g., normal pressure hydrocephalus).

| Dememtia = **mem**ory impairment |
| Deli**rium** = change in senso**rium** |

A useful mnemonic for etiologies is **DEMENTIAS:**

- **D**egenerative diseases (Parkinson's, Huntington's)
- **E**ndocrine (thyroid, parathyroid, pituitary, adrenal)
- **M**etabolic (alcohol, fluid electrolytes, B_{12} deficiency, glucose, hepatic, renal, Wilson's disease)
- **E**xogenous (heavy metals, carbon monoxide, drugs)
- **N**eoplasia
- **T**rauma (subdural hematoma)
- **I**nfection (meningitis, encephalitis, abscess, endocarditis, HIV, syphilis, prion diseases, Lyme disease)
- **A**ffective disorders (depression may cause pseudodementia)
- **S**troke/Structure (multi-infarct dementia (Neuro.25), ischemia, vasculitis, normal pressure hydrocephalus)

History/PE

Patients present with **deterioration of cognitive functions,** including memory impairment, aphasia, apraxia, agnosia, and disturbances in abstract thought, planning, organizing, and sequencing. Symptoms typically occur in the presence of a clear sensorium.

Avoid benzodiazepines in demented patients.

Differential

Depression (pseudodementia), delirium, schizophrenia, amnestic disorder, mental retardation, substance intoxication, traumatic brain injury.

Personality disorders—

MEDIC
Maladaptive
Enduring
Deviates from normal
Inflexible
Causes an impairment in social functioning

Treatment

Treat reversible causes. Provide **environmental clues** and supportive intervention. Use low-dose **antipsychotics** for agitation. **Avoid benzodiazepines,** as they will often worsen disinhibition and confusion.

UCV *Neuro.17, 23, 34, 36, Psych.2*

PERSONALITY DISORDERS

Personality disorders typically become evident by late adolescence or early adulthood. They tend to be stable over time and affect all facets of interpersonal relationships. Their prevalence is 10% in the general population, 30% among psychiatric outpatients, and 40% among psychiatric inpatients.

Evaluation

Differentiate from axis I disorders. Ask about attitudes toward self and others, moral and religious attitudes and standards, variability of mood, leisure activities and interests, fantasy life, and reaction patterns to stress. Consider psychological testing (Minnesota Multiphasic Personality Inventory [MMPI], Bender Gestalt, Rorschach) as an aid in diagnosis.

Treatment

Treat with **psychotherapy** and **pharmacotherapy.** Recognize and treat comorbid axis I disorders. For specific personality disorders, see Table 2.14–4.

[UCV] *Psych.44, 45, 46*

SEXUAL ABUSE

Sexual abuse has become more common in recent years; the incidence is now 200,000 cases per year in the United States. The abuser is commonly known to the victim. Incidence is highest at ages 9–12 years. Risk factors include single-parent households, marital problems, substance abuse, and crowded living conditions.

History/PE

Precocious sexual behavior, **genital or anal trauma, STDs,** or UTIs. Sexual abuse may predispose patients to psychiatric problems, including anxiety, phobias, and depression.

Treatment

When sexual abuse is suspected, the physician must intervene to protect the abused and **report the case to the appropriate authority.**

[UCV] *Psych.13*

TABLE 2.14–4. Signs and Symptoms of Personality Disorders

Cluster	Examples	Characteristics	Clinical Dilemma	Clinical Strategy
Cluster A	Paranoid Schizoid Schizotypal	Eccentric, strange, fearful of social relationships, paranoid, suspicious, social isolation, odd beliefs, shy, withdrawn, impoverished personal relationships.	Patient is suspicious of doctor and does not trust doctor.	Use clear, honest attitude, noncontrolling, nondefensive, **no humor;** keep distance.
Cluster B	Borderline Histrionic Narcissistic Antisocial	Emotional, dramatic, erratic, self-indulgent, hostile, aggressive, exploitive relationships, attention seeking.	Patient will change rules on doctor. Clingy and demands attention. Feels that he or she is special. Will manipulate doctor and staff ("splitting").	Firm: **Stick to treatment plan** and don't waffle. Fair: Don't be punitive or derogatory. Consistent: Don't change the rules on them.
Cluster C	Obsessive–compulsive Avoidant Dependent Passive–aggressive	Fearful, anxious, adheres to rules and regulations, anxiety, repressed, unable to express affect.	Patient may subtly sabotage his or her own treatment. Very controlling.	**Avoid power struggles.** Give clear treatment recommendations, but do not push the patient into a decision.

ADHD affects approximately 3% of children. Boys are affected more frequently than girls.

History/PE

Children must exhibit ADHD symptoms in more than one setting (e.g., home and school).

- **Inattention:** Patients exhibit **poor attention span** for schoolwork or play; do not listen when spoken to; have **difficulty following instructions;** lose items necessary for completion of school tasks; and are forgetful and **easily distracted.**
- **Hyperactivity/impulsivity:** Patients are **fidgety** and unexpectedly leave their desks; run around inappropriately; cannot play quietly; are often "on the go"; talk excessively; blurt out answers before questions have been completed; **do not wait for their turn;** and **interrupt others.**

Differential

Normal active child, medication side effects, head trauma, learning disabilities, major depression, bipolar disorder, anxiety disorder, cyclothymic disorder, conduct disorder, oppositional-defiant disorder.

Evaluation

To be diagnosed with ADHD, a child must exhibit six inattention symptoms and six hyperactivity symptoms before the age of 7, and these symptoms must cause **significant social and academic impairment.**

Treatment

Initial treatment involves reducing caffeine intake. Sugar and food additives are not etiologic factors.

Initial treatment should be conservative and nonpharmacologic. Reduce caffeine intake (sugar and food additives are not considered etiologic factors). Treatment for refractory/severe cases includes:

- **Psychostimulants: Methylphenidate,** dextroamphetamine, and pemoline. Adverse effects include stunted growth, tics, insomnia, irritability, and decreased appetite.
- **Antidepressants:** Nortriptyline, imipramine, bupropion.

UCV *Psych.11*

A repetitive and persistent pattern of inappropriate conduct that lasts at least **six months** in which patients < 18 years of age ignore or violate the rights of others.

HIGH-YIELD FACTS

Psychiatry

History/PE

Conduct disorder may be **aggressive** (e.g., **violence, destruction,** or **theft**) or **nonaggressive** (e.g., violation of rules, **lying**). The **undersocialized variant** affects individuals who cannot form social bonds with others. The **socialized** variant shows bonding, often with loyal groups that support deviant behavior (e.g., **urban gangs**).

Treatment

Address emotional conflicts and sociocultural factors.

UCV *Psych.14*

Oppositional-defiant disorder is associated with loss of temper and defiance but not theft or lying.

First-line pharmacotherapy for depression.	SSRIs
Antidepressant associated with hypertensive crisis.	MAO inhibitors
Patient presents with agitation and pressured speech. He has not slept for three days and just lost $20,000 gambling.	Bipolar disorder, manic episode
A 17-year-old female presents with paralysis of left arm since she heard about the death of her boyfriend in a car crash. No medical cause can be found.	Conversion disorder
A 35-year-old male presents with recurrent episodes of palpitations, diaphoresis, and feelings of impending doom.	Panic disorder
A 21-year-old male presents with social withdrawal, worsening grades, flattened affect, and concrete thinking for the past nine months.	Schizophrenia
Most worrisome side effect of clozapine.	Agranulocytosis
A 19-year-old female presents with enlarged parotid glands, normal body weight, and complaints of "feeling fat."	Bulimia
Pharmacotherapy for alcohol withdrawal symptoms	Benzodiazepines
Medications to avoid in patients with history of alcohol withdrawal seizures?	Neuroleptics
A 13-year-old male with a history of theft, vandalism, and violence toward family pets.	Conduct disorder

The following clinical questions and accompanying answers are reproduced, with permission, from Mancini-Mezzacappa GM, *PreTest: Psychiatry*, 9th ed., New York: McGraw-Hill, 2001.

Questions

1. A 25-year-old man's teaching career has been abruptly terminated by a psychiatric illness. During a psychiatric evaluation he is asked the meaning of the proverb "People in glass houses should not throw stones." The patient replies, "They will break the windows." This response is an example of

   a. Idiosyncratic thinking
   b. Concrete thinking
   c. Formal operation
   d. Loose associations
   e. Autistic thinking

Items 2 and 3

Match the symptoms with the most appropriate diagnosis.

   a. Conversion disorder
   b. Specific phobia
   c. Agoraphobia
   d. Narcissistic personality disorder
   e. Body dysmorphic disorder
   f. Schizophrenia
   g. Borderline personality disorder
   h. Dissociative amnesia

2. The career of a young executive who needs to travel often for his business is much impaired because, due to his overwhelming fear of flying, he refuses all the jobs that require traveling by plane.

3. A young woman who has ambivalent feelings about separating from her family wakes up paralyzed on the morning she is scheduled to go back to college.

4. A 27-year-old woman has been sad for the past two weeks. She is fatigued and has a hard time concentrating at work. Just a few weeks earlier she was energetic and enthusiastic, and was able to work 10–12 hours a day with little sleep and go dancing at night. Her husband wants a divorce because he is tired of "these constant ups and downs." The most accurate diagnosis is

   a. Borderline personality disorder
   b. Seasonal mood disorder
   c. Dissociative identity disorder
   d. Cyclothymic disorder
   e. Recurrent major depression

Answers

1. **The answer is b.** Patients who present with concrete thinking have lost the ability to form abstract concepts, such as metaphors, and focus instead on actual things and facts. Concrete thinking is the norm in children and is seen in cognitive disorders (mental retardation, dementia) and schizophrenia.

2–3. **The answers are 2-b, 3-a.** Fear of flying is one of the many presentations of specific phobias. Phobic individuals have an excessive or unreasonable fear of an object, an animal, or a situation. When exposed to the feared stimulus, they experience severe anxiety that can reach the level of panic attack. Characteristically, phobic patients go to great lengths to avoid whatever they fear and this phobic avoidance can greatly interfere with functioning.

   Conversion disorder is characterized by the sudden appearance of often dramatic neurological symptoms that are not associated with the usual diagnostic signs and test results. Conversion disorder occurs in the context of a psychosocial stressor or an insoluble interpersonal or intrapsychic conflict. The psychological distress is not consciously acknowledged but it is expressed through a metaphorical body dysfunction. In the vignette example, the young woman who was torn between leaving home and becoming independent found a temporary solution in her paralysis, which prevented her from leaving her home without having to consciously acknowledge her conflict.

4. **The answer is d.** Cyclothymic disorder is characterized by recurrent periods of mild depression alternating with periods of hypomania. This pattern has to have been present for at least two years (one year for children and adolescents) before the diagnosis can be made. During these two years, the symptom-free intervals should not be longer than two months. Cyclothymic disorder usually starts during adolescence or early adulthood and tends to have a chronic course. The marked shifts in mood of cyclothymic disorder can be confused with the affective instability of borderline personality disorder or may suggest a substance abuse problem.

Pulmonary

Obstructive vs. restrictive lung disease

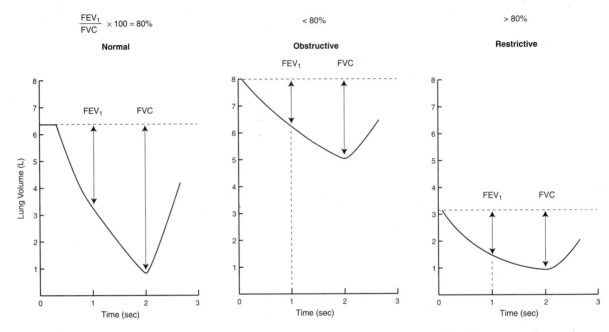

Note: Obstructive lung volumes > normal (increased TLC, increased FRC, increased RV); restrictive lung volumes < normal. In both obstructive and restrictive, FEV_1 and FVC are reduced, but in obstructive, FEV_1 is more dramatically reduced, resulting in a decreased FEV_1/FVC ratio.

HIGH-YIELD FACTS

Pulmonary Medicine

Asthma drugs

Nonspecific beta-agonists **Isoproterenol:** relaxes bronchial smooth muscle (beta-2). Adverse effect is tachycardia (beta-1).

Beta-2-agonists **Albuterol:** relaxes bronchial smooth muscle (beta-2). Use during acute exacerbation. Adverse effects are tremor and arrhythmia.

Methylxanthines **Theophylline:** mechanism unclear—may cause bronchodilation by inhibiting phosphodiesterase, enzyme involved in degrading cAMP (controversial).

Muscarinic antagonists **Ipratropium:** competitive block of muscarinic receptors preventing bronchoconstriction.

Cromolyn Prevents release of mediators from mast cells. Effective only for the prophylaxis of asthma. Not effective during an active asthmatic attack. Toxicity is very rare.

Corticosteroids **Beclomethasone, prednisone:** Prevent production of leukotrienes from arachidonic acid by blocking phospholipase A_2. Are drugs of choice in a patient with status asthmaticus (in combination with albuterol).

Antileukotrienes **Zileuton:** blocks synthesis by lipoxygenase.
Zafirlukast: blocks leukotriene receptors.

Treatment strategies in asthma

HIGH-YIELD FACTS

Pulmonary Medicine

Lung volumes

1. Residual volume (RV) = air in lung at maximal expiration
2. Expiratory reserve volume (ERV) = air that can still be breathed out after normal expiration
3. Tidal volume (TV) = air that moves into lung with each quiet inspiration, typically 500 mL
4. Inspiratory reserve volume (IRV) = air in excess of tidal volume that moves into lung on maximum inspiration
5. Vital capacity (VC) = TV + IRV + ERV
6. Functional reserve capacity (FRC) = RV + ERV (volume in lungs after a normal expiration)
7. Inspiratory capacity (IC) = IRV + TV
8. Total lung capacity = TLC = IRV + TV + ERV + RV

Vital capacity is everything but the residual volume.

A capacity is a sum of ≥ 2 volumes.

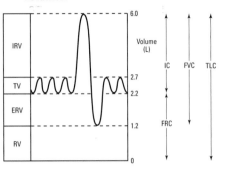

Pulmonary Medicine

HIGH-YIELD FACTS

CYSTIC FIBROSIS (CF)

An **autosomal-recessive** disorder caused by mutations in the CFTR gene (chloride channel) and characterized by widespread exocrine gland dysfunction. CF is the most common severe genetic disease in the United States (and is most common in **Caucasians**). It was previously considered a childhood disease, but life expectancy has increased so that many CF patients are treated well into adulthood.

History/PE

- **Respiratory:** Recurrent pulmonary infections (especially with *Pseudomonas* and *S. aureus*), cyanosis, digital clubbing, cough, dyspnea, **bronchiectasis,** hemoptysis, chronic sinusitis.
- **Gastrointestinal:** Fifteen percent of infants present with **meconium ileus**. Patients usually have greasy stools and flatulence. **Malabsorption syndromes, failure to thrive,** pancreatitis, rectal prolapse, esophageal varices, and biliary cirrhosis may be seen.
- **Other: Abnormal glucose tolerance,** type II diabetes, "salty taste," unexplained hyponatremia. Ninety-five percent of males are **infertile.** Fifty percent of patients present with failure to thrive or respiratory compromise.

Evaluation

Sweat chloride test > 60 mEq/L under age 20; > 80 mEq/L in adults; genetic testing.

Treatment

Pulmonary manifestations are managed by **DNase,** chest physical therapy, **bronchodilators, anti-inflammatory agents,** and **antibiotics.** Administer pancreatic enzymes and fat-soluble vitamins A, D, E, and K for malabsorption. Patients with severe disease (but who can tolerate surgery) may be candidates for lung or pancreas transplants.

UCV *Ped.11*

PLEURAL EFFUSION

Abnormal accumulation of fluid in the pleural space. Pleural effusions are classified as **transudative** or **exudative.**

History

Often **asymptomatic,** but patients may present with **dyspnea** and **pleuritic chest pain.**

PE

Decreased breath sounds, dullness to percussion, and **decreased** tactile fremitus.

Consolidation = decreased breath sounds + increased fremitus.
Effusion = decreased breath sounds + decreased fremitus.

Differential

Transudative and exudative pleural effusions may be differentiated as follows:

	Pleural/Serum Protein	Pleural/Serum LDH
Transudate	< 0.5	< 0.6
Exudate	> 0.5	> 0.6

- **Transudative effusion: Intact capillaries** lead to protein-poor pleural fluid that is an ultrafiltrate of plasma. Common causes of pleural fluid transudates include **CHF, nephrotic syndrome, cirrhosis,** and protein-losing enteropathy.
- **Exudative effusion:** Inflammation leads to **leaky capillaries,** resulting in protein-rich pleural fluid. Common causes of exudative pleural effusions include **malignancy, TB,** bacterial **infection** (parapneumonic effusion and empyema), viral infection, pulmonary emboli with infarct, collagen vascular disease, pancreatitis, hemothorax, chylothorax, and traumatic tap.

Evaluation

- CXR shows **blunting of the costophrenic angles.** A decubitus CXR will determine whether the fluid is free flowing or loculated.
- Pleural fluid analysis:
  - LDH and protein help distinguish transudate from exudate.
  - Gram stain.
  - CBC with differential and culture for evidence of infection or trauma (increased RBCs).
  - Increased amylase suggests malignancy or pancreatitis.
  - Cytology may reveal malignant cells.
- Needle biopsy of pleura diagnoses TB effusion.
- Definitive diagnosis is made by **thoracocentesis** or open biopsy.

Treatment

- **Transudative:** Treat the underlying condition. Perform therapeutic thoracocentesis if the patient is dyspneic.
- **Malignant:** Consider pleurodesis (injection of an irritant into the pleural cavity to scar the two pleural layers together) in symptomatic patients who are unresponsive to chemotherapy and radiation therapy. Alternatives include therapeutic thoracocentesis, pleuroperitoneal shunting, and surgical pleurectomy.
- **Parapneumonic:** Pleural effusion in the presence of **pneumonia.** If there is evidence of empyema (pH < 7.2, glucose < 40 mg/dL, positive Gram stain), initiate **chest tube** drainage.
- **Hemothorax:** Chest tube.

PULMONARY EMBOLISM (PE)

Occlusion of the pulmonary vasculature, typically by a blood clot. Ninety-five percent of emboli originate from DVTs in the deep leg veins. Pulmonary thromboembolism often leads to pulmonary infarction, right heart failure, and hypoxia. Risk factors for DVT and subsequent pulmonary thromboembolism include **Virchow's triad:**

- **Stasis** (immobility, CHF, obesity, surgery, increased CVP).
- **Endothelial injury** (e.g., trauma, surgery, recent fracture, previous DVT).
- **Hypercoagulable states** (e.g., pregnancy/postpartum, OCP use, and coagulation disorders such as protein C/protein S deficiency, factor V Leiden, malignancy, and severe burns).

History/PE

Presenting symptoms include sudden-onset dyspnea, **pleuritic chest pain, low-grade fever,** cough, and, rarely, hemoptysis or hypotension and syncope. Signs include **tachypnea; tachycardia;** erythematous, **edematous, tender, warm lower extremity;** and positive Homans' sign (calf pain on forced dorsiflexion; neither sensitive nor specific). Loud P2 and prominent jugular a waves with **right heart** failure are also seen.

Consider PE in any dyspneic hospitalized patient.

Evaluation

- ABGs reveal **respiratory alkalosis** (due to hyperventilation), with PO_2 < 80 mm (90% sensitive). The alveolar-arterial gradient may be elevated with arterial hypoxemia.
- CXR is usually normal but may show a pleural effusion, **Hampton's hump** (wedge-shaped infarct), or **Westermark's sign** (oligemia in the embolized lung zone). **Dyspnea, tachycardia, and a normal CXR** in a hospitalized and/or bedridden patient should raise suspicion of pulmonary thromboembolism.
- **V/Q scan** may reveal segmental area(s) of mismatch. Results are reported with a designated probability of pulmonary thromboembolism (low, medium, high) and are interpreted on the basis of clinical suspicion. Patients must be willing and able to cooperate for the study.
- **Pulmonary angiogram** is the gold standard but is more invasive (Figure 2.15–1).
- Helical (spiral) CT (with IV contrast) is sensitive for PE in the proximal pulmonary arteries but less so in the distal segmental arteries.
- EKG is not diagnostic and will most often show **sinus tachycardia.** The "classic" pattern of acute right heart strain with an S in lead I and T-wave inversion in V3 is uncommon.

See Figure 2.15–2 for the diagnostic algorithm.

Treatment

- Treat with **heparin** bolus and then weight-based continuous infusion. Start **warfarin** for long-term anticoagulation, usually 3–6 months of therapy unless the underlying predisposing factor persists (then indefinitely). Follow INR; maintain between 2 and 3.
- An **IVC filter** is indicated if anticoagulation is contraindicated or if the patient has recurrent emboli while anticoagulated.
- Thrombolysis is indicated only in severe cases.
- **Prevent DVTs** in bedridden and surgical patients with intermittent pneumatic compression of the lower extremities, **low-dose subcutaneous heparin,** and **early ambulation.**

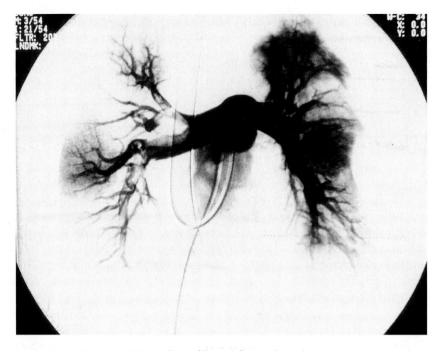

FIGURE 2.15–1. Pulmonary embolus. A large filling defect in the pulmonary artery is evident on pulmonary angiogram.

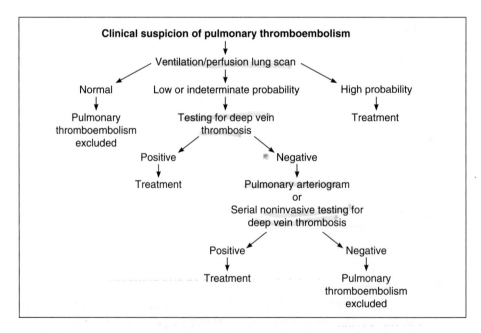

FIGURE 2.15–2. Diagnostic approach to pulmonary embolism. (From Tierney LM, *Current Medical Diagnosis & Treatment*, 39th ed., New York: McGraw-Hill, 2000: p. 326, Fig. 9–2.)

- Low-molecular-weight heparin (LMWH), which is administered subcutaneously and does not require monitoring of bleeding times, has a reduced risk of complications such as GI bleeding. LWMH is now accepted as an alternative means of anticoagulation on an outpatient basis.

UCV *EM.22, 46*

PNEUMOTHORAX

A collection of air in the pleural space that can lead to pulmonary collapse.

- **Primary spontaneous** pneumothorax is thought to occur with the rupture of subpleural apical blebs (usually in tall, thin young males).
- **Secondary** causes of pneumothorax include COPD, TB, trauma, *Pneumocystis carinii* pneumonia, and iatrogenesis (thoracocentesis, subclavian line placement, positive-pressure mechanical ventilation, or bronchoscopy).
- **Tension** pneumothorax occurs when a pulmonary or chest wall defect acts as a one-way valve, drawing air into the pleural space during inspiration but trapping air during expiration. Etiologies include penetrating trauma, infection, CHF, and positive-pressure mechanical ventilation. Tension pneumothorax is a life-threatening condition that proceeds to shock and death unless it is immediately recognized and treated.

History

Unilateral pleuritic chest pain and dyspnea.

Tension pneumothorax is a medical emergency.

PE

Tachypnea, **diminished/absent breath sounds, hyperresonance,** and **decreased tactile fremitus.** Suspect tension pneumothorax if you see respiratory distress, falling O_2 saturation, hypotension, distended neck veins, and **tracheal deviation.**

Differential

MI, pulmonary emboli, pneumonia, pericardial tamponade, pleural effusion.

Evaluation

CXR often shows a visceral pleural line and/or **lung retraction** from the chest wall (best seen in end-expiratory films; see Figure 2.15–3).

Treatment

Small pneumothoraces may reabsorb spontaneously. Large, symptomatic pneumothoraces require **chest tube** placement and/or **pleurodesis.**

Tension pneumothorax is an emergency requiring **immediate needle decompression** in the second intercostal space at the midclavicular line. Do not wait for a CXR! After initial decompression, insert a chest tube.

UCV *IM2.47, Surg.51*

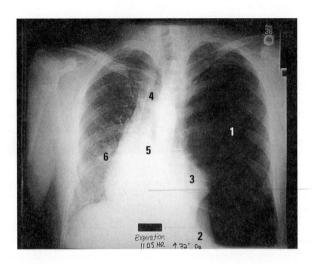

FIGURE 2.15–3. Tension pneumothorax. Note the hyperlucent lung field (1), hyperexpanded lower diaphragm (2), collapsed lung (3), tracheal deviation (4), mediastinal shift (5), and compression of the opposite lung (6) on anteroposterior CXR.

ACUTE RESPIRATORY DISTRESS SYNDROME (ARDS)

ARDS occurs in the setting of aspiration, infection, shock, or sepsis.

Acute respiratory failure with refractory **hypoxemia, decreased lung compliance,** and **noncardiogenic pulmonary edema.** Its underlying pathogenesis is thought to be endothelial injury. ARDS commonly occurs in the setting of aspiration, infection, multiple blood transfusions, lung injury, shock, or sepsis.

History/PE

Acute onset (12–48 hours) of respiratory distress, tachypnea, fever, crackles, and rhonchi.

Differential

Cardiogenic pulmonary edema, pneumonia, bronchiolitis obliterans with organizing pneumonia.

Evaluation

Criteria for diagnosis are as follows:

- Acute onset of respiratory distress.
- $PaO_2:FiO_2$ ratio $\leq$ 200 mmHg.
- Bilateral pulmonary infiltrates on CXR.
- No evidence of cardiac origin (normal capillary wedge pressure $\leq$ 18 mmHg).

Patients have severe hypoxemia refractory to oxygen therapy and decreased lung compliance.

Treatment

There is no standard successful treatment. The goal is to treat the underlying disease and to maintain adequate perfusion and O_2 delivery to organs. Use **mechanical ventilation** with low PEEP, increased inspiratory times, and FiO_2 with a goal of $SaO_2 \geq 90\%$. Support cardiac output with inotropes and cautious fluid administration. Steroids may be beneficial but have been shown to increase mortality in patients with sepsis and ARDS. Overall mortality is > 50%.

UCV *IM2.42*

ASTHMA

Reversible airway obstruction secondary to bronchial **hyperreactivity,** acute airway **inflammation, mucous plugging,** and smooth muscle hypertrophy of the airways. Triggers include allergens (dust, animal hair, odors), URIs, cold air, exertion, and stress.

Asthma triggers include allergens, URIs, cold air, exercise, and stress.

History

Cough, dyspnea, **episodic wheezing,** and/or chest tightness. Historical features suggesting severe asthma include a history of frequent ER visits, intubations, and PO steroid use. Symptoms are often worse at night or early in the morning.

PE

Tachypnea, tachycardia, **prolonged expiratory duration** (decreased I/E ratio), decreased O_2 saturation (late sign), decreased breath sounds, wheezing, hyperresonance, **accessory muscle use,** and possibly pulsus paradoxus.

Differential

- **Children:** Aspiration, bronchiolitis, bronchopulmonary dysplasia, CF, GERD, vascular rings, pneumonia.
- **Adults:** CHF, COPD, GERD, pulmonary embolism, foreign body, tumor, sleep apnea, anaphylaxis.

"All that wheezes is not asthma."

Evaluation

ABGs may reveal **mild hypoxia** and **respiratory alkalosis;** a normalizing pCO_2 in acute exacerbation warrants close observation, as it may indicate fatigue of ventilatory muscles and impending respiratory failure. **Peak flow** is diminished during acute exacerbation. Spirometry demonstrates decreased 1-second forced expiratory volume (FEV_1). **CBC** may demonstrate eosinophilia. CXR may show **hyperinflation.** Definitive diagnosis (when the patient is not acutely ill) can be made with the bronchial hyperresponsiveness (BHR) test with a **methacholine challenge.**

Rising pCO_2 may indicate fatigue and impending respiratory failure.

Treatment

- **Acute management** includes **oxygen, bronchodilators** (beta-agonist and/or ipratropium), and **steroids (inhaled; if refractory, IV).**
- **Chronic management** includes regularly inhaled **bronchodilators**

TABLE. 2.15–1. Medications for chronic treatment of asthma

Severity	Frequency of Symptoms	Treatment
Mild intermittent	Infrequent, > 2 times/week.	Metered-dose (beta-agonist) inhaler (MDI) for symptomatic relief.
Mild persistent	Daily, with occasional nighttime occurrence.	MDI and inhaled corticosteroids. May also add another long-term treatment (cromolyn sodium or leukotriene antagonist).
Moderate/severe persistent	Multiple daily symptoms, frequent nighttime occurrence.	Multiple medications, including systemic steroids. Close monitoring by a pulmonologist.

and/or **steroids,** systemic steroids, **cromolyn,** or **theophylline.** New guidelines support the use of anti-inflammatory agents if the patient is symptomatic > 2 times per week or has nocturnal symptoms ≥ 2 times per month. **Zafirlukast** and other leukotriene antagonists are oral agents that may serve as adjuncts to inhalant therapy (see Table 2.15–1).

- Patients should avoid allergens or any potential exacerbating factor.

UCV *EM.45, IM2.42, Ped.54*

CHRONIC OBSTRUCTIVE PULMONARY DISEASE (COPD)

A chronic, progressive disease characterized by a decrease in lung function with airflow obstruction. COPD is generally due to chronic bronchitis or emphysema. **Chronic bronchitis** is a productive cough lasting at least three months per year for two consecutive years. **Emphysema** is a pathologic diagnosis of terminal airway destruction due to smoking (centrilobular) or inherited alpha-1-antitrypsin deficiency (panlobular). Most patients have components of both, and **nearly all are smokers.** COPD is the fourth most common cause of death in the United States.

History/PE

Often minimal or nonspecific until disease is advanced (with loss of > 50% of lung function).

- **Emphysema ("pink puffer"):** Decreased breath sounds, minimal cough, **dyspnea,** pursed lips, hypercarbia/hypoxia late, barrel chest.
- **Chronic bronchitis ("blue bloater"):** Rhonchi, productive cough, cyanotic but with **mild** dyspnea, hypercarbia/hypoxia early, frequently overweight with peripheral edema.

PE may show barrel chest from high lung volumes, use of accessory chest muscles, JVD, end-expiratory wheezing, or muffled breath sounds.

Differential

Asthma, bronchiectasis, CHF, CF.

Evaluation

CXR classically shows decreased markings with flat diaphragms, **hyperinflated lungs,** and a thin-appearing heart and mediastinum; parenchymal **bullae** or subpleural **blebs** may be noted and are pathognomonic of emphysema (Figure 2.15–4). Spirometry is diagnostic, showing decreased FEV_1 and a decreased FEV_1:FVC ratio with increased TLC (compare to restrictive lung disease, where the FEV_1:FVC ratio is normal or increased). Peak flows are decreased. An ABG during an acute exacerbation will show **hypoxemia** with **acute respiratory acidosis** (increased pCO_2; however, patients have baseline increased pCO_2). Obtain blood cultures if the patient is febrile or has a productive cough. Gram stain and culture sputum.

Treatment

- **Acute exacerbations:** Oxygen, **inhaled beta-agonists** (albuterol) and **anticholinergics** (ipratropium), **IV steroids,** and **antibiotics.**
- **Chronic:** **Smoking cessation,** supplemental oxygen, inhaled beta-agonists (albuterol), anticholinergics (ipratropium) and steroids, **pneumococcal and flu vaccines.** ~~Atrovent (best choice)~~

Complications

- **Chronic respiratory failure:** Chronic hypoxemia with a compensated respiratory acidosis (high pCO_2).
- **Cor pulmonale:** Right heart failure secondary to pulmonary hypertension. *IM1.5*
- **Pneumonia.**
- **Bronchogenic carcinoma.**

UCV *IM2.45, 46*

"CO_2 retainers" occasionally do worse with supplemental O_2 because they lose their hypoxemic drive to breathe and acutely increase their pCO_2.

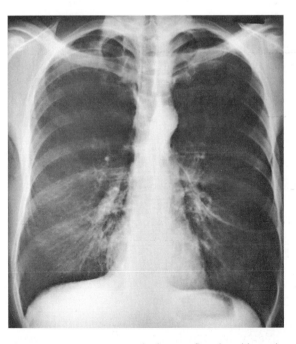
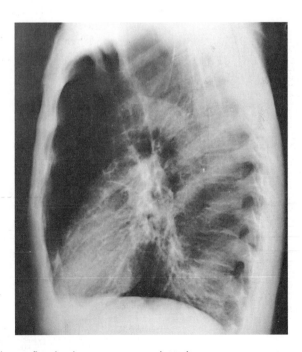

FIGURE 2.15–4. COPD. Note the hyperinflated and hyperlucent lungs, flat diaphragms, increased AP diameter, narrow mediastinum, and large upper lobe bullae on (A) anteroposterior and (B) lateral chest x-rays. (Reproduced, with permission, from Stobo JD, *Principles and Practice of Medicine*, 23rd ed., Stamford, CT: Appleton & Lange, 1997: p. 135, Fig. 2.3–2.)

Sleep apnea may be obstructive or central. Patients with obstructive apnea have recurrent episodes of partial or complete closure of the upper airway during sleep, during which respiratory efforts continue. Patients with central (nonobstructive) apnea have episodic cessation of both airflow and respiratory efforts due to loss of central drive. Mixed apnea, with both obstructive and central elements, may also occur. Risk factors include male sex (four times greater incidence in males), obesity, and use of sedatives during sleep.

The cause is unknown but may include abnormalities with the feedback control of breathing during sleep or decreased sensitivity of upper airway muscles or muscles of inspiration to stimulation. Anatomic abnormalities of the upper airway are also a possible cause.

History/PE

Daytime sleepiness and fatigue, impaired concentration, loud snoring, gasping or choking during sleep, and recurrent arousals from sleep. Patients may be otherwise normal, with normal PFTs.

Evaluation

Diagnosis is made by **sleep studies** that document the number of arousals or episodes of decreased oxygen saturation.

Treatment

- For obstructive sleep apnea, treat via weight loss and avoidance of sedating/hypnotic medications.
- Treat the underlying condition, which may include tonsillar hypertrophy, GERD or myxedema of hypothyroidism, or hypertension (which is frequently associated). For chronic disease, continuous positive airway pressure is helpful.
- Surgery can improve obstruction caused by enlarged tonsils, nasal polyps, macroglossia, or micrognathia.
- Tracheostomy may be necessary to completely bypass the obstruction.

UCV *Surg.9*

A systemic disease of unknown etiology characterized by noncaseating granulomas. In the United States, sarcoid is most common in **black females** and usually presents in the third or fourth decade of life.

History/PE

Fever, cough, malaise, weight loss, dyspnea, and **arthritis,** commonly of the knees and ankles. The lungs, liver, eyes, skin (erythema nodosum), nervous system, heart, and kidney may be affected.

Differential

TB, lymphoma, histoplasmosis, coccidioidomycosis, idiopathic pulmonary fibrosis, pneumoconioses, HIV, berylliosis.

Evaluation

Sarcoidosis is a **diagnosis of exclusion** (steroid treatment for sarcoid will exacerbate TB or other infections).

- CXR shows **bilateral hilar lymphadenopathy** and/or pulmonary infiltrates.
- Biopsy (transbronchial is best) of involved regions reveals noncaseating granulomas.
- PFTs show decreased volumes and diffusion capacity (a restrictive pattern).
- Other findings may include **elevated serum ACE levels** (neither sensitive nor specific), **hypercalcemia,** hypercalciuria, elevated alkaline phosphatase (with liver involvement), and lymphopenia.
- Kveim skin test is often positive (performed by injecting protein from human sarcoid tissue) but is rarely done.

Treatment

Systemic **corticosteroids.**

UCV *IM2.48*

> **Features of sarcoid—**
>
> **GRUELING**
> **G**ranulomas
> **R**heumatoid arthritis
> **U**veitis
> **E**rythema nodosum
> **L**ymphadenopathy
> **I**nterstitial fibrosis
> **N**egative TB test
> **G**ammaglobulinemia

PNEUMOCONIOSES

Occupational lung injury affecting the pulmonary interstitium. Typically, interstitial lung disease (ILD) develops after long-term, high-concentration exposure to particles that are inhaled and induce inflammation and fibrosis. These sorts of conditions are becoming rare in developed countries owing to the enforcement of safety regulations, and physicians who diagnose these conditions should alert the appropriate agency (e.g., OSHA). The risk of developing clinically evident disease increases with the level and duration of exposure (see Table 2.15–2).

ILD presents with cough, sputum, and exertional dyspnea. Crackles and fine wheezing may be heard on chest auscultation. CXR may show linear or nodular opacification. **High-resolution CT scan** is used in patients with a normal CXR who are suspected of having pneumoconiosis.

There is no cure for pneumoconiosis. Treatment generally involves supportive therapy and oxygen supplementation. Patients should quit smoking, as it can have an additive detrimental effect.

UCV *IM2.46*

HIGH-YIELD FACTS

Pulmonary Medicine

TABLE. 2.15–2. Pneumoconioses

Agent	Exposure History	Aids to Diagnosis	Complications
Asbestosis IM2.43	Work involving manufacture of tile or brake linings, insulation, construction, demolition, or building maintenance. Disease presents 15–20 years after initial exposure.	CXR: **linear opacities** at lung bases and pleural plaques. Biopsy: **asbestos bodies.**	Increased risk of mesothelioma, particularly in smokers.
Coal mine dust	Work in underground coal mines.	CXR: For simple coal workers' pneumoconiosis, small (< 1 cm) **nodular opacities** in upper lung zones. Spirometry consistent with restrictive disease.	Progressive massive fibrosis with increased morbidity and mortality.
Silicosis IM2.49	Miners, sandblasters, quarries, work with abrasives, stone, pottery, glass, or silica flour.	CXR: For simple silicosis, small (< 1 cm) **nodular opacities** in upper lung zones. Spirometry consistent with restrictive disease.	**Increased risk of *Mycobacterium tuberculosis*;** perform annual TB skin test. Progressive massive fibrosis.
Beryllium	High-technology fields such as aerospace, nuclear power, telecommunications, and electronics; ceramics, foundries, plating, dental materials, tool and die manufacturing.	CXR: diffuse infiltrates, hilar adenopathy.	Need for chronic corticosteroid treatment.

UCV

SOLITARY PULMONARY NODULE

Forty percent of solitary pulmonary nodules are malignant.

A lung nodule < 5 cm in size that is discovered on CXR or CT. Solitary pulmonary nodules have a 40% likelihood of being malignant.

Etiologies

Granuloma (e.g., old or active TB infection, fungal infection, foreign body reaction), carcinoma, **hamartoma,** metastasis (usually multiple), bronchial adenoma (95% carcinoid tumors), **pneumonia.**

(hormone serotonin)
5-HIAA)
pellagra (↓ niacin)

412

Evaluation

Obtain old x-rays if available and perform a CT scan to determine the nature, location, progression, and extent of the nodule. Proceed to biopsy or resection if diagnosis is still in doubt.

Benign lesions may be distinguished from malignant lesions by the following means:

- **Characteristics favoring carcinoma:** Age > 45–50 years; lesions new or larger in comparison to old films; absence of calcification or **irregular calcification;** size > 2 cm; irregular margins.
- **Characteristics favoring a benign lesion:** Age < 35 years; no change from old films; **central/uniform/laminated calcification;** smooth margins; size < 2 cm; regular margins.

Older age of patient and larger size of nodule favor malignancy.

Treatment

- A nodule in a patient > 35 years old should be **resected** unless there is radiologic proof that the lesion has not changed in size or appearance in at least two years.
- If the patient is young, if the lesion is unchanged, or if the patient objects, the lesion can be followed with a **second study in 3–6 months** (resect lesions that change in size or character).
- Surgical excision is preferred over biopsy. In some cases, surgeons opt for thoracoscopic biopsy with conversion to open resection if necessary.

LUNG CANCER

Risk factors include **smoking** (all types except bronchoalveolar carcinoma) and exposure to secondhand smoke, **asbestos,** and other environmental agents.

History

Patients can present with **hemoptysis, cough,** dyspnea, chest pain, and systemic symptoms (fatigue, malaise, weight loss). Some patients are **asymptomatic** and present with a lung nodule noted on CXR/CT.

Lung cancer is the leading cause of cancer death.

PE

Physical examination is usually unremarkable but may reveal abnormalities on respiratory exam (crackles, atelectasis). Other findings include **Horner's syndrome** (miosis, ptosis, anhidrosis) in patients with Pancoast's tumor and many **paraneoplastic syndromes** (Table 2.15–3).

Differential

TB/other granulomatous diseases, fungal disease (aspergillus, histoplasmosis), lung abscess, metastasis, benign tumor (bronchial adenoma), hamartoma.

TABLE 2.15–3. Paraneoplastic Syndromes in Lung Cancer

Classification	Syndrome	Histologic Type of Cancer
Endocrine and metabolic	**Cushing's syndrome**	Small cell
	SIADH	Small cell
	Hypercalcemia	Squamous cell
	Gynecomastia	Large cell
Connective tissue and osseous	Hypertrophic pulmonary osteoarthropathy	Squamous cell, adenocarcinoma, large cell
Neuromuscular	Peripheral neuropathy (sensory, sensorimotor)	Small cell
	Subacute cerebellar degeneration	Small cell
	Myasthenia **(Eaton–Lambert syndrome)**	Small cell
	Dermatomyositis	All
Cardiovascular	Thrombophlebitis	Adenocarcinoma
	Nonbacterial verrucous (marantic) endocarditis	
Hematologic	Anemia	All
	DIC	
	Eosinophilia	
	Thrombocytosis	
Cutaneous	Acanthosis nigricans	All
	Erythema gyratum repens	

(Adapted, with permission, from Tierney LM, *Current Medical Diagnosis and Treatment*, 39th ed., New York: McGraw-Hill, 2000: p. 310, Table 9–16.)

Evaluation

Lung cancer is usually first noted as a nodule on CXR and is best seen with **lung CT. Bronchoscopy with biopsy** or brushing or **fine needle aspiration** under CT guidance can usually establish the diagnosis. Mediastinoscopy may be necessary for biopsy of hilar nodes. Thoracoscopic biopsy may be performed, with conversion to open thoracotomy if the lesion is found to be malignant.

Treatment

- Although there are multiple types of lung cancer (large cell, bronchoalveolar, adenocarcinoma, squamous, small cell), they can be grouped into **non–small cell** (NSCLC) and **small cell** (SCLC) for the purposes of treatment.
- **NSCLC** should be treated with **surgical resection** if possible. The decision is based on the size of the lesion, the presence of metastases (metastatic disease is usually not resected unless there is only a single brain met), and the patient's age, general health, and lung function.

Lung cancer—

SPHERE of complications
Superior vena caval syndrome
Pancoast's tumor
Horner's syndrome
Endocrine (paraneoplastic)
Recurrent laryngeal symptoms (hoarseness)
Effusions (pleural or pericardial)

Follow surgery with radiation/chemotherapy (depends on stage). Unresectable disease should be treated with radiation and chemotherapy.

- SCLC is not considered resectable and often responds initially to **radiation** and **chemotherapy** but usually recurs, carrying a much **lower median survival rate** than NSCLC.
- Treat oncologic emergencies (e.g., SVC syndrome) with radiation.
- Treat metastases (brain, liver, bone) palliatively. Risk for brain metastasis is very high.

Prevention

Smoking cessation (nothing else, including CXR screening, has been shown to help).

UCV *Surg.50*

Causes of an exudative effusion.	Malignancy, TB, bacterial or viral infection, PE with infarct, and pancreatitis are some causes
Criteria for exudative effusion.	Pleural: serum protein > 0.5 Pleural: serum LDH > 0.6
Risk factors for DVT. *Virchow's triad →*	Stasis, endothelial injury and hypercoagulability
Acid–base disorder in PE.	Respiratory alkalosis
Acute-onset tachypnea, pleuritic chest pain in tall, thin young men.	Spontaneous pneumothorax
Hypoxemia and pulmonary edema with normal pulmonary capillary wedge pressure.	ARDS *↓ lung Compliance / non cardiac pul. edema*
Dyspnea, lateral hilar lymphodenopathy on CXR; increased ACE, hypercalcemia.	Sarcoidosis
FEV_1:FVC ratio in persons with obstructive pulmonary disease, versus normal.	Decreased
Cor pulmonale.	Right heart failure secondary to pulmonary hypertension
Lung disease of coal miners.	Coal workers' pneumoconiosis
Increased risk of what infection with silicosis?	M. *tuberculosis*
Treatment for tension pneumothorax.	Immediate decompression using a needle in the second intercostal space; chest tube placement
Infant with failure to thrive, frequent pulmonary infections, greasy stools. Diagnostic test?	Sweat chloride > 60 mEq/L = cystic fibrosis (children)
Treatment for mild, persistent asthma.	Inhaled beta-agonists and inhaled corticosteroids
Normalizing pCO_2 in a patient having an asthma exacerbation may indicate?	Fatigue and impending respiratory failure
Duration of anticoagulation therapy following PE.	3–6 months
Pulmonary lesion of sarcoidosis.	Noncaseating granulomas

Questions reproduced, with permission, from Reteguiz J, *PreTest: Physical Diagnosis*, 4th ed., New York: McGraw Hill, 2001.

Questions

1. A 39-year-old woman presents with the sudden onset of pleuritic chest pain and shortness of breath. She has been in good health until three days ago, when she noticed some swelling of her left lower extremity. She is not a smoker and denies any recent trauma. On physical examination, she is afebrile but has a respiratory rate of 32/min. Her heart rate is 120/min and her blood pressure is normal. An accentuated (loud) S2 is heard on heart auscultation. The left lower extremity is swollen, tender to palpation, and erythematous. Dorsiflexion of the left foot (**Homans' sign**) causes severe calf discomfort. Lung examination and chest radiograph are normal. Arterial blood analysis on room air shows a PC_{O_2} of 30 mmHg and a P_{O_2} of 58 mmHg. Which of the following is the most appropriate next diagnostic step?
   a. Transesophageal echocardiogram
   b. Transthoracic echocardiogram
   c. Cardiac catheterization
   d. Ventilation/perfusion scan
   e. D-dimer assay

   and brochiectasis,

2. A 14-year-old boy presents with a <u>history of chronic sinusitis</u> and frequent pneumonias. On physical examination, the patient has normal vital signs and is afebrile. He has mild frontal maxillary sinus tenderness with palpation. Transillumination of the sinuses is normal. Heart sounds are best heard on the right side of the chest. The boy is coughing copious amounts of yellowish sputum. Which of the following is the most likely diagnosis?
   a. Cystic fibrosis
   b. Kartagener syndrome
   c. Pulmonary dysplasia
   d. Tuberculosis
   e. Pulmonary hypertension

3. A 70-year-old man with a history of chronic obstructive pulmonary disease (COPD) presents complaining of worsening shortness of breath for the last several days. He is coughing large amounts of yellow-colored sputum and is receiving <u>no relief from his β_2-agonist and ipratropium aerosolized pumps</u>. On physical examination, the patient's respiratory rate is 40/min and his heart rate is 110/min. His blood pressure is 150/85 mmHg. The patient is afebrile. He is using his accessory muscles of respiration (sternocleidomastoids and intercostals) to assist in breathing. Lung examination reveals inspiratory and expiratory diffuse wheezing. Which of the following is the most likely diagnosis?
   a. Acute exacerbation of COPD
   b. α_1-antitrypsin deficiency
   c. Chronic bronchitis
   d. Exacerbation of asthma
   e. Pneumonia

4. A man is stabbed and arrives at the emergency room within 30 minutes. You notice that the trachea is deviated away from the side of the chest with the puncture. The most likely lung finding on physical examination of the traumatized side is which of the following?
   a. Increased fremitus
   b. Increased breath sounds
   c. Dullness to percussion
   d. Hyperresonant percussion   *Tension pneu*
   e. Wheezing
   f. Stridor

Answers

1. **The answer is d.** The most frequent presenting clinical sign of **pulmonary embolus (PE)** is shortness of breath. Patients may also present with pleuritic chest pain, hemoptysis, and tachycardia. An excellent clue to the diagnosis of PE is deep venous thrombosis (DVT), but absence of signs of DVT does not exclude the diagnosis of PE. Embolus from a thrombus in the lower extremities (DVT) is the most common cause of PE. Common settings for PE include prolonged immobilization, use of oral contraceptives, obesity, recent surgery, burns, severe trauma, congestive heart failure, malignancy, pregnancy, sickle cell anemia, polycythemias, inherited deficiencies of the anticoagulating proteins (protein C, protein S, antithrombin III), and the Leiden factor V mutation. Chest radiograph in PE may be normal but may demonstrate a peripheral wedge-shaped density above the diaphragm **(Hampton's hump),** focal oligemia **(Westermark sign),** or abrupt occlusion of a vessel **(cutoff sign).** A loud S2 is often heard in disorders that cause pulmonary hypertension, such as pulmonary embolism. The next best step in making the diagnosis would be to order a ventilation/perfusion (V/Q) scan. If the V/Q scan results are of low or indeterminate probability, the patient may need further studies, such as pulmonary arteriogram or venous ultrasonography of the lower extremity. **D-dimer assays** will result in future changes to existing diagnostic strategies for pulmonary embolism, but the marker is still in the investigative stages (the absence of this product is evidence against thromboembolism). **Helical (spiral) CT** scans are comparable to V/Q scans and may be the first step in diagnosing pulmonary embolus.

2. **The answer is b. Kartagener syndrome** is the inheritable disorder of dextrocardia, chronic sinusitis (with the formation of nasal polyps), and bronchiectasis. Patients may also present with **situs inversus.** The disorder is due to a defect that causes the cilia within the respiratory tract epithelium to become immotile. Cilia of the sperm are also affected.

3. **The answer is a. COPD** is defined as a condition where there is chronic obstruction to airflow due to chronic bronchitis or emphysema. An exacerbation of COPD occurs when the patient develops the acute onset of marked dyspnea and tachypnea requiring the use of accessory muscles that is unresponsive to medications. α_1-antitrypsin deficiency should be suspected in nonsmokers who present with COPD of the lung bases in their fifties without any predisposing history, such as occupational exposure to support the diagnosis. α_1-antitrypsin deficiency is rare in African Americans and Asian–Pacific Islanders.

4. **The answer is d.** The patient has a **tension pneumothorax,** which is evidenced by the trachea deviating away from the side of the traumatized lung. This occurs secondary to trauma or during mechanical ventilation. Breath sounds will be faint or distant, percussion will be hyperresonant, and fremitus will be decreased. The increased air on the affected side is in the pleural space, not in the lung. As an attempt is made to inflate the lung, air moves into the pleural space from the puncture site, resulting in a collapsed lung with a large pleural space. The contralateral lung is also at risk for collapse. Any time the trachea is deviated from the involved side, it is considered a medical emergency and the tension pneumothorax must be relieved or the patient will die from hypoxemia or inadequate cardiac output.

Renal/Genitourinary

Acid–base physiology

	pH	Pco$_2$	[HCO$_3^-$]	Cause	Compensatory response
Metabolic acidosis	↓	↓	↓	Diabetic ketoacidosis; diarrhea; lactic acidosis; salicylate OD; acetazolamide OD	Hyperventilation
Respiratory acidosis	↓	↑	↑	COPD; airway obstruction	Renal [HCO$_3^-$] reabsorption
Respiratory alkalosis	↑	↓	↓	High altitude; hyperventilation	Renal [HCO$_3^-$] secretion
Metabolic alkalosis	↑	↑	↑	Vomiting	Hypoventilation

Henderson–Hasselbalch equation: $pH = pKa + \log \dfrac{[HCO_3^-]}{0.03\ Pco_2}$

Key: ↑ ↓ = primary disturbance; ↓ ↑ = compensatory response.

Diuretics: site of action

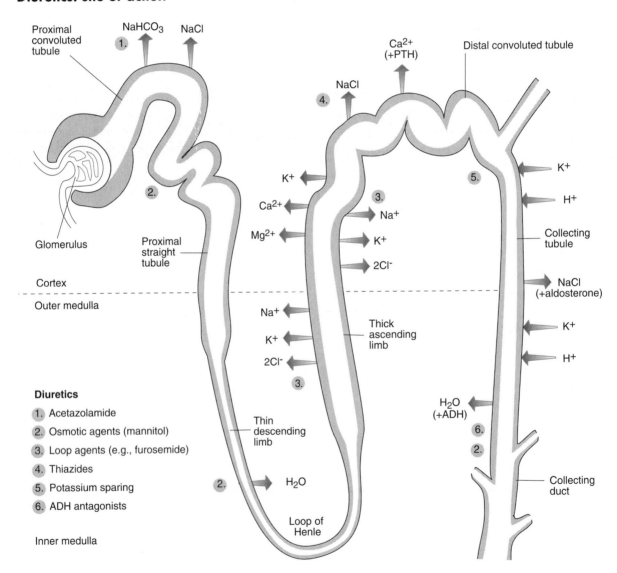

Diuretics

1. Acetazolamide
2. Osmotic agents (mannitol)
3. Loop agents (e.g., furosemide)
4. Thiazides
5. Potassium sparing
6. ADH antagonists

(Adapted, with permission, from Katzung BG, *Basic and Clinical Pharmacology*, 7th ed., Stamford, CT: Appleton & Lange, 1997: p. 243.)

Renal tubular acidosis is a net decrease in either tubular hydrogen secretion or bicarbonate reabsorption that produces a non-anion-gap metabolic acidosis. There are three main types:

- **Type 1:** Defective hydrogen ion secretion. Increased urinary pH.
- **Type 2:** Decreased bicarbonate reabsorption. Increased urinary pH until bicarbonate wasting reaches a steady state and no longer causes a rise in urinary pH.
- **Type 4:** Aldosterone resistance or deficiency impairs distal Na^+ reabsorption and K^+ secretion. Results in hyperkalemia. The most common type of RTA.

Table 2.16–1 further distinguishes the three main types of RTA.

TABLE 2.16–1. Types of RTA

	Type 1 (Distal)	Type 2 (Proximal)	Type 4 (Distal)
Defect	Defective H+ secretion ↓	↓ HCO_3 reabsorption	Inadequate aldosterone
Serum K	Low	Low	High
Urinary pH	> 5.3	< 5.3	< 5.3
Etiology (most common)	Hereditary, amphotericin, collagen vascular disease, cirrhosis, nephrocalcinosis	Hereditary, sulfonamides, carbonic anhydrase inhibitors, Fanconi syndromes	Hyporeninemic hypoaldosteronism with diabetes, HTN, or chronic interstitial nephritis; aldosterone resistance
Treatment	$HCO_3 + K^+$	$HCO_3 + K^+$, thiazide	Fludrocortisone, K^+ restriction, HCO_3

(Etiologies are derived from multiple referenced articles in *Primary Care Pearls and References*, Oxford, U.K: Blackwell Science, 1996, p. 225. The table format is derived from *Guide to Inpatient Medicine*, Baltimore, MD: Williams &Wilkins, 1997, p. 225.)

UCV *IM2.37*

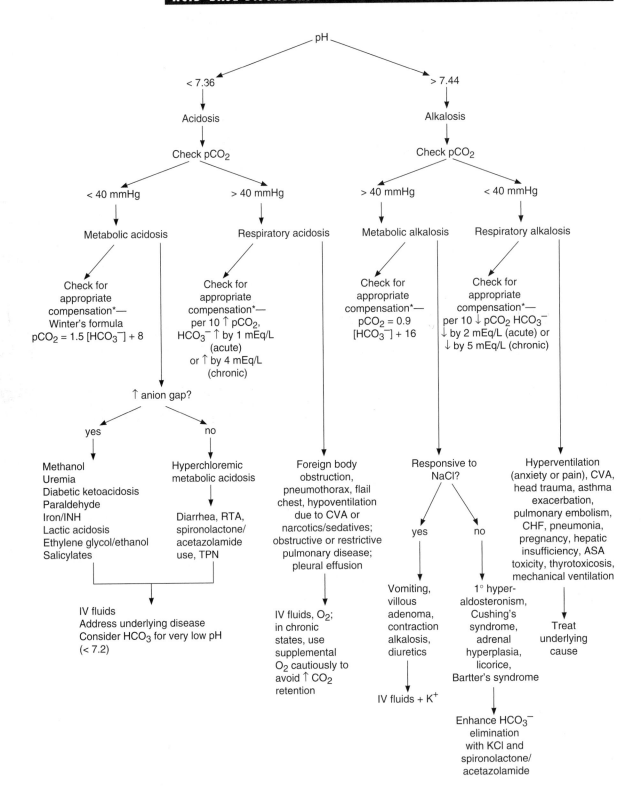

*Hint: compensatory mechanisms will not correct all the way to a normal pH. If pCO_2 and HCO_3^- are abnormal in the setting of a normal pH, a mixed disturbance is present.

FIGURE 2.16–1. Evaluation of acid–base disorders.

HYPERNATREMIA

Serum sodium > 145 mEq/L.

History/PE

Patients may report oliguria and polyuria (depending on the etiology) and thirst. Other symptoms include mental status changes, weakness, focal neurologic deficits, and seizures.

Evaluation

Assess volume status by clinical exam. Measure urine volume and osmolality. Hypervolemic hypernatremia suggests increased aldosterone or excess sodium (e.g., IV saline). Minimal volume (approximately 500 mL/d) of maximally concentrated (> 400 mOsm/kg) urine suggests adequate renal response without adequate free water replacement due to decreased intake, diuretics, glycosuria, or third spacing. Large volumes of dilute urine suggest diabetes insipidus (central or nephrogenic).

Treatment

Treat underlying causes and replace free water deficit with hypotonic saline. The deficit should be replaced gradually over 48–72 hours to prevent neurologic damage secondary to swelling.

HYPONATREMIA

Serum sodium < 135 mEq/L.

History/PE

Asymptomatic or may present with **confusion,** muscle cramps, nausea, and **lethargy.** Hyponatremia can progress to seizures, status epilepticus, or coma.

Evaluation

Hyponatremia can be classified by serum osmolality, volume status (by clinical exam), and urinary sodium. Osmolality can be further classified as:

- **High** (> 295): Hyperglycemia, hypertonic infusion.
- **Normal** (280–295): Pseudohyponatremia, hyperlipidema, hyperproteinemia.
- **Low** (< 280): Hypotonic. See Table 2.16–2.

TABLE 2.16–2. Evaluation of Hypotonic Hyponatremia

Variable	Hypervolemic	Euvolemic	Hypovolemic
Renal salt wasting, FeNa > 1%	Renal failure	SIADH, hypothyroidism, renal failure, drugs	Diuretics, RTA, adrenal insufficiency, ACE inhibitors
Renal salt conservation, FeNa < 1%	Nephrosis, CHF, cirrhosis	Polydipsia	Vomiting, diarrhea, third spacing, dehydration
Treatment	Salt and water restriction	Salt and water restriction	Replete volume with normal saline

HYPERKALEMIA

Serum potassium > 5.0 mEq/L.

History/PE

Verify hyperkalemia with a repeat blood draw.

Asymptomatic or may present with nausea, vomiting, **intestinal colic, areflexia, weakness,** flaccid paralysis, and paresthesias. Causes include:

- **Spurious:** Hemolysis (e.g., during phlebotomy), fist clenching during blood draw, leukocytosis, thrombocytosis.
- **Decreased excretion:** Renal insufficiency, drugs (spironolactone, triamterene, **ACE inhibitors,** trimethoprim, NSAIDs), mineralocorticoid deficiency.
- **Cellular shifts:** Tissue injury, acidosis, insulin deficiency, drugs (succinylcholine, digitalis, beta-agonists, arginine).
- **Iatrogenic.**

Evaluation

EKG findings may include **tall peaked T waves,** PR prolongation followed by loss of P waves, wide QRS complex that can progress to **torsades de pointes** (Figures 2.16–2 and 2.16–3), ventricular fibrillation, and cardiac arrest.

Treatment

- First verify hyperkalemia with a **repeat blood draw** unless the suspicion was already high.

UCV *IM1.14*

FIGURE 2.16–2. Hyperkalemia. Electrocardiographic manifestations include peaked T waves, PR prolongation, and a widened QRS complex. (Reproduced, with permission, from Cogan MG, *Fluid and Electrolytes,* 1st ed., Stamford, CT: Appleton & Lange, 1991: p. 170, Fig. 9–4.)

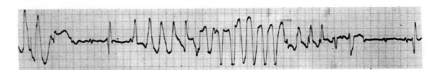

FIGURE 2.16–3. Torsades de pointes. The QRS axis gradually shifts so that the complex appears as a twisting strip; this is a pleomorphic ventricular tachycardia often caused by QT prolongation from electrolyte abnormalities or drugs. (Reproduced, with permission, from Stobo J, *The Principles and Practice of Medicine,* 23rd ed., Stamford, CT: Appleton & Lange, 1996: p. 81, Fig. 1–9–5.)

- Values > 6.5–7.0 mEq/L and/or EKG changes require emergent treatment.

The mnemonic **C BIG K** is useful for the treatment of hyperkalemia:

- Use **C**alcium gluconate for cardiac membrane stabilization.
- Shift potassium into cells (an immediate, short-term solution) with sodium **B**icarbonate, **I**nsulin and **G**lucose, or albuterol.
- **K**ayexalate and **loop diuretics** (furosemide) will remove potassium from the body.
- **Dialysis** is an option for patients with renal failure or in severe, refractory cases.

UCV *IM2.34*

HYPOKALEMIA

Serum potassium < 3.5 mEq/L.

History/PE

May present with fatigue, **muscle weakness, muscle cramps, ileus,** hyporeflexia, paresthesias, and flaccid paralysis if severe.

Evaluation

Twenty-four-hour urine may distinguish renal losses from GI losses. EKG may show **T-wave flattening** and ST depression followed by AV block and subsequent cardiac arrest. **U waves** may be present. Consider RTA in the setting of metabolic acidosis.

Etiologies

Diarrhea, alkalosis, Bartter's syndrome, hypomagnesemia, chronic laxative abuse, vomiting, drugs (diuretics, insulin, gentamicin, digitalis, amphotericin, carbenicillin), RTA, mineralocorticoid excess, DKA.

Treatment

Treat the underlying disorder. Administer oral and/or IV **potassium replacement.** Magnesium deficiency will make potassium repletion more difficult; replete Mg^{2+} as well.

Mg deficiency makes K⁺ repletion difficult.

HYPERCALCEMIA

Serum calcium > 10.5 mg/dL. Most cases are caused by hyperparathyroidism or malignancy. The major causes can be remembered with the mnemonic **CHIMPANZEES:**

- **C**alcium supplementation
- **H**yperparathyroidism (common)
- **I**atrogenic (thiazides)/**I**mmobility
- **M**ilk alkali syndrome
- **P**aget's disease
- **A**ddison's disease/**A**cromegaly
- **N**eoplasm (common, especially squamous cell cancers, myeloma)

- Zollinger–Ellison syndrome (MEN I)
- Excess vitamin A
- Excess vitamin D
- Sarcoidosis

History/PE

Clinical presentation involves "**bones** (fractures), **stones** (renal), abdominal **groans** (anorexia, vomiting, constipation), and psychic **overtones**" (weakness, fatigue, altered mental status).

Evaluation

Evaluation should include EKG (may show **short QT interval**), total/ionized calcium, albumin, phosphate, PTH (IRMA), vitamin D, and TSH.

Treatment

"Loops (furosemide) Lose calcium."

Treat with **IV hydration** (watch for CHF) followed by **furosemide diuresis.** Calcitonin, pamidronate, etidronate, glucocorticoids, plicamycin, and dialysis are used in severe or refractory cases. **Avoid thiazide diuretics** (increase tubular reabsorption of calcium).

HYPOCALCEMIA

Serum calcium < 8.5 mg/dL.

History

Abdominal/muscle cramps, dyspnea, **tetany,** and convulsions.

PE

Serum calcium may be falsely low in hypoalbuminemia.

Facial spasm with tapping over facial nerve **(Chvostek's sign)** and carpal spasm seen with arterial occlusion by a blood pressure cuff **(Trousseau's sign).** EKG may show a **prolonged QT interval** (a variety of drugs do this).

Etiologies

Hypoparathyroidism (postsurgery, idiopathic), malnutrition, hypomagnesemia, acute pancreatitis, medullary thyroid cancer (excess calcitonin).

Treatment

Treat the underlying disorder. Administer oral **calcium supplements;** give IV calcium if symptoms are severe.

Serum magnesemia < 1.5 mEq/L.

History/PE

Symptoms generally relate to the concurrent hypocalcemia and hypokalemia and include anorexia, nausea, vomiting, muscle cramps, and muscle weakness. At very low levels, symptoms include paresthesias, irritability, confusion, lethargy, seizures, and arrhythmias.

Etiologies

- **Decreased intake:** Malnutrition, **alcoholism,** malabsorption, short bowel syndrome, TPN.
- **Increased loss:** Diuretics, diarrhea, vomiting, renal insufficiency, Conn's syndrome.
- **Miscellaneous: Diabetic ketoacidosis,** pregnancy, pancreatitis.

Evaluation

Labs may show concurrent hypocalcemia and hypokalemia. EKG may show prolonged PR and QT intervals.

Treatment

IV, IM, and oral supplements are available. Hypokalemia and hypocalcemia will not correct without magnesium correction.

ACUTE RENAL FAILURE

Acute renal failure (ARF) is an abrupt decrease in renal function leading to the retention of creatinine and BUN. ARF is categorized as **prerenal, intrinsic,** or **postrenal.** Prerenal failure is caused by decreased renal plasma flow. Intrinsic renal failure results from injury within the nephron unit. Postrenal failure is caused by urinary outflow obstruction. Table 2.16–3 outlines the causes of acute renal failure according to subtype.

TABLE 2.16–3. Causes of Acute Renal Failure

Prerenal	Renal (Intrinsic)	Postrenal
Hypovolemia (dehydration, hemorrhage)	ATN	Prostate disease
Cardiogenic shock	Acute interstitial nephritis	Kidney stones
Sepsis	Glomerulonephritis	Pelvic tumors
Drugs (NSAIDs)	Nephrotic syndrome	Recent pelvic surgery
Renal artery stenosis	Thromboembolism	

Adapted from Stobo JD, *The Principles and Practice of Medicine*, 23rd ed., Stamford, CT: Appleton & Lange, 1996: p. 383.

History

Patients may present with malaise, fatigue, oliguria, anorexia, and nausea secondary to **uremia.**

PE

Pericardial friction rub, asterixis, hypertension, or decreased urine output. Hypovolemia and orthostasis suggest a prerenal etiology. Fever and rash support an acute interstitial nephritis. Patients with postrenal etiologies may have an enlarged prostate or a distended bladder.

Evaluation

Obtain **UA** (RBCs, casts, WBCs), **urine electrolytes,** and serum electrolytes. Pass a urinary catheter to rule out obstruction. **Renal ultrasound** may rule out obstruction or chronic renal failure. The fractional excretion of Na (FeNa) can be useful in identifying prerenal failure. It is calculated as follows:

$$FeNa = (U_{Na}/P_{Na}) / (U_{Cr}/P_{Cr})$$

FeNa < 1% suggests a prerenal etiology.

A FeNa < 1%, U_{Na} < 20, or BUN/creatinine ratio > 20 suggests a prerenal etiology.

Table 2.16–4 lists the potential findings on microscopic urine examination.

Treatment

- Balance fluids and electrolytes.
- Adjust/discontinue offending medications in interstitial nephritis.
- Dialyze if indicated.
- Give corticosteroids/cytotoxic agents for glomerulonephritis.

Indications for dialysis—

AEIOU
Acidosis
Electrolyte abnormalities (K > 6.5 mEq/L)
Ingestions
Overload (fluid)
Uremic symptoms (pericarditis, encephalopathy)

TABLE 2.16–4. Findings on Microscopic Urine Examination in Renal Failure

Urine Sediment (UA)	Etiology
Hyaline casts	Prerenal
Red cell casts, red cells	Glomerulonephritis (intrinsic)
White cells, white cell casts, +/– eosinophils	Allergic tubulointerstitial nephritis (intrinsic) _pyelo_
Granular casts, renal tubular cells	Acute tubular necrosis (intrinsic)

NEPHRITIC SYNDROME

Nephritic syndrome is defined as acute onset of **hematuria** and proteinuria (small amounts) with decreased renal function. It is the clinical manifestation of acute glomerular inflammation. See Table 2.16–5 for a summary of major etiologies of nephritic syndrome.

History/PE

Patients may present with oliguria, macroscopic hematuria (smoky-brown urine), hypertension, and **edema in low-pressure regions** such as the periorbital and scrotal areas.

TABLE 2.16–5. Causes of Nephritic Syndrome

	Description	History and PE	Labs and Histology	Treatment
Postinfectious glomerulonephritis	Often associated with recent **streptococcal infection** (group A beta-hemolytic), but may follow a variety of infections	Oliguria, edema, hypertension, smoky-brown urine	Low serum C3, ↑ ASO titer, lumpy-bumpy immuno-fluorescence	Supportive Px: Very good
IgA nephropathy (Berger's disease)	Associated with URI or GI infection; etiology unknown Most common worldwide glomerulonephritis	Gross hematuria	Increased serum IgA level, renal biopsy is standard for diagnosis	Glucocorticoids for acute flares Px: 20% progress to end-stage renal disease
Wegener's granulomatosis	Granulomatous inflammation of the respiratory tract with necrotizing vasculitis of small and medium-sized vessels	Fever, malaise, weight loss, hematuria, respiratory symptoms with nodular lesions that cavitate and bleed	Presence of **cANCA,** cell-mediated immune response is present	High-dose cortico-steroid and cytotoxic agents Px: Frequent relapses after remission
Goodpasture's syndrome	Glomerulonephritis with pulmonary hemorrhage; peak incidence in men in their mid-20s	**Hemoptysis,** dyspnea, possible respiratory failure	Iron-deficiency anemia, hemosiderin-filled macrophages in sputum, pulmonary infiltrates on CXR	Plasma exchange therapy, pulsed steroids Px: Variable; may progress to end-stage renal failure

IM2.57

HIGH-YIELD FACTS

Renal/Genitourinary

431

Evaluation

UA will show hematuria and proteinuria. Patients have a reduced GFR with elevated BUN and creatinine. Complement, ANA, ANCA, and anti-GBM antibody levels should be measured to assess the underlying etiology. Renal biopsy may be useful for histologic evaluation.

Treatment

Treatment of hypertension, fluid congestion, and uremia through salt and water restriction; diuretics and dialysis if needed. **Corticosteroids** are useful in reducing glomerular inflammation.

NEPHROTIC SYNDROME

Nephrotic syndrome is defined as proteinuria (> 3.5 g/day), generalized edema, hyperlipiduria, hyperlipidemia, and hypoalbuminemia. In adults, approximately one-third of all cases of nephrotic syndrome occur with a systemic disease such as lupus, diabetes, or amyloidosis. Other common causes are presented in Table 2.16–6.

History/PE

Patients present with **generalized edema** and may report "foamy urine" secondary to proteinuria. In severe cases, dyspnea and ascites may develop. Pa-

TABLE 2.16–6. Causes of Nephrotic Syndrome

	Description	History/PE	Labs and Histology	Treatment
Minimal change disease IM2.36	Common in children; generally idiopathic	Tendency toward infections and thrombotic events	Lipid-laden renal cortices, fusion of epithelial foot processes	Steroids; excellent prognosis
Focal segmental glomerular sclerosis	Idiopathic or secondary to drug use, HIV infection	Hypertension, typical nephrotic presentation; typical patient is young black male	Microscopic hematuria, requires renal biopsy—sclerosis in capillary tufts of deep JG apparatus	Supportive care, prednisone, cytotoxic therapy for refractory patients
Membranous glomerulonephritis	Most common adult nephropathy; immune complex disease	Associated with hepatitis B, syphilis, and malaria	"Spike and dome" appearance due to excess basement membrane, granular deposits of IgG and C3	Prednisone and cytotoxic therapy in severe disease

tients have an increased susceptibility to infection as well as venous thrombosis and pulmonary embolism.

Evaluation

Urinalysis will show **proteinuria** (> 3.5 g/day) and lipidemia. Blood chemistry will show **decreased albumin** (< 3 g/dL) and low serum protein. Renal biopsy is used to diagnose the underlying etiology in some cases.

Treatment

Protein and salt restriction, diuretic therapy, diet modification and antihyperlipidemics. Cytotoxic drug therapy may be helpful in severe/refractory disease. **Anticoagulation therapy** reduces the risk of DVT and renal vein thrombosis.

NEPHROLITHIASIS

Nephrolithiasis most commonly occurs in males in the third and fourth decades of life. Risk factors include a positive family history, **low fluid intake,** gout, postcolectomy/ileostomy, specific enzyme disorders (e.g., glyoxylate carboxylase deficiency, xanthine oxidase deficiency), RTA, certain medications (e.g., acetazolamide, allopurinol, chemotherapeutic agents, calcium carbonate, methoxyflurane, loop diuretics, vitamin D), and hyperparathyroidism. Table 2.16–7 further details the various forms of nephrolithiasis.

TABLE 2.16–7. Types of Nephrolithiasis

Type	Frequency	Etiology/Characteristics
Calcium oxalate	75%	Most common cause is **idiopathic hypercalciuria.** Form in alkaline urine. Radiopaque.
Calcium phosphate	8%	Think **primary hyperparathyroidism.** Radiopaque.
$Mg\text{-}NH_4\text{-}PO_4$ (struvite)	9%	Synonymous with struvite or triple phosphate stones. Associated with *Proteus, Pseudomonas, Providencia, Klebsiella* **UTIs.** Form in alkaline urine. Radiopaque; often form **staghorn** calculi.
Uric acid	7%	The pH is < 5.5. Can be dissolved by alkalinizing urine. **Radiolucent.** Occur in gout and high purine turnover states.
Cysteine	1%	Amino acid transport defect. COLA: cysteine, ornithine, lysine, arginine. Radiopaque; often form **staghorn** calculi.

History/PE

Acute-onset, colicky, severe flank pain that may radiate to the testes or vulva. Nausea and vomiting are also seen. Patients are unable to get comfortable and shift position frequently (as opposed to those with peritonitis).

Evaluation

Lab studies may show either gross or **microscopic hematuria** and an **altered urinary pH.** Obtain **plain film** of the abdomen and possibly **renal ultrasound.** An **IVP** can be used to confirm the diagnosis (it will show nonfilling of contrast; Figure 2.16–4). **Helical CT scans** may help diagnose other potential etiologies of flank pain.

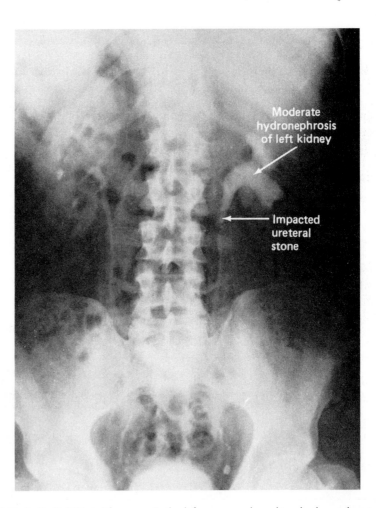

FIGURE 2.16–4. Nephrolithiasis. The stone in the left ureter and resulting hydronephrosis are evident on excretory urogram. (Reproduced, with permission, from Saunders C, *Current Emergency Diagnosis & Treatment*, 4th ed., Stamford, CT: Appleton & Lange, 1992: p. 554, Fig. 31–2.)

Treatment

Hydration, analgesia. Further treatment is based on the size of the stone. Kidney stones < 5 mm in diameter can pass through the urethra. Kidney stones < 3 cm in diameter can be treated with **extracorporeal shock wave lithotripsy** or percutaneous nephrolithotomy. Preventive measures include **hydration** and **thiazide diuretics** for calcium stones.

UCV EM.30

POLYCYSTIC KIDNEY DISEASE

Autosomal-dominant polycystic kidney disease (ADPKD) is **the most common form** of this disorder. One-half of ADPKD patients will have end-stage renal failure (ESRF) by age 60. Autosomal-recessive polycystic kidney disease (ARPKD) is less common but more severe, presenting in infants and young children and leading to death in the first few years of life.

History/PE

Symptoms rarely occur before the age of 20. **Pain and hematuria** are the most common presenting symptoms. Sharp, localized pain may result from cyst rupture, infection, or passage of renal calculi. Other findings include hypertension, nephrolithiasis, cerebral aneurysms, and mitral valve prolapse. Patients may also have large, palpable kidneys on abdominal examination.

Evaluation

Diagnosis can be based on ultrasound or CT scan. Multiple cysts will be present throughout the renal parenchyma, and renal enlargement will be visualized.

Treatment

Treatment is aimed at **preventing complications and symptomatology.** BP control and early management of UTIs are critical. Dialysis or renal transplantation is indicated in ESRF.

SIADH

An important cause of hyponatremia due to **nonosmotically stimulated ADH release.** SIADH is associated with CNS disease (head injury, tumor, nausea), pulmonary disease (sarcoid), ectopic tumor production/paraneoplastic syndrome (small cell carcinoma), drugs (antipsychotics, antidepressants), or surgery.

Evaluation

Diagnosis is based on urine osmolality > 50–100 mOsm/kg in the setting of serum hyposmolarity. **Urinary sodium is ≥ 20 mEq/L.** A water-loading test can be performed to evaluate free water excretion.

SIADH may be due to CNS disease, pulmonary disease, paraneoplastic syndromes, or drugs.

435

Treatment

Treat with **fluid restriction.** Address the underlying cause. If the patient is symptomatic owing to hyponatremia, give hypertonic saline followed by furosemide. Lasting correction depends on treatment of the underlying disease. In chronic SIADH, demeclocycline can help normalize serum sodium.

UCV *IM1.28*

DIABETES INSIPIDUS (DI)

Can be central or nephrogenic in origin. In **central DI,** there is a failure of the posterior pituitary to secrete ADH. Causes include tumor, infection, and autoimmune disease. In **nephrogenic DI,** the kidneys fail to respond to circulating ADH. Causes include chronic renal diseases and drugs (lithium, demeclocycline, colchicine).

History/PE

Patients have polydipsia and polyuria and excrete large volumes of dilute urine. They may present with hypernatremia and dehydration.

Differential

Psychogenic polydipsia, Cushing's syndrome, glucocorticoid treatment, Parkinson's disease, sarcoidosis.

Evaluation

Patients with DI continue to excrete a high volume of dilute urine during a water deprivation test. **In central DI, an ADH challenge after water deprivation will reduce urine output and increase urine osmolarity.** MRI may show a pituitary or hypothalamic mass.

Treatment

- **Central DI: DDAVP** or desmopressin acetate is administered as a synthetic analog of ADH.
- **Nephrogenic DI: Salt restriction and increased water intake are the primary treatment.** The underlying disease process must be addressed.

BENIGN PROSTATIC HYPERPLASIA (BPH)

A benign enlargement of the prostate that is a normal part of the aging process. Enlargement of the prostate may partially obstruct the urethra and cause urinary symptoms. BPH most commonly presents **after the age of 50.**

History/PE

BPH consists of obstructive and/or irritative symptoms.

- **Obstructive:** Hesitancy, weak stream, intermittent stream, incomplete emptying, urinary retention, and terminal dribbling.
- **Irritative:** Nocturia, daytime frequency, urge incontinence, dysuria, and opening hematuria.

On digital rectal exam, the prostate may be uniformly enlarged and have a rubbery feel (hard or irregular lesions raise the suspicion of cancer). However, BPH most commonly occurs in the central zone of the prostate and may not be detected on exam.

Differential

Calculi, bladder tumor, neurogenic bladder, prostatitis, prostatic cancer, urethral stricture, urethritis.

Evaluation

Potentially dangerous causes of urinary symptomatology must be ruled out before considering BPH.

- **Digital rectal examination** to detect masses.
- Ultrasound-guided biopsy of suspicious lesions.
- **UA and/or culture** to rule out infection/hematuria (cystitis, prostatitis).
- **Creatinine levels** to determine if there is obstructive uropathy and subsequent renal insufficiency.
- Imaging of the upper tract is recommended only for patients with preexisting urinary tract disease or complications.
- PSA testing and cystoscopy are not regarded as helpful in monitoring BPH.

Treatment

- **Watchful waiting:** Observe and monitor mild symptoms.
- **Medical therapy: 5-α-reductase inhibitors** (finasteride) and **alpha-receptor blockers** (terazosin) are useful in reducing mild to moderate symptoms.
- **Surgery:** Use in men with moderate to severe symptoms. **TURP** (transurethral resection of the prostate) or open prostatectomy in severe cases.

UCV *Surg.35*

PROSTATE CANCER

Prostate cancer is the most common cancer in men and the second leading cause of cancer death in men. Risk factors include advanced age and a positive family history.

History

Prostate cancer is usually **asymptomatic** but may present with **urinary retention,** a decrease in force of the urinary stream, lymphedema (metastases), weight loss, and **back pain** (spinal metastases and/or perineural invasion).

PE

Physical findings can include a **palpable nodule** or area of induration on **digital rectal exam.** Early carcinoma is usually not detectable on physical exam.

Differential

BPH, prostatitis (e.g., bacterial, TB), urethral stricture, neurogenic bladder.

Evaluation

Diagnosis is suggested by clinical findings and/or a markedly **elevated PSA** (mild elevations in PSA may be seen with BPH). Diagnosis is made with **biopsy** (transrectal ultrasound guided); tumors are graded by the **Gleason histologic system.** Look for metastases with bone scan and CXR.

Treatment

- Although many cases of prostate cancer are latent and do not progress without treatment, a significant number do lead to metastases (local perineural invasion and bone metastases) and death. Appropriate treatment is controversial.
- **Radical prostatectomy** may result in **incontinence** and/or **impotence** (nerve-sparing surgery decreases the risk of side effects).
- Radiation therapy (brachytherapy) is used in some centers.
- Some patients, especially those of advanced age, choose follow-up with serial PSA/examination/ultrasound.
- Follow PSA in all patients post-treatment.
- Treat **metastatic disease** with **androgen ablation** (GnRH agonists or orchiectomy/flutamide) and chemotherapy.

Prevention

- Screening with PSA is common, although its utility is controversial.
- All males > age 40 should have an annual **digital rectal exam.**

UCV *Surg.37*

BLADDER CANCER

Bladder cancer is the second most common urologic cancer and **the most frequent malignant tumor of the urinary tract.** It is more prevalent in men and occurs most commonly in the sixth and seventh decades. Risk factors include smoking, chronic bladder infections, calculous disease, and exposure to aniline dye.

History/PE

Gross hematuria is the most common presenting symptom in bladder cancer. Microscopic hematuria is often present as well. Other urinary symptoms such as frequency, urgency, and dysuria can occur, but most patients are asymptomatic in the early stages of disease.

Evaluation

UA is the most basic evaluation performed and often shows hematuria (macro- or microscopic). IVP is used to examine the upper urinary tracts and possible defects in bladder filling. **Cystoscopy is diagnostic.** Ultrasound, endorectal MRI, and pelvic CT scan can also be employed.

Treatment

Treatment depends on staging.

- **Superficial cancers** are treated with complete transurethral resection and use of intravesical chemotherapy.
- **Large, high-grade recurrent lesions and carcinoma in situ** are treated with intravesical chemotherapy.
- **Invasive cancers** that have not metastasized require aggressive surgery, XRT, or a combination of both.
- **Patients with distant metastases** receive chemotherapy as monotherapy.

UCV *Surg.36*

MALE INFERTILITY

Infertility is defined as the inability to achieve pregnancy in one year of normal sexual activity without contraception. **Infertility affects 15% of couples, and male factors are responsible 40% of the time.**

History/PE

A full history of both partners is essential. History should address **drug effects,** prior testicular insults, surgeries, infections, poor coital technique, and psychosocial issues. On PE, look for anatomic defects of the penis (hypospadias, epispadias) and testicles (varicocele).

Differential

- Hypothalamic, pituitary, testicular, and androgen disorders
- Hyperthyroidism, hypothyroidism, and adrenal disorders
- Disorders of the vas deferens, seminal vesicles, and prostate

Evaluation

Basic lab studies, including CBC, UA, testing for STDs, thyroid function tests, and testing for antisperm antibodies, must be performed. An ejaculate analysis is the hallmark of fertility workups. Semen should be examined within 1–2 hours after collection. **Normal semen volumes range between 1.5 and 5 mL.** Abnormal sperm concentrations are < 20 million/mL. Imaging can also be used to detect a subclinical varicocele.

Treatment

- **Education:** Inform the patient about proper timing for intercourse in relation to the female reproductive cycle.
- Endocrine therapy can be used in patients with pituitary diseases.
- Surgery is employed to correct varicoceles or obstruction of the vas deferens.
- Assisted reproductive techniques such as **intrauterine insemination** and in vitro fertilization can be used with low sperm counts.

Peaked T waves on an EKG.	Hyperkalemia
Carpal spasm upon inflation of blood pressure cuff.	Hypocalcemia
First-line treatment for moderate hypercalcemia.	IV hydration and loop diuretics (e.g., furosemide)
FeNa < 1% indicates what category of renal failure?	Prerenal
A 49-year-old male presents with acute-onset flank pain and microscopic hematuria. What is the most likely diagnosis?	Nephrolithiasis
The presence of red cell casts in urine sediment.	Glomerulonephritis
Eosinophils in urine sediment.	Allergic interstitial nephritis
Waxy casts in urine sediment.	Nephrotic syndrome
Drowsiness, asterixis, nausea, and a pericardial friction rub.	Uremic syndrome
First-line medical treatment of BPH.	Alpha-blockers (e.g., prazosin)
Low urine specific gravity in the presence of high serum osmolality.	Diabetes insipidus
Overly rapid correction of hyponatremia.	Central pontine myelinolysis
Salicylate ingestion results in what type of acid–base disorder?	Anion gap acidosis
Acid–base disturbance commonly seen in pregnant women.	Respiratory alkalosis

HIGH-YIELD FACTS

Renal/Genitourinary

441

The following clinical questions and accompanying answers are reproduced, with permission, from Berk SL, *PreTest: Medicine*, 9th ed., New York: McGraw-Hill, 2001.

Questions

1. A 70-year-old male with a history of urinary tract infection and congestive heart failure was admitted to the hospital for sepsis and pulmonary edema. He was treated with clindamycin and tobramycin and also received intravenous furosemide. After several days, the signs of sepsis improved, but the BUN rose to 60 mg/dL and the creatinine to 5.0 mg/dL. The blood pressure was stable at 120/70, pulse 70, and there were no postural changes. Weight was unchanged throughout the hospital course. The most likely cause of the patient's deteriorating renal function is
   a. Prerenal azotemia
   b. Acute tubular necrosis
   c. Interstitial nephritis
   d. Hypercalcemic nephropathy

2. The best evidence to support the diagnosis of acute tubular necrosis in this patient would be
   a. Urine Na$^+$ of 25 mEq/L
   b. Renal tubular epithelial cells and muddy brown casts in urine sediment
   c. A negative renal ultrasound
   d. An intravenous pyelogram showing abnormalities of the medulla

3. Under what circumstances would this patient require acute hemodialysis?
   a. BUN and creatinine do not return to normal after three days
   b. The patient produces less than 200 cc of urine a day following the development of ATN
   c. The patient develops hyperkalemia with peaked T waves and widening of the QRS complex
   d. Urine sodium is more than 40 mEq/L

4. A 70-year-old is found to be hypotensive in his home. He appears volume-depleted. Initial blood gases show a pH of 7.2, Pco$_2$ (mmHg) 35. Other electrolytes are

Na$^+$ 136 mEq/L	Cl$^-$ 114
K$^+$ 4.0	HCO$_3$ 14

   The primary acid–base disorder in this patient is
   a. Respiratory acidosis
   b. Metabolic acidosis
   c. Respiratory alkalosis
   d. Metabolic alkalosis with compensation

5. A 30-year-old male with HIV disease presents with complaints of flank pain and hematuria that have occurred suddenly. The patient, while being examined, is writhing in pain. A urinalysis shows many red blood cells without casts, and few white blood cells. The most likely diagnosis in this patient is
   a. Urolithiasis
   b. Streptococcal glomerulonephritis
   c. Bladder tumor
   d. Pyelonephritis

Answers

1. **The answer is b.** Since there is no clinical evidence of prerenal azotemia, it is most likely that this patient's acute renal failure is secondary to aminoglycoside toxicity and acute tubular necrosis.

2. **The answer is b.** The urine sediment in acute tubular necrosis is usually abnormal, with renal tubular epithelial cells, debris, and muddy brown casts. The high urine sodium, particularly if the patient has been getting a diuretic, is less specific. An ultrasound would rule out obstruction as a cause of renal failure, but would not be helpful in distinguishing prerenal from intrinsic renal failure. An IVP is contraindicated in the setting of acute renal failure.

3. **The answer is c.** Hyperkalemia with cardiotoxicity is an indication for acute hemodialysis. The BUN and creatinine would not be expected to return to normal within days, and the patient may remain oliguric for several days or longer. The urine sodium is not a measure of recovery in ATN.

4. **The answer is b.** The pH of 7.2 shows this to be a severe acidosis. The P_{CO_2} is less than 40 mmHg; hence there is no CO_2 retention to suggest respiratory acidosis. The patient has a metabolic acidosis.

5. **The answer is a.** The patient presents with clinical features of a renal stone, which is supported by the findings of red blood cells in the urine sediment. Red blood cell casts would be expected in glomerular disease, white blood cells in pyelonephritis. The patient's symptoms are not consistent with bladder cancer.

Selected Topics in Emergency Medicine

Table 2.17–1 below summarizes some major drug side effects.

TABLE 2.17–1. Drug Side Effects

Drug	Side Effects
Penicillin/beta-lactams	Hypersensitivity reactions
Vancomycin	Nephrotoxicity, ototoxicity, "red man syndrome" (histamine release; not an allergy)
Aminoglycosides	Ototoxicity, nephrotoxicity
Tetracyclines	Tooth discoloration, photosensitivity, Fanconi's syndrome
Chloramphenicol	Aplastic anemia, gray baby syndrome
Fluoroquinolones	Cartilage damage in children
Metronidazole	Disulfiram reaction, vestibular dysfunction
INH	Neuropathies, hepatotoxicity, seizures with overdose
Rifampin	Induction of liver enzymes, orange-red body secretions
Amphotericin	Fever/chills, nephrotoxicity
–azoles (fluconazole, etc.)	Inhibition of liver p450 enzymes
Amantadine	Ataxia
AZT	Thrombocytopenia, anemia
Antipsychotics	Sedation, akathisia, tardive dyskinesia, neuroleptic malignant syndrome
Clozapine	Agranulocytosis
TCAs	Sedation, anticholinergic effects, seizures and arrhythmias in overdose
SSRIs	Anxiety, sexual dysfunction
MAOIs	Hypertensive crisis with tyramine (cheese and wine)
Benzodiazepines	Sedation, dependence
Carbamazepine	Induction of p450, agranulocytosis, aplastic anemia
Phenytoin	Nystagmus, diplopia, ataxia, gingival hyperplasia, hirsutism
Valproic acid	Neural tube defects
Halothane	Hepatotoxicity
HCTZ	Hypokalemia, hyperuricemia, hyperglycemia
Furosemide	Ototoxicity, hypokalemia, nephritis

TABLE 2.17-1. (continued). Drug Side Effects

Drug	Side Effects
Clonidine	Dry mouth, severe rebound hypertension
Methyldopa	Positive Coombs' test
Reserpine	Depression
Prazosin	First-dose hypotension
Beta-blockers	Asthma exacerbation, masking of hypoglycemia, impotence
Hydralazine	Lupus syndrome
Calcium channel blockers	Peripheral edema, constipation, cardiac depression
ACE inhibitors	Cough, rash, proteinuria, angioedema, taste changes
Nitroglycerin	Hypotension, tachycardia, headache, tolerance
Digoxin	GI disturbance, yellow visual changes, arrhythmias
Quinidine	Cinchonism (headache, tinnitus), thrombocytopenia, dysrhythmias (e.g., torsades de pointes)
Amiodarone	Pulmonary fibrosis, peripheral deposition (bluish), arrhythmias, hypo/hyperthyroidism
Procainamide	Lupus syndrome
Bile acid resins	GI upset, malabsorption of vitamins and medications
HMG-CoA reductase inhibitors	Myositis, reversible ↑ LFTs
Niacin	Cutaneous flushing
Gemfibrozil	Myositis, reversible ↑ LFTs
Cyclophosphamide	Myelosuppression, hemorrhagic cystitis
Cisplatin	Nephrotoxicity, acoustic nerve damage
Doxorubicin	Cardiotoxicity
Corticosteroids	Mania (acute), immunosuppression, bone mineral loss, thin skin, easy bruising, myopathy (chronic)

- phenytoin: gingival hyperplasia, hirsutism (↑ hair)
- valproic acid: wt gain (↓) hair loss

Table 2.17–2 summarizes drug withdrawal symptoms and treatment.

TABLE 2.17–2. Management of Drug Withdrawal

Drug	Withdrawal	Treatment
Alcohol	Tremor (6–12 hours), tachycardia, hypertension, agitation, seizures (within 48 hours), hallucinations, **delirium tremens** (severe autonomic instability, including tachycardia, hypertension, delirium, and death) within 2–7 days. Mortality is 15–20%.	Benzodiazepines, haloperidol for hallucinations. Thiamine, folate, and multivitamin replacement (will not affect withdrawal, but most alcoholics are malnourished).
Opioids	Anxiety, insomnia, anorexia, sweating/piloerection, fever, rhinorrhea, nausea, stomach cramps, diarrhea.	Clonidine and/or buprenorphine for moderate withdrawal. Methadone for severe symptoms. Naltrexone for patients drug-free for 7–10 days.
Cocaine/amphetamines	Depression, hyperphagia, hypersomnolence.	Bromocriptine.
Barbiturates	Anxiety, seizures, delirium, tremor.	Mainstay of treatment is with benzodiazepines.
Benzodiazepines	Rebound anxiety, seizures, tremor, insomnia.	Mainstay of treatment is with benzodiazepines (same as alcohol withdrawal). Watch out for delirium tremens.

Table 2.17–3 describes some common drug interactions.

TABLE 2.17–3. Drug Interactions

Interaction/Reaction	Drugs
Induction of p450 enzymes	Barbiturates, phenytoin, carbamazepine, rifampin
Inhibition of p450 enzymes	Cimetidine, ketoconazole
Metabolism by p450 enzymes	Benzodiazepines, amide anesthetics, metoprolol, propranolol, nifedipine, phenytoin, quinidine, theophylline, warfarin, barbiturates
Raising of serum levels of digoxin	Quinidine, amiodarone, calcium channel blockers
Competition for albumin binding sites	Warfarin, aspirin, phenytoin
Blood dyscrasias	Ibuprofen, quinidine, methyldopa, chemotherapeutic agents
Hemolysis in G6PD-deficient patients	Sulfonamides, INH, aspirin, ibuprofen, primaquine
Gynecomastia	Cimetidine, ketoconazole, spironolactone
Stevens–Johnson syndrome	Ethosuximide, sulfonamides
Photosensitivity	Tetracycline, amiodarone, sulfonamides
Lupus-like syndrome	Procainamide, hydralazine, INH

HIGH-YIELD FACTS

Emergency Medicine

Table 2.17–4 summarizes the treatment for various substance overdoses.

TABLE 2.17–4. Specific Antidotes

Toxin	Antidote/Treatment
Acetaminophen	N-acetylcysteine
Anticholinesterases, organophosphates	Atropine, pralidoxime
Iron salts	Deferoxamine
Methanol, ethylene glycol (antifreeze)	Ethanol, fomepizole, dialysis
Lead	CaEDTA, dimercaprol, succimer
Arsenic, mercury, gold	Dimercaprol, succimer
Copper, arsenic, lead, gold	Penicillamine
Antimuscarinic, anticholinergic agents	Physostigmine
Cyanide	Nitrite, sodium thiosulfate
Salicylates	Alkalinize urine, dialysis
Heparin	Protamine
Methemoglobinemia	Methylene blue
Opioids	Naloxone
Benzodiazepines	Flumazenil
Tricyclic antidepressants	Sodium bicarbonate for QRS prolongation, diazepam or lorazepam for seizures, cardiac monitor for arrhythmias
Warfarin	Vitamin K, FFP
Carbon monoxide	100% O_2, hyperbaric O_2
Digitalis	Stop dig, normalize K, lidocaine, anti-dig Fab
Beta-blockers	Glucagon
tPA, streptokinase	Aminocaproic acid
PCP	Nasogastric suction
Theophylline/phenobarbital	Activated charcoal
Cocaine/amphetamines	Supportive, avoid beta-blockers

UCV EM.39, 40, 47, 48, 49

A **hypoxemic poisoning syndrome** seen in patients exposed to automobile exhaust, smoke inhalation, barbecues in poorly ventilated locations, or old appliances.

History/PE

Hypoxemia, flushed, **cherry-red skin,** confusion, and **headaches.** Coma or seizure occurs in severe cases. Chronic low-level exposure may mimic **flulike symptoms** with generalized myalgias, nausea, and headaches. **Suspect smoke inhalation in the presence of singed nose hairs, facial burns, hoarseness, wheezing, or carbonaceous sputum.**

Evaluation

Check ABG; normal serum carboxyhemoglobin level is < 5% in nonsmokers and < 10% in smokers. Look for evidence of smoke inhalation, including carbon deposits and mucosal edema on laryngoscopy or bronchoscopy. Check an EKG in the elderly and in patients with a history of cardiac disease.

Pulse oximetry will be falsely elevated in CO poisoning.

Treatment

Treat with 100% oxygen (**hyperbaric oxygen** for pregnant patients and those with neurologic symptoms or severely elevated carboxyhemoglobin) to facilitate displacement of CO from hemoglobin. Patients with **smoke inhalation** may require early intubation, since upper airway edema can rapidly progress to complete obstruction.

UCV *EM.47*

Evaluation/Treatment

Airway patency and adequacy of ventilation take precedence over other treatment (the A of the "ABCs" of CPR). Start with supplemental oxygen by nasal cannulae or face mask for conscious patients. Try a chin-lift or jaw-thrust maneuver to reposition the tongue (the most common cause of airway obstruction in an unconscious patient). An oropharyngeal airway (in unconscious patients) or a nasopharyngeal airway (in responsive patients) can aid bag mask ventilation. Intubate patients with apnea, decreased mental status (protect airway from aspiration of blood/vomitus), impending airway compromise (significant maxillofacial trauma, inhalation injury in fires), and severe closed head injury (to hyperventilate) or if there is failure to adequately oxygenate with a face mask. In traumas, patients should be immediately intubated if the patency of the airway is in doubt. A surgical airway (cricothyroidotomy) may be necessary in patients with significant maxillofacial trauma or who cannot be intubated. Remember to maintain C-spine stabilization in trauma patients, but **never allow this concern to delay airway management.**

Intubate patients with apnea, inability to protect their airway, impending airway compromise, and inadequate oxygenation.

Acute-onset abdominal pain that may require immediate surgical intervention. The approach to the patient with an acute abdomen is as follows:

History

- **Character of pain:** Sharp pain implies parietal (peritoneal) pain; dull, diffuse pain is commonly visceral (organ) pain. Note location (and whether it shifts or radiates), onset (sudden vs. gradual), severity, the exacerbating and ameliorating factors, and temporal nature (constant vs. colicky).
- GI and systemic symptoms (e.g., anorexia, nausea/emesis); ask about constipation, bloody diarrhea, or hematochezia.
- Hematuria (GU disorders), STD risk factors (PID is a common cause of acute abdominal pain in women), and fever/chills.
- Note the patient's menstrual history, family history (acute intermittent porphyria, familial Mediterranean fever), and past medical and surgical history (vasculitis, SLE, sickle cell disease).

PID is a common cause of acute abdominal pain in women.

PE

- Low BP and high HR are signs of shock or impending shock. High fever in the presence of abdominal pain is a concern.
- **Abdominal distention** suggests a surgical abdomen.
- Manipulate the lower extremity to elicit abdominal pain (suggestive of appendicitis), and check for **CVA tenderness** (pyelonephritis).

All abdominal pain is not GI pain (PID, pyelonephritis).

Differential

Figure 2.17–1 differentiates the causes of acute abdominal pain by quadrant.

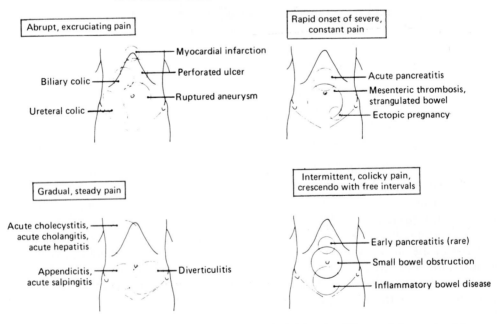

Abrupt, excruciating pain
- Myocardial infarction
- Perforated ulcer
- Ruptured aneurysm
- Biliary colic
- Ureteral colic

Rapid onset of severe, constant pain
- Acute pancreatitis
- Mesenteric thrombosis, strangulated bowel
- Ectopic pregnancy

Gradual, steady pain
- Acute cholecystitis, acute cholangitis, acute hepatitis
- Appendicitis, acute salpingitis
- Diverticulitis

Intermittent, colicky pain, crescendo with free intervals
- Early pancreatitis (rare)
- Small bowel obstruction
- Inflammatory bowel disease

FIGURE 2.17–1. Acute abdomen. The location and character of pain are helpful in the differential diagnosis of the acute abdomen. (Reproduced, with permission, from Way L, *Current Surgical Diagnosis & Treatment*, 10th ed., Stamford, CT: Appleton & Lange, 1994: p. 444, Fig. 21–3.)

Evaluation

Evaluation should include CBC/electrolytes, amylase, ABG if the patient is hypoxic or unstable, lactate, LFTs, PT/PTT, UA/culture, and stool guaiac. **All women of childbearing age should have a β-HCG test to rule out ectopic/uterine pregnancy.** Obtain abdominal plain x-rays followed by appropriate studies based on clinical suspicion. Contrast studies are often performed, but do not use barium if a lower bowel obstruction (LBO) is suspected, as it may worsen the patient's condition. If RUQ pain is present, perform an ultrasound/HIDA scan to detect cholecystitis. Paracentesis may be diagnostic if there is ascites.

In patients with acute abdomen, always assess for surgical emergencies.

Treatment

Determine whether emergent surgical intervention is necessary (Table 2.17–5). Discontinue oral feeds; insert NG tube if obstruction is suspected or in cases of impending surgery; provide analgesia and supportive care (IV fluids). Type and cross all patients.

TABLE 2.17–5. Indications for Urgent Operation in Patients with Acute Abdomen

Physical findings

    Involuntary guarding or rigidity, especially if spreading

    Increasing or severe localized tenderness

    Tense or progressive distention

    Tender abdominal or rectal mass with high fever or hypotension

    Rectal bleeding with shock or acidosis

    Equivocal abdominal findings along with

        Septicemia (high fever, marked or rising leukocytosis, mental changes, or increasing glucose intolerance in a diabetic patient)

        Bleeding (unexplained shock or acidosis, falling hematocrit)

        Suspected ischemia (acidosis, fever, tachycardia)

        Deterioration on conservative treatment

Radiologic findings

    Pneumoperitoneum

    Gross or progressive bowel distention

    Free extravasation of contrast material

    Space-occupying lesion on scan with fever

    Mesenteric occlusion on angiography

Endoscopic findings

    Perforated or uncontrollably bleeding lesion

Paracentesis findings

    Blood, bile, pus, bowel contents, or urine

PELVIC FRACTURES

If there is blood at the urethral meatus, do not insert a Foley catheter.

Patients often present after a motor vehicle accident. Evaluate with x-rays of the hip and pelvis. Pelvic fractures should be discovered during the secondary trauma survey (after ABCs) and may present as instability when the pelvis is "rocked" or compressed. Hypotension and shock suggest **exsanguinating hemorrhage** requiring emergent operative therapy or embolization of bleeding vessels. MAST (Military Anti-Shock Trousers) can be used in the field to maintain adequate BP/perfusion. A stable pelvic hematoma found on CT should not be explored; follow with serial hematocrit/hemoglobin and clinical exams. Patients with uncontrolled pelvic hemorrhage require fracture stabilization with **external pelvic fixation.** If this fails to control hemorrhage, embolization of the injured pelvic vessels is necessary. Pelvic fractures may be associated with **bladder rupture** or urethral injury. Thus, if there is blood at the urethral meatus (do not insert a Foley catheter!), the next critical step in management is to obtain a **retrograde urethrogram** to rule out GU injury.

COMPARTMENT SYNDROME

Elevated pressure within a confined space that compromises nerve, muscle, and soft tissue perfusion, most often in the lower leg or forearm. Etiologies include fractures, crush injuries, burns, and reperfusion following arterial repair in an ischemic extremity.

History/PE

Signs of compartment syndrome—

6 P's:
Pain
Pallor
Pulselessness
Paresthesias
Paralysis
Poikilothermia

Pain out of proportion to physical findings; **pain with passive extension** of the finger/toes; **weakness and paresthesias;** tense compartment on palpation; **pulselessness** and **paralysis** (late findings); and **Volkmann's contracture** of the wrist and fingers secondary to vascular insufficiency (seen after supracondylar fractures). *or improper use of tourniquet.*

Dupuytren's Contracture: flexion deformity of fingers or toe due to shortening thickening + fibrosis of palmar or plantar fascia

Evaluation

This is a clinical diagnosis. Measure compartment pressures (which are usually elevated to > 30 mmHg) if diagnosis is uncertain.

Arterial pulses are often normal early in presentation.

Treatment

A **surgical emergency** that requires **immediate fasciotomy** to decrease compartmental pressures and restore tissue perfusion.

AORTIC DISRUPTION

A **rapid deceleration injury** seen in high-speed motor vehicle accidents, falls from great heights, or ejection from vehicles. Since complete aortic rupture is rapidly fatal (85% of cases die at the scene), trauma patients with an aortic injury usually have a contained hematoma within the adventitia.

Evaluation/Treatment

Obtain an immediate CXR, which may reveal a **widened mediastinum, pleural cap,** deviation of the trachea to the right, and obliteration of the aortic knob. Be suspicious if there are first/second rib fractures. Laceration usually occurs at the ligamentum arteriosum. **Aortography is the gold standard for evaluation.** Evaluation via CT remains controversial, although spiral CT has improved the utility of CT. TEE should be performed on patients going to the OR.

Aortic disruption is often associated with first and second rib fractures.

PENETRATING WOUNDS

Evaluation/Treatment

- **Neck:** Intubate early. Surgically explore penetrating injuries to **zone 2.** Evaluation can include aortography, tracheobronchoscopy, and esophagoscopy for zone 1/zone 3 injuries (see Figure 2.17–2).
- **Chest:** Unstable patients with penetrating thoracic injuries require immediate **intubation** and bilateral **chest tubes.** Thoracotomy may be necessary for patient in extremis or if a patient remains unstable despite resuscitative efforts. Leave any impaled objects in place until the patient is taken to the OR, since such objects may tamponade further blood loss. Beware of pneumothorax, hemothorax, cardiac tamponade, aortic disruption, diaphragmatic tear, and esophageal injury.
- **Abdomen:** Patients with a gunshot wound to the abdomen require an **exploratory laparotomy.** Patients with stab wounds who are hemodynamically unstable or who are demonstrating peritoneal signs or evisceration also need an exploratory laparotomy. The remainder of patients with abdominal stab wounds should undergo local wound exploration, serial physical examinations, and diagnostic peritoneal lavage or abdominal CT. The **spleen is the most common abdominal organ injured in blunt trauma** (*Surg.35*).
- **Wound irrigation** and **tissue debridement,** not antibiotic therapy, is the most important step in the treatment of contaminated wounds.

Leave any impaled objects in place until the person is taken to the OR.

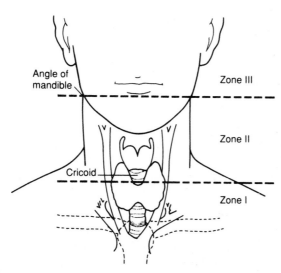

FIGURE 2.17–2. Zones of the neck. (Reproduced, with permission, from Way L, *Current Surgical Diagnosis & Treatment,* 10th ed., Stamford, CT: Appleton & Lange, 1994: p. 223, Fig. 13–9.)

Class of drugs that may cause syndrome of muscle rigidity, hyperthermia, autonomic instability, and extrapyramidal symptoms.	Antipsychotics (neuroleptic malignant syndrome)
Antibiotics that lead to cartilage damage in children.	Fluoroquinolones
Antihypertensive that may create a lupus-like syndrome.	Hydralazine
Side effects of corticosteroids.	Acute mania, immunosuppression, osteoporosis, thin skin, easy bruising, myopathies
Treatment for delirium tremens.	Benzodiazepines
Treatment for acetaminophen overdose.	N-acetylcysteine
Treatment for opioid overdose.	Naloxone
Treatment for iron overdose.	Deferoxamine
Symptoms of CO poisoning.	Acutely, confusion, cherry-red flushed skin, coma, seizure; chronically, may mimic flulike symptoms
Treatment for CO poisoning.	100% O_2; hyperbaric O_2 in severe cases or in pregnant patients
Blood in the urethral meatus of a trauma patient may indicate . . .	Pelvic fracture with bladder rupture or urethral injury
Gold standard for diagnosis of aortic disruption.	Aortography
Radiologic findings indicating need for surgery in acute abdominal pain.	Free air in the abdomen; severe bowel distention; extravasation of contrast; space-occupying lesion (CT scan); mesenteric occlusion (angiography)

Clinical Images

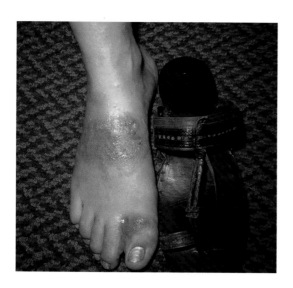

Contact dermatitis. Erythematous papules, vesicles, and serous weeping localized to areas of contact with the offending agent are characteristic. (Reproduced, with permission, from Hurwitz RM, *Pathology of the Skin: Atlas of Clinical–Pathological Correlation,* 1st ed. Stamford, CT: Appleton & Lange, 1991: p. 3, Fig. 1–5.)

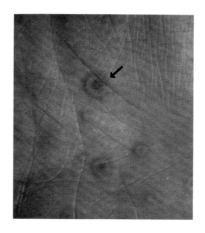

Erythema multiforme. The classic target lesion has a dull red center, pale zone, and darker outer ring (arrow). This acute self-limited reaction may occur with infection, antibiotic use, exposure to radiation or chemicals, or malignancy. (Reproduced, with permission, from Bondi EE, *Dermatology: Diagnosis and Therapy,* 1st ed., Stamford, CT: Appleton & Lange, 1991: p. 392, Fig. 19.)

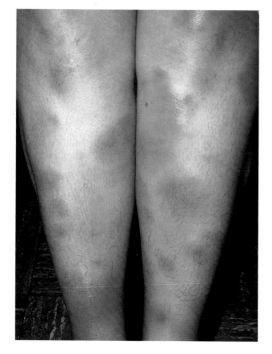

Erythema nodosum. The erythematous plaques and nodules are commonly located on pretibial areas. Lesions are painful and indurated and heal spontaneously without ulceration. (Reproduced, with permission, from Hurwitz RM, *Pathology of the Skin: Atlas of Clinical–Pathological Correlation,* 1st ed., Stamford, CT: Appleton & Lange, 1991: p. 132, Fig. 10–1A.)

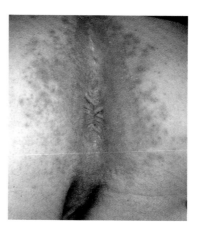

Candidial intertrigo. Erythematous areas surrounded by satellite pustules are restricted to warm, moist intertriginous areas. (Reproduced, with permission, from Bondi EE, *Dermatology: Diagnosis and Therapy,* 1st ed., Stamford, CT: Appleton & Lange, 1991: p. 390, Fig. 11.)

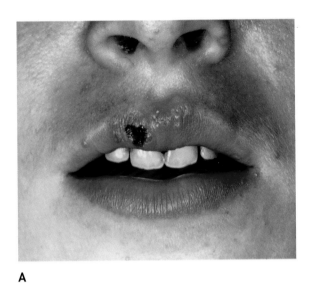

A

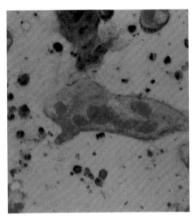

B

Herpes simplex. (A) Primary infection. Grouped vesicles on an erythematous base on the patient's lips and oral mucosa may progress to pustules before resolving. (B) Tzanck smear. The multinucleated giant cells from vesicular fluid provide a presumptive diagnosis of HSV infection. However, the Tzanck smear cannot distinguished between HSV and VZV infection. (Reproduced, with permission, from Hurwitz RM, *Pathology of the Skin: Atlas of Clinical–Pathological Correlation*, 1st ed., Stamford, CT: Appleton & Lange, 1991: p. 145, Fig. 11–9 and Bondi EE, *Dermatology: Diagnosis and Therapy*, 1st ed., Stamford, CT: Appleton & Lange, 1991: p. 396, Fig. 47.)

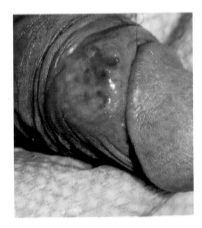

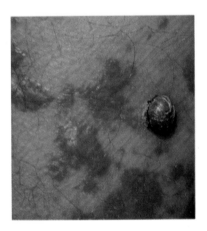

Primary syphilis. The chancre, which appears at the site of infection, is an ulcerated papule with a smooth, clean base; raised, indurated borders; and scant discharge. (Reproduced, with permission, from Bondi EE, *Dermatology: Diagnosis and Therapy*, 1st ed., Stamford, CT: Appleton & Lange, 1991: p. 394, Fig. 33.)

Kaposi's sarcoma. Manifests as red to purple nodules and surrounding pink to red macules. The latter appear most often in immunosuppressed patients. (Reproduced, with permission, from Bondi EE, *Dermatology: Diagnosis and Therapy*, 1st ed., Stamford, CT: Appleton & Lange, 1991: p. 393, Fig. 25.)

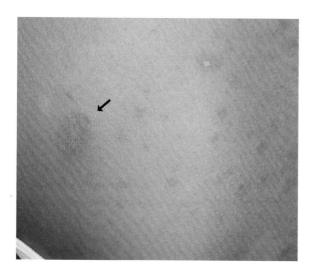

Pityriasis rosea. The round to oval erythematous plaques are often covered with a fine white scale ("cigarette paper") and are often found on the trunk ("Christmas tree distribution") and proximal extremities. The plaques are often preceded by a larger herald patch (arrow). (Reproduced, courtesy of the Yale Department of Dermatology.)

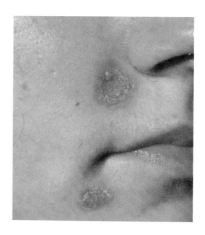

Impetigo. Dried pustules with superficial golden-brown crust are most commonly found around the nose and mouth. (Reproduced, with permission, from Bondi EE, *Dermatology: Diagnosis and Therapy*, 1st ed., Stamford, CT: Appleton & Lange, 1991: p. 390, Fig. 12.)

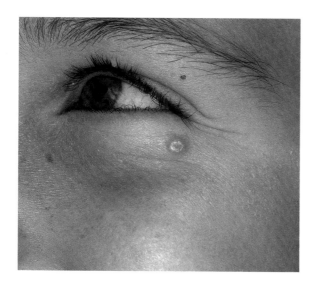

Molluscum contagiosum. The dome-shaped, fleshy, umbilicated papule on the child's eyelid is characteristic. (Reproduced, with permission, from Hurwitz RM, *Pathology of the Skin: Atlas of Clinical–Pathological Correlation*, 1st ed., Stamford, CT: Appleton & Lange, 1991: p. 149, Fig. 11–19.)

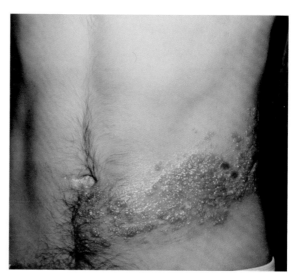

Herpes zoster. The unilateral dermatomal distribution of the grouped vesicles on an erythematous base is characteristic. (Reproduced, courtesy of the Yale Department of Dermatology.)

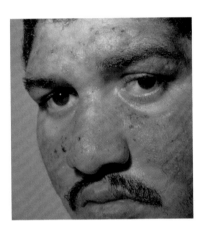

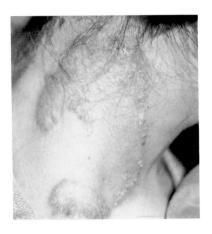

Malar rash of systemic lupus erythematosus. The malar rash is a red to purple continuous plaque extending across the bridge of the nose and to both cheeks. (Reproduced, with permission, from Bondi EE, *Dermatology: Diagnosis and Therapy,* 1st ed., Stamford, CT: Appleton & Lange, 1991: p. 395, Fig. 38.)

Tinea corporis. Ring-shaped, erythematous, scaling macules with central clearing are characteristic. (Reproduced, with permission, from Bondi EE, *Dermatology: Diagnosis and Therapy,* 1st ed., Stamford, CT: Appleton & Lange, 1991: p. 389, Fig. 4.)

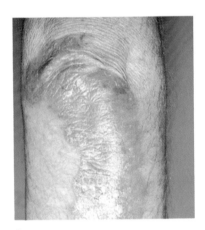

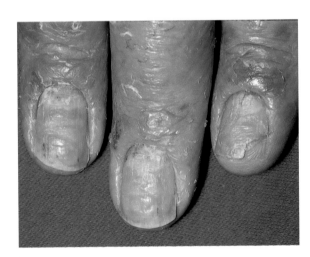

A

B

Psoriasis. (A) Skin changes. The classic sharply demarcated dark red plaques with silvery scales are commonly located on extensor surfaces (e.g., elbows, knees). (B) Nail changes. Note the pitting, onycholysis, and oil spots. (Reproduced, with permission, from Bondi EE, *Dermatology: Diagnosis and Therapy,* 1st ed., Stamford, CT: Appleton & Lange, 1991: p. 389, Fig. 1 and Hurwitz RM, *Pathology of the Skin: Atlas of Clinical–Pathological Correlation,* 1st ed., Stamford, CT: Appleton & Lange, 1991: p. 15, Fig. 1–55.)

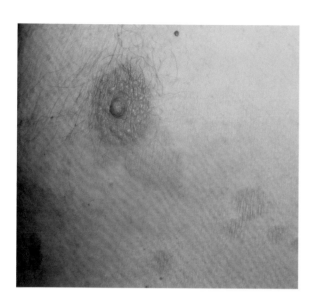

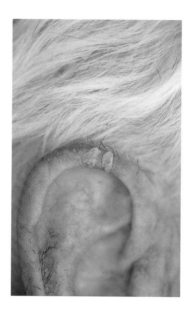

Tinea versicolor. These pinkish scaling macules commonly appear on the chest and back. Lesions may also be lightly pigmented or hypopigmented depending on the patient's skin color and sun exposure. (Reproduced, courtesy of the Yale Department of Dermatology.)

Actinic keratosis. The discrete patch has an erythematous base and rough white scaling. Actinic keratosis is a premalignant lesion that may progress to squamous cell carcinoma. It is most commonly found in sun-exposed areas. (Reproduced, with permission, from Hurwitz RM, *Pathology of the Skin: Atlas of Clinical–Pathological Correlation*, 1st ed., Stamford, CT: Appleton & Lange, 1991: p. 354, Fig. 31–3.)

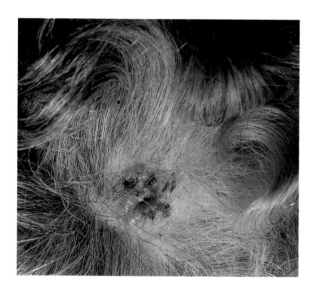

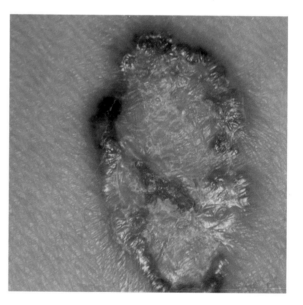

Squamous cell carcinoma. Note the crusting and ulceration of this erythematous plaque. Most lesions are exophytic nodules with erosion or ulceration. (Reproduced, with permission, from Hurwitz RM, *Pathology of the Skin: Atlas of Clinical–Pathological Correlation*, 1st ed., Stamford, CT: Appleton & Lange, 1991: p. 360, Fig. 31–20.)

Basal cell carcinoma. Note the pearly, translucent surface (often covered with fine telangiectasias), rolled border, and central ulceration. (Reproduced, courtesy of the Yale Department of Dermatology.)

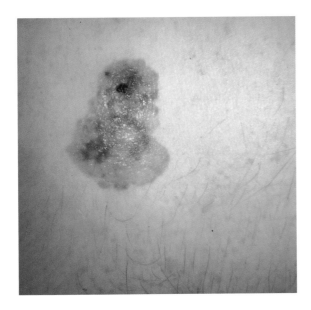

Melanoma. Note the **a**symmetry, **b**order irregularity, **c**olor variation, and large **d**iameter of this plaque. (Reproduced, with permission, from Hurwitz RM, *Pathology of the Skin: Atlas of Clinical–Pathological Correlation*, 1st ed., Stamford, CT: Appleton & Lange, 1991: p. 432, Fig. 36–8.)

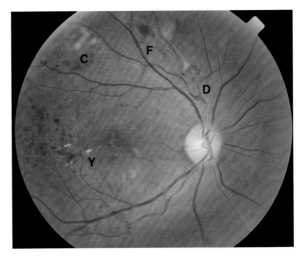

Nonproliferative diabetic retinopathy. Flame hemorrhages (F), dot-blot hemorrhages (D), cotton-wool spots (C), and yellow exudate (Y) result from small vessel damage and occlusion. (Reproduced, courtesy of the Washington University Department of Ophthalmology.)

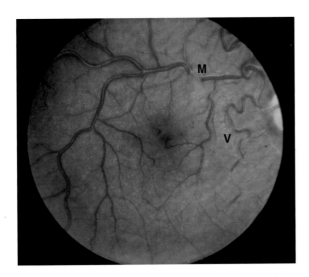

Hypertensive retinopathy. Note the tortuous retinal veins (V) and venous microaneurysms (M). Other findings include hemorrhages, retinal infarcts, detachment of the retina, and disk edema. (Reproduced, courtesy of the Washington University Department of Ophthalmology.)

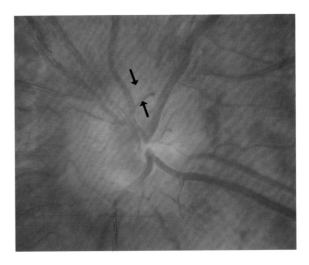

Papilledema. Look for blurred disk margins due to edema of the optic disk (arrows). (Reproduced, courtesy of the Washington University Department of Ophthalmology.)

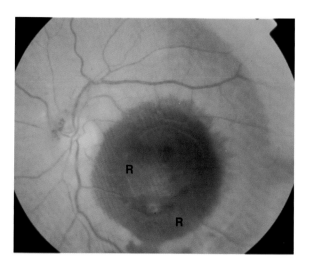

Subretinal hemorrhage. Note the preretinal blood and overlying retinal vessels (R). Subretinal hemorrhages may be seen in any condition with abnormal vessel proliferation (e.g., diabetes, hypertension) or in trauma. (Reproduced, courtesy of the Washington University Department of Ophthalmology.)

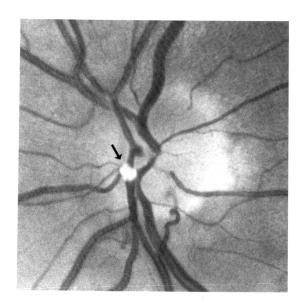

Cholesterol emboli. Cholesterol emboli (Hollenhorst plaque; arrow) usually arise in atherosclerotic carotid arteries and often lodge at the bifurcation of retinal arteries. (Reproduced, with permission, from Vaughan D, *General Ophthalmology*, 14th ed., Stamford, CT: Appleton & Lange, 1995: p. 299, Fig. 15–6.)

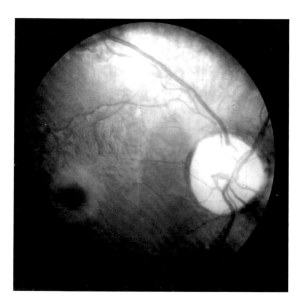

Tay–Sachs. Cherry-red spot. The red spot in the macula may be seen in Tay–Sachs disease, Niemann–Pick disease, central retinal artery occlusion, and methanol toxicity. (Reproduced, with permission, from Vaughan D, *General Ophthalmology*, 14th ed., Stamford, CT: Appleton & Lange, 1995: p. 293, Fig. 14–29.)

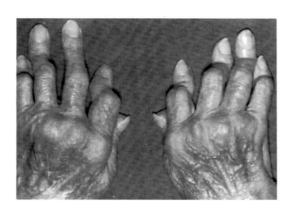

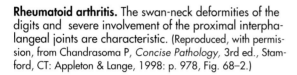

Rheumatoid arthritis. The swan-neck deformities of the digits and severe involvement of the proximal interphalangeal joints are characteristic. (Reproduced, with permission, from Chandrasoma P, *Concise Pathology*, 3rd ed., Stamford, CT: Appleton & Lange, 1998: p. 978, Fig. 68–2.)

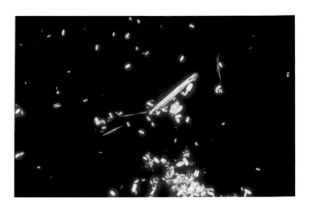

Gout. Negatively birefringent crystals. (Reproduced, with permission, from Milikowshi C, *Color Atlas of Basic Histopathology*, 1st ed., Stamford, CT: Appleton & Lange, 1997: p. 546.)

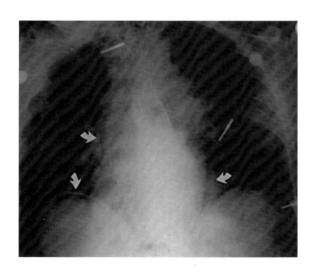

Pneumomediastinum. The lucency outlining the left heart border on chest x-ray suggests air in the mediastinum. (Reproduced, with permission, from Goldfrank LR, *Toxic Emergencies*, 6th ed., Stamford, CT: Appleton & Lange, 1998: p. 285, Fig. 8–2A.)

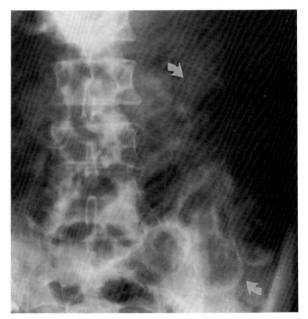

Pneumoperitoneum. The lucency outlining small bowel on abdominal x-ray indicated the abnormal presence of air. (Reproduced, with permission, from Goldfrank LR, *Toxic Emergencies*, 6th ed., Stamford, CT: Appleton & Lange, 1998: p. 285, Fig. 8–2B.)

Database of Clinical Science Review Resources

Comprehensive
Internal Medicine
Neurology
OB/GYN
Pediatrics
Preventive Medicine
Psychiatry
Surgery
Miscellaneous
Commercial Review
  Courses
Publisher Contacts

This section is a database of current clinical science review books, sample examination books, and commercial review courses marketed to medical students studying for the USMLE Step 2. Selected Step 3 resources that have been used by medical students and found to have appropriate content have also been included. At the end of this section there is a list of publishers and independent bookstores with addresses and phone numbers. For each book, we list the **Title** of the book, the **First Author** (or editor), the **Current Publisher,** the **Copyright Year,** the **Edition,** the **Number of Pages,** the **ISBN Code,** the **Approximate List Price,** the **Format** of the book, and the **Number of Test Questions.** Most entries also include Summary Comments that describe their style and utility for studying. Finally, each book receives a **Rating.** The books are sorted into a comprehensive section as well as into sections corresponding to the seven clinical disciplines (internal medicine, neurology, OB/GYN, pediatrics, preventive medicine, psychiatry, and surgery). Within each section, books are arranged first by Rating, then by Title, and finally by Author.

For this third edition of *First Aid for the USMLE Step 2,* the database of review books has been completely revised, with in-depth summary comments on more than 100 books and software. A letter rating scale with ten different grades reflects the detailed student evaluations. Each book receives a rating as follows:

A+	Excellent for boards review.
A A–	Very good for boards review; choose among the group.
B+ B B–	Good, but use only after exhausting better sources.
C+ C C–	Fair, but many better books in the discipline, or low-yield subject material.
N	Not rated.

The **Rating** is meant to reflect the overall usefulness of the book in preparing for the USMLE Step 2 examination. This is based on a number of factors, including:

- The cost of the book.
- The readability of the text.
- The appropriateness and accuracy of the book.
- The quality and number of sample questions.
- The quality of written answers to sample questions.
- The quality and appropriateness of the illustrations (e.g., graphs, diagrams, photographs).
- The length of the text (longer is not necessarily better).
- The quality and number of other books available in the same discipline.
- The importance of the discipline on the USMLE Step 2 examination.

Please note that **the rating does not reflect the quality of the book for purposes other than reviewing for the USMLE Step 2 examination.** Many books with low ratings are well written and informative but are not ideal for boards preparation. We have also avoided listing or commenting on the wide variety of general textbooks available in the clinical sciences.

Evaluations are based on the cumulative results of formal and informal surveys of hundreds of medical students from medical schools across the country. The summary comments and overall ratings represent a consensus opinion, but there may have been a large range of opinion or limited student feedback on any particular book.

Please note that the data listed are subject to change because:

- Publishers' prices change frequently.
- Individual bookstores often charge an additional markup.
- New editions come out frequently, and the quality of updating varies.
- The same book may be reissued through another publisher.

We actively encourage medical students and faculty to submit their opinions and ratings of these clinical science review books so that we may update our database. (See How to Contribute, p. xv.) In addition, we ask that publishers and authors submit review copies of clinical science review books, including new editions and books not included in our database, for evaluation. We also solicit reviews of new books or suggestions for alternate modes of study that may be useful in preparing for the examination, such as flashcards, computer-based tutorials, commercial review courses, and World Wide Web sites.

Disclaimer/Conflict of Interest Statement

No material in this book, including the ratings, reflects the opinion or influence of the publisher. All errors and omissions will gladly be corrected if brought to the attention of the authors through the publisher. Please note that the *Underground Clinical Vignette* series are publications by the authors of this book.

NMS Review for USMLE Step 2
Gruber

$36.95   Test/900 q

Lippincott Williams & Wilkins, 1999, 2nd edition, 506 pages, ISBN
0683302833

Comprehensive review book in question-and-answer format. **Pros:** The
level of difficulty, content, and style of questions closely approximate
those seen on the Step 2 exam. Clear, concise, excellent coverage of high-
yield topics. Complete explanations. **Cons:** Lacks illustrations or images.
Summary: Best single source of Step 2-style questions with appropriate
format and content. Highly recommended.

Boards & Wards
Ayala

$27.95   Review

Blackwell Science, 2000, 1st edition, 363 pages, ISBN 0632044934

A concise book packed with key information across the various fields of
medicine. **Pros:** Very high yield. Good use of tables and charts. **Cons:**
Small print; few explanations. Not tremendously in-depth though it covers many topics. Few images. **Summary:** Good comprehensive review although it lacks some details.

Cracking the Boards
Mariani

$29.95   Review

Random House, Inc., 1999, 1st edition, 282 pages, ISBN 0375750932

Clinical vignette review organized by specialty. **Pros:** Well organized, with
uniform format throughout book and lots of charts. Appropriate emphasis
on treatment. **Cons:** Very few images. **Summary:** Useful review that follows Step 2's emphasis on clinical vignettes.

Medical Student Pearls of Widsom
USMLE Parts I and II
Plantz

$32.00   Review

Boston Medical Publishing, 1998, 1st edition, 331 pages, ISBN
1890369101

Pros: Does a good job approximating the questions on Step 2 of the
boards, with similar clinical emphasis and distribution across various specialties. **Cons:** Lacks illustrations, including images to aid in diagnosis.
Summary: Easy to read, compact review designed for self testing.

NMS Review for USMLE Step 2
Gruber

$49.95   Software/900 q

Lippincott Williams & Wilkins, 2000, V3.0, ISBN 0781729440

Comprehensive question bank with complete explanations (see review of
NMS Review for USMLE Step 2 book). **Pros:** Added benefit of mimicking
the computer-based testing format of the actual boards. **Cons:** Some find
the interface awkward or confusing. **Summary:** Quality questions in
boards-type setting, though a little difficult to navigate.

REVIEW RESOURCES

Comprehensive

PreTest Clinical Vignettes for the USMLE Step 2 $24.95   Test/400 q
McGraw-Hill

McGraw-Hill, 2001, 2nd edition, 309 pages, ISBN 0071364536

Vignette-style question book with answers, organized by subject. A collection of the "best of" from the Pretest question books. **Pros:** Broad coverage of Step 2 topics. Good variety. Detailed explanations. **Cons:** Some questions are too picky or lack the appropriate emphasis for boards review. **Summary:** Good source of practice questions, strongest of the PreTest series.

 Step 2 Exam, General Clinical Sciences $32.00   Test/800 q
Alario

Mosby–Year Book, 1999, 1st edition, 417 pages, ISBN 081513715X

Board-type questions in both integrated and topic-based test sections. **Pros:** Questions have appropriate content and level of difficulty. Explanations of both correct and incorrect answers are provided. **Cons:** Very little use of images (radiographic, patient photos, pathology, or EKG). **Summary:** Decent practice questions approximating the boards.

 Advanced Life Support for the USMLE Step 2 $18.95   Review
Flynn

Lippincott Williams & Wilkins, 1999, 2nd edition, 142 pages, ISBN 0781719763

Brief outline format with high-yield topics described in tables or illustrations. **Pros:** Very quick, easy read. Emphasis on high-yield facts. Amusing cartoons highlight key concepts. A great last-minute review. **Cons:** Not adequate for in-depth review. **Summary:** A worthwhile review for the night before the exam.

 A&L's Flash Facts for the USMLE Steps 2 and 3 $26.50   Test 200 q
Kaiser

McGraw-Hill, 1997, 1st edition, 220 pages, ISBN 0838526063

More than 200 clinically based questions presented on flashcards. Answers and discussions are on the reverse side of each card. **Pros:** Quick case-based review. Covers high-yield topics in core specialties. Focuses on key aspects of management and diagnosis. Useful for on-the-go review. **Cons:** Style may not suit all students. Expensive for a limited number of topics. Awkward reference system. No index. **Summary:** High-quality material, but expensive and limited in scope. Use with other comprehensive resources.

REVIEW RESOURCES

Comprehensive

B+ **A&L's Review for the USMLE Step 2** $39.95   Test/1060 q
Chan

McGraw-Hill, 1999, 3rd edition, 361 pages, ISBN 0838503411

Review questions organized by specialty and two comprehensive practice exams. **Pros:** Overall question content good, with broad coverage of high-yield topics. Well illustrated. **Cons:** Vignettes are brief. Questions do not reflect Step 2 style and format. **Summary:** Good overall review questions on high-yield topics that lends itself well to focused specialty review. Good buy for the number of questions.

B+ **Crush the Boards:** $28.00   Review
The Ultimate USMLE Step 2 Review
Brouchert

Hanley & Belfus, 2000, 1st edition, 224 pages, ISBN 1560533668

Comprehensive review of many high-yield topics organized by specialty. **Pros:** Good emphasis of key points. Conversational style that is easy to read. Good use of charts and diagrams. **Cons:** Almost pure text, with few images. Some information is vague, and not clearly organized. No practice questions or vignettes. **Summary:** Should probably be supplemented with other review material and practice tests.

B+ **Mosby's Ace the Boards: Specialty** $41.95   Review/100+ q
Clinical Sciences Step 3
Donnelly

Mosby–Year Book, 1996, 1st edition, 483 pages, ISBN 0815127561

Review by specialty with short vignettes at the end of each chapter. **Pros:** Well organized and to the point. Not a quick read. Appropriate emphasis on risk factors and management. Good explanations to answers. **Cons:** Confusing icons and rampant boldfacing. Illustrations on insert separated from corresponding text. Expensive, even considering the included disk. **Summary:** Well written but dense text.

B+ **Rx: Prescription for the Boards USMLE Step 2** $32.95   Review
Feibusch

Lippincott Williams & Wilkins, 1998, 2nd edition, 496 pages, ISBN 0781714273

Comprehensive text review based on the USMLE content outline. **Pros:** Comprehensive coverage of high-yield core and specialty topics, including outpatient medicine, dermatology, ophthalmology, ENT, and toxicology. Well-designed format. **Cons:** Some topics lack the necessary details. Facts outlining the next step in management are often not discussed. **Summary:** Good single source for Step 2 review. Occasionally sparse coverage of topics. Requires a time commitment.

B	**A&L's Outline Review for the USMLE Step 2**	**$36.95**	Review

Goldberg

McGraw-Hill, 1999, 3rd edition, 749 pages, ISBN 0838503543

General outline of major clinical topics. "Cram facts" are scattered throughout. **Pros:** Information is presented by symptoms, diagnosis, pathology, and treatment. Many classic photos. Covers most relevant topics. **Cons:** Coverage varies widely from topic to topic. Difficult to extract key points. Time consuming. **Summary:** Big, well-illustrated book that is sometimes light on meaningful content.

B	**A&LERT USMLE Step 2**	**$65.00**	Software/1200+ q

Appleton & Lange

McGraw-Hill, 1998, 1st edition, ISBN 0838584470

Computerized test bank based on *Appleton & Lange's Review of the USMLE Step 2*. Users can take timed exams that are scored automatically. **Pros:** Quick way to review selected topics with use of search function and bookmarks. Allows user to simulate a timed exam. Questions and answers may be printed out for further review. **Cons:** Some questions are too specific. Vignettes are relatively short and do not accurately reflect the length of questions on the exam. Interface does not reflect the new CBT. **Summary:** Good-quality questions, although interface differs from the actual CBT.

B	**Medical Boards Step 2 Made Ridiculously Simple**	**$24.95**	Review

Carl

MedMaster, 1999, 1st edition, 356 pages, ISBN 0940780283

General review of topics for step 2 exam. Outline format with tables and brief discussions of topics. **Pros:** Quick review. Useful in areas that might otherwise be overlooked, e.g., ophthalmology, dermatology, ENT. **Cons:** Often lacks substantive details. **Summary:** Highlights most high-yield topics. Should not be used as sole source for review.

B	**MEPC USMLE Step 2 Review**	**$32.95**	Test/1000+ q

Jacobs

McGraw-Hill, 1996, 410 pages, ISBN 0838562701

Question-and-answer format with explanations. **Pros:** Relatively quick review. Numerous photographs of classics findings. Appropriate coverage of high-yield topics. Answers highlight important buzzwords. **Cons:** Discussions of answers are sometimes brief. Relatively simple vignettes do not reflect the current boards format. **Summary:** Fair source of additional questions that may be read quickly. Well illustrated.

B USMLE Step 2 Clinical Sciences, Books 1–5

Luder

$14.00
(each)

Test/315 q
315 q, 315 q, 220 q

Book 1: Maval Medical Education, 1997, 3rd edition, 82 pages, ISBN 1884083579

Book 2: Maval Medical Education, 1995, 3rd edition, 67 pages, ISBN 1884083587

Book 3: Maval Medical Education, 1996, 3rd edition, 63 pages, ISBN 1884083595

Books 4 & 5: Maval Medical Education, 1996, 3rd edition, 62 pages, ISBN 1884083609

Individual mini-exam format with discussion of questions and answers. **Pros:** Good clinical content with some clinical vignettes. Features many classic pathologic images and radiographs. **Cons:** Many questions are too easy and do not reflect boards format. Occasional factual mistakes and typographical errors are found in answer key. Some questions have letter answers only. Relatively expensive for the number of questions. **Summary:** Good content review, but questions are too easy. Relatively expensive.

B USMLE Step 2, Clinical Sciences Book 6

Luder

$25.00

Test/540 q

Maval Medical Education, 1996, 3rd edition, 128 pages, ISBN 1884083560

Individual mini-exam format with discussion of questions and answers. **Pros:** Good clinical content with some clinical vignettes. Features many classic pathologic images and radiographs. **Cons:** Many questions are too easy and do not reflect boards format. Occasional factual mistakes and typographical errors are found in answer key. Some questions have letter answers only. Relatively expensive for the number of questions. **Summary:** Good content review, but questions are too easy.

B USMLE Step 2: The Stanford Solutions to the NBME Computer-Based Sample Test Questions

Kush

$18.95

Test/150 answers

Planet Med Publishing, 1999, 1st edition, 152 pages, ISBN 1893730255

Detailed answers to questions provided on NBME sample test. **Pros:** An inexpensive review with good discussion of topics and page references to standard textbooks of medicine. Answers are very thoroughly explained. **Cons:** Questions are not reprinted in the book, giving no reference for the answers provided. **Summary:** By nature, not a systematic or well-organized review, but a welcome solution for many students who take the NBME practice test and would like explanations for the answers. A supplement to initial practice testing.

B **USMLE Step 2 Secrets** $33.00 Review

Brouchert

Hanley & Belfus, 2000, 1st edition, 257 pages, ISBN 1560534516

Typical *Secrets* series format, with question-and-answer, organized by specialty. **Pros:** Concise review of many high-yield topics. Good use of clinical images, including patient photos, blood smears, and radiographs. **Cons:** No clinical vignettes, simply lists of questions that might be posed on the wards. Does not follow Step 2 format and may leave out important information. Expensive. **Summary:** Overall, good content for self-quizzing and study, but does not substitute for a formal review or practice tests.

B− **A&L's Review for the USMLE Step 3** $36.95 Test/1000 q

Jacobs

McGraw-Hill, 1997, 2nd edition, 313 pages, ISBN 0838503055

Review questions organized by specialty in addition to two 150-question comprehensive practice exams. (A new edition is due out in 2001.) **Pros:** Overall question content is good, with broad coverage of high-yield topics. Organized by specialty for focused review. Explanations are generally complete. Some classic illustrations. **Cons:** Vignettes are brief and few. Questions are frequently straight-recall-oriented rather than clinically based. Not well illustrated. **Summary:** Average source of questions that do not reflect Step 2 style and format.

B− **A&LERT USMLE Step 2 Deluxe** $95.00 Software/3400 q

Appleton & Lange

McGraw-Hill, 1998, 1st edition, ISBN 0838503748

This question bank includes questions from *Appleton & Lange's Review of the USMLE Step 2* and from A&L's MEPC series. Otherwise identical to *A&LERT: USMLE Step 2*. **Pros:** Large collection of questions will keep you busy. **Cons:** Includes lower-yield "second-tier" questions that do not accurately reflect USMLE style. **Summary:** Worth considering if you need a large collection of computerized questions.

B− **Insider's Guide to the USMLE Step 2** $35.95 Review/450 q

Stang

Saunders, 1999, 1st edition, 426 pages, ISBN 0721682790

Contains case-based questions with explanations and includes suggested review topics. **Pros:** "Pop quizzes" after each section encourage retention. Practice test has detailed explanations to answers. **Cons:** Sparse information; may serve as a study guide rather than a review book. **Summary:** Well-organized though not very detailed comprehensive review.

B⁻ Step 2 of the Boards Part A

$129.00 Audio Review

Gold Standard Board Preparation Systems

Gold Standard, 1997–1999, 15 tapes

Audio review organized into the following topics: Differential Diagnosis, Drugs of Choice, Urgent Care, Surgery, Pediatrics, OB/GYN, Advanced Cardiac Life Support, Cardiology and EKGs, and Diabetes and Hypertension. Can be ordered at (740) 592-4124. **Pros:** Offers a novel study method. Question-and-answer format keeps the listener engaged. **Cons:** Lacks adequate emphasis on diagnosis and management. Focuses on low-yield topics, sometimes overly simplistic. Disorganized, no outline to search tapes for a particular topic. Expensive. **Summary:** Useful as supplemental review source but relatively expensive with some focus on low-yield material.

B⁻ Clinical Science Question Bank for the USMLE Step 2

$28.00 Test/500 q

Zaslau

FMSG, 1997, 1st edition, 135 pages, ISBN 1886468168

Review-question book with five 100-question exams. Includes lengthy clinical vignettes as well as figures and images. **Pros:** Questions focus on high-yield topics. **Cons:** Questions are of variable quality and do not reflect boards style and format. Some questions lack explanations. Illustrations are not representative of Step 2. Relatively expensive. **Summary:** Covers appropriate topics, but many questions are poorly written.

B⁻ Mosby's Ace the Boards: General Clinical Sciences Step 2

$41.95 Review/1000+ q

Bollet

Mosby–Year Book, 1996, 1st edition, 530 pages, ISBN 0815107234

General, detailed review of Step 2. Features questions in book and on disk. **Pros:** Comprehensive review of most major Step 2 topics. Explanations to questions are generally complete. **Cons:** Very dense, overly detailed text makes for difficult reading. Few clinical vignette questions in non–boards style. Poorly illustrated. **Summary:** Comprehensive review is too dense and detailed for boards review of wards preparation.

B⁻ REA's Interactive Flashcards USMLE Step 2

$8.95 Flashcard

Fogiel

REA, 1998, 1st edition, 500 pages, ISBN 0878911685

"Flashcard" review in book format. **Pros:** Cheap. Has fill-in-the-blank format. **Cons:** Cannot remove pages to use as flashcards. Fairly random questions. Some picky and low-yield questions. **Summary:** Not very helpful as a sole source of review given non–boards-style questions and low-yield topics.

Comprehensive

B⁻ **Step 2 Virtual Reality** $20.00 Test/320 q
Zaslau

FMSG, 1998, 1st edition, 170 pages, ISBN 1886468249

Two practice exams with discussions of correct and incorrect responses:
Pros: Lengthy question stems approximate those of Step 2. Questions also
reflect emphasis on management and treatment decisions. Generally
good-quality content. **Cons:** Not very much material covered. Explanations of incorrect answers are very superficial. **Summary:** Expensive for a
limited number of good-quality questions.

B⁻ **Classic Presentations and Rapid Review** $25.00 Review
for USMLE Step 2
O'Connell

J&S, 1999, 1st edition, 215 pages, ISBN 1888308052

Light overview organized by specialty, with emphasis on "classic" presentations of commonly seen conditions. In bulleted-point format. **Pros:**
Good for last-minute studying. **Cons:** Not comprehensive nor consistent
in the material provided on each topic. Information is not very in-depth.
No clinical images, EKGs, or clinical case examples. **Summary:** A quick
and superficial review.

C⁺ **Step 2 Success** $26.00 Test/720 q
Zaslau

FMSG, 1995, 1st edition, 224 pages, ISBN 1886468060

Simulated full-length exam for Step 2. **Pros:** Many clinical vignettes.
Cons: Questions are generally too easy. Some focus on low-yield topics.
Some weak explanations. Poorly illustrated. Expensive for the number of
questions. **Summary:** Below-average questions that do not reflect the
boards style and format.

C **USMLE Success** $38.00 Review/540 q
Zaslau

FMSG, 1996, 3rd edition, 280 pages, ISBN 1886468095

General overview for Steps 1, 2, and 3 in outline format. Contains simulated exams for both Step 1 and Step 2. **Pros:** Many clinical vignette
questions with appropriate emphasis on diagnosis and management. Quick
read. **Cons:** Scanty facts, outdated book recommendations. Poorly written
explanations. Few illustrations. Expensive for amount and quality of material. **Summary:** Inadequate source for any Step review. Questions may be
helpful, but explanations are poorly written.

Clinical Science Review Success $22.00   Review

Zaslau

FMSG, 1997, 1st edition, 132 pages, ISBN 188646815X

General overview of core clinical rotations. Notes are printed straight
from the author's PowerPoint presentation. There is added information on
the Match and residency. **Pros:** Overview of high-yield topics may be
quickly reviewed. "Most common" list may be useful for quick cramming.
Cons: Mostly superficial coverage. PowerPoint printout is difficult to read.
Summary: Inadequate, superficial, poorly formatted content review with
an expensive price tag.

 A&L's Practice Tests: USMLE Step 2 $36.95   Test/900 q

Goldberg

McGraw-Hill, 1999, 1st edition, 350 pages, ISBN 0838503721

Not yet reviewed or rated.

 Underground Clinical Vignettes: 8 Volume Set $135.00   Review

Bhushan

Blackwell Science, 1999, 1st edition, ISBN 1890061468

All eight Step 2 titles shrink wrapped. New edition expected in late 2001,
featuring an extensive color atlas supplement.

Blueprints in Medicine

$29.95   Review/89 q

Young

Blackwell Science, 2000, 2nd edition, 247 pages, ISBN 0632044845

Text review of internal medicine organized by common diseases and common symptoms. Question-and-answer section, with explanations. **Pros:** Well-organized, concise review. Engaging, easy reading. Symptom approach is helpful for boards review. Good charts and diagrams. **Cons:** Few illustrations. Not a quick read. Has some superfluous details. **Summary:** Very good primary boards for internal medicine though poorly illustrated.

PreTest Medicine

$21.95   Test/500 q

Berk

McGraw-Hill, 2001, 9th edition, 238 pages, ISBN 0071359605

Question-and-answer format organized by medical subspecialty. **Pros:** Organization by subspecialty helps pinpoint weak areas. Decent number of vignette-style questions, with detailed explanations. **Cons:** Many questions are more detailed than level needed for the boards. Few illustrations. **Summary:** Solid source of challenging review questions.

Underground Clinical Vignettes: Internal Medicine, Vol. I

$18.95   Review

Bhushan

Blackwell Science, 1999, 1st edition, 100 pages, ISBN 1890061204

Clinical vignette review of common topics in internal medicine. **Pros:** Well organized by focus points: pathogenesis, epidemiology, management, complications, and associated diseases. Well illustrated. **Cons:** Not comprehensive, use as a supplement to review. **Summary:** Organized and easy-to-read supplement to studying. New fully revised editions expected in late 2001 with links to a color atlas supplement, new "mini-cases" and updated treatments.

Underground Clinical Vignettes: Internal Medicine, Vol. II

$18.95   Review

Bhushan

Blackwell Science, 1999, 1st edition, 100 pages, ISBN 1890061255

Clinical vignette review of common topics in internal medicine. **Pros:** Well organized by focus points: pathogenesis, epidemiology, management, complications, and associated diseases. Well illustrated. **Cons:** Not comprehensive, use as a supplement to review. **Summary:** Organized and easy-to-read supplement to studying. New fully revised editions expected in late 2001 with links to a color atlas supplement, new "mini-cases" and updated treatments.

B+ A&L's Review of Internal Medicine $34.95 Test/1100+ q

Goldlist

McGraw-Hill, 1999, 2nd edition, 260 pages, ISBN 0838503551

General review with questions and answers divided by subspecialty. **Pros:** Well-written vignette questions reflect boards format. Representative of the content of the boards. Complete explanations. Well illustrated. **Cons:** Questions are shorter and some non-vignette questions are more straight-forward than those on the exam. **Summary:** Very good source of questions that accurately reflect the multi-step nature of boards questions.

B+ High-Yield Internal Medicine $18.95 Review

Nirula

Lippincott Williams & Wilkins, 1997, 1st edition, 197 pages, ISBN 0683180444

Core review of internal medicine in outline format. **Pros:** Focus is on high-yield diseases and symptoms. Quick and easy read. **Cons:** Some mistakes in formulas. Needs more illustrations. No index. **Summary:** Good, fast review presented in a format that allows for quick and repetitive readings.

B+ Saint-Frances Guide to Inpatient Medicine $23.95 Review

Lippincott Williams & Wilkins, 1997, 1st edition, 533 pages, ISBN 0683075470

General review of high-yield medicine topics in outline format. **Pros:** Very readable, concise, and well organized with mnemonics and "hot keys" emphasized. **Cons:** Brief coverage of some important topics. Lacks images. Requires a time commitment. **Summary:** Solid medicine review that sits somewhere between Wards and Step 2 prep.

B+ Underground Clinical Vignettes: Emergency Medicine $18.95 Review

Bhushan

Blackwell Science, 1999, 1st edition, 100 pages, ISBN 1890061271

Clinical vignette review of emergency medicine topics. **Pros:** Well organized by focus points: pathogenesis, epidemiology, management, complications, and associated diseases. Well illustrated. **Cons:** Not comprehensive; use as a supplement to review. **Summary:** Organized and easy-to-read supplement to studying. New fully revised editions expected in late 2001 with links to a color atlas supplement, new "mini-cases" and updated treatments.

B Medicine Recall $28.00 Review

Bergin

Lippincott Williams & Wilkins, 1997, 1st edition, 928 pages, ISBN 0683180983

Standard *Recall* series question–answer format, organized by medical specialty. **Pros:** Addresses a broad range of high-yield clinical topics. Good format for self-quizzing. Appropriate level of detail. **Cons:** No vignettes, no images, requires a time commitment. **Summary:** Style may be more conducive to wards than to boards preparation. Use as a supplement to other resources.

B   **Internal Medicine Pearls** $45.00   Review

Heffner

Lippincott Williams & Wilkins, 2000, 2nd edition, 275 pages, ISBN 1560534044

Detailed clinical vignettes with laboratory and radiographic findings, followed by a discussion and emphasis of clinically important "pearls." **Pros:** High-quality, realistic vignettes. Questions focus on decision-making and management. **Cons:** Selected topics, not comprehensive. Discussions may be too detailed for purposes of review. **Summary:** A good clinically focused supplement for review.

B   **Outpatient Medicine Recall** $28.00   Review

Franko

Lippincott Williams & Wilkins, 1998, 1st edition, 350 pages, ISBN 0683180185

Question–answer format typical of *Recall* series books, focused on outpatient management. **Pros:** Well written material, good for self-testing. **Cons:** Not as concise or focused as other boards resources. No vignettes or images. **Summary:** Style is not ideal for boards review, but may be a useful adjunct.

B   **Physical Diagnosis Secrets** $38.00   Review

Mangione

Lippincott Williams & Wilkins, 1999, 1st edition, 350 pages, ISBN 1560531649

Secrets series question-and-answer format. **Pros:** Concise review of many high-yield topics. Good use of clinical images. **Cons:** No clinical vignettes, simply lists of questions that might be posed on the wards. Does not have a structured format and may leave out important information. Expensive for amount of material. **Summary:** Overall, good content for self-quizzing and study, but does not substitute for a formal review or practice tests.

B–   **Medical Secrets** $39.00   Review

Zollo

Lippincott Williams & Wilkins, 1997, 2nd edition, 525 pages, ISBN 156053172X

Question–discussion style typical of the *Secrets* series. **Pros:** Covers a great deal of clinically relevant information. **Cons:** Lengthy and detailed for USMLE review. No images or vignettes. **Summary:** May be most appropriate for wards use. Not a focused review.

B- Step 2 of the Boards Part B

Gold Standard Board Preparation Systems

Gold Standard, 27 tapes

$199.00 Audio Review

Audio review of internal medicine with tapes in Pulmonary, Hematology, Genitourinary, Heart Failure, Cardiac Arrhythmias, Gastrointestinal, and Endocrinology. Can be ordered at (740) 592-4124. **Pros:** Offers a novel way to review medicine. Question-and-answer style of tapes makes listening interactive. Tapes well organized with specific subject labels. **Cons:** Expensive relative to other options for internal medicine review. Focuses on some low-yield topics while neglecting some important material. Requires time commitment. **Summary:** Expensive audio review with some focus on low-yield topics.

C+ Oklahoma Notes Family Medicine

Hirsch

Springer-Verlag, 1996, 2nd edition (revised), 290 pages, ISBN 0387946381

$19.95 Review/100 q

Outline review of family medicine. **Pros:** Quick read. Relatively inexpensive. **Cons:** Incomplete test with some errors. No emphasis on risk factors or management. Few to no tables or diagrams. Questions are really hokey (trust us). Letter answers only. **Summary:** Poor review for family medicine with inadequate details and poorly written (but entertaining) questions.

C+ Oklahoma Notes Internal Medicine

Jarolim

Springer-Verlag, 1996, 2nd edition, 424 pages, ISBN 0387946365

$19.95 Review/358 q

General topics in internal medicine reviewed in brief outline format typical for this series. **Pros:** Inexpensive. Broad coverage of topics. Includes questions. **Cons:** Very little emphasis on treatment and management. No tables or illustrations. Questions at the end of the book have letter answers only without explanations. **Summary:** Mediocre medicine review text.

N PreTest Physical Diagnosis

Reteguiz & Avendano

McGraw-Hill, 2001, 4th edition, 328 pages, ISBN 0071360980

$21.95 Test/500 q

General review questions for physical diagnosis organized by organ system. Not yet reviewed or rated.

N Saint-Frances Guide to Outpatient Medicine

Frances

Lippincott Williams & Wilkins, 2000, 1st edition, 713 pages, ISBN 0781726123

$23.95 Review

General review questions for physical diagnosis organized by organ system. Not yet reviewed or rated.

B+ **PreTest Neurology** $21.95 Test/500 q

Elkind

McGraw-Hill, 2001, 4th edition, 292 pages, ISBN 0070525285

Question-and-answer review of neurology. **Pros:** Thorough coverage of neurology topics with good number of clinical vignettes. Good emphasis on common topics. **Cons:** Some questions may be more detailed than level needed for boards. Poorly illustrated. **Summary:** Good source of topic review.

B+ **Underground Clinical Vignettes: Neurology** $18.95 Review

Bhushan

Blackwell Science, 1999, 1st edition, 100 pages, ISBN 1890061263

Clinical vignette review of high-yield topics in neurology. **Pros:** Well organized by focus points: pathogenesis, epidemiology, management, complications, and associated diseases. Well illustrated. **Cons:** Not comprehensive, use as a supplement to review. **Summary:** Organized and easy-to-read supplement to studying. New fully revised editions expected in late 2001 with links to a color atlas supplement, new "mini-cases" and updated treatments.

B **Neurology Pearls** $39.00 Review

Waclawik

Lippincott Williams & Wilkins, 2000, 1st edition, 250 pages, ISBN 1560532610

Detailed clinical vignettes, including laboratory and test results and radiographic findings, followed by a discussion of the diagnosis and emphasis on important "pearls." **Pros:** High-quality vignettes on many important neurologic conditions. **Cons:** Requires an investment in time. A number of entries are devoted to closure disease entities. **Summary:** Challenging clinical scenarios to supplement a more structured topic review.

B **Neurology Recall** $28.00 Review

Miller

Lippincott Williams & Wilkins, 1997, 1st edition, 360 pages, ISBN 0683182161

Brief question–answer format. **Pros:** Many important facts reviewed, useful for self-quizzing. **Cons:** Not a comprehensive review. Concepts are not integrated. **Summary:** Good for review of some high-yield concepts, but not a stand-alone resource for this topic.

B **Neurology Secrets** $38.00   Review

Rolak

Lippincott Williams & Wilkins, 1998, 2nd edition, 450 pages, ISBN
1560532513

Secrets series question-and-answer format. **Pros:** Concise review of many
high-yield topics. Good use of clinical images. **Cons:** No clinical vignettes, simply lists of questions that might be posed on the wards. Does
not have a structured format and may leave out important information.
Expensive for amount of material. **Summary:** Overall, good content for
self-quizzing and study, but does not substitute for a formal review or practice tests.

C+ **Oklahoma Notes Neurology** $19.95   Review/100 q
and Clinical Neuroscience

Brumback

Springer-Verlag, 1996, 2nd edition, 186 pages, ISBN 0387946357

General topics in clinical neurology reviewed in brief outline format.
Pros: Some illustrations. Inexpensive. Easy read. **Cons:** Outline has poor
coverage of risk factors and management. Clinical vignette questions are
too easy. **Summary:** Limited review of neuroscience topics with no emphasis on differential diagnosis, risk factors, or management.

Blueprints in Obstetrics and Gynecology   **$29.95**   Review/149 q

Callahan

Blackwell Science, 2000, 2nd edition, 207 pages, ISBN 0632044845

Text review with tables and illustrations. Includes a short exam with explanations. **Pros:** Strong emphasis on high-yield topics with concise text, clear diagrams, and many classic illustrations. Easy read. **Cons:** Some overly detailed material included. Lengthy text. **Summary:** Overall, very good choice for boards and wards preparation, although some not for last-minute Step 2 review.

B+ **Underground Clinical Vignettes: OB/GYN**   **$18.95**   Review

Bhushan

Blackwell Science, 1999, 1st edition, 100 pages, 1890061239

Clinical vignette review of frequently tested diseases in obstetrics and gynecology. **Pros:** Well organized by focus points: pathogenesis, epidemiology, management, complications, and associated diseases. Well illustrated. **Cons:** Not comprehensive; use as a supplement to review. **Summary:** Well organized and easy-to-read practice vignettes. New fully revised editions expected in late 2001 with links to a color atlas supplement, new "mini-cases" and updated treatments.

B **NMS Obstetrics and Gynecology**   **$30.00**   Review/500 q

Beck

Lippincott Williams & Wilkins, 1997, 4th edition, 510 pages, ISBN 0683180150

Detailed outline of OB/GYN with few tables and diagrams. **Pros:** Comprehensive review for both wards and boards. Final exam is relatively good with complete explanations. **Cons:** Dense and lengthy OB/GYN review. Many questions do not reflect boards format. Lacks illustrations. **Summary:** Complete review with questions and discussion. May be too ambitious for exam prep alone, may be most helpful if used throughout clerkship.

B **PreTest Obstetrics and Gynecology**   **$21.95**   Test/500 q

Evans & Ginsburg

McGraw-Hill, 2001, 9th edition, 263 pages, ISBN 0071359613

Question-and-answer review with detailed explanations for OB/GYN. **Pros:** Organization by subtopic may be useful for studying weak areas. Good content emphasis. Generally well illustrated. **Cons:** Some questions are too difficult or detailed. Vignette-based questions are short and simplistic compared to Step 2 content, which recently has had an emphasis on this topic. **Summary:** Decent source of questions to supplement topic study.

B– BRS Obstetrics and Gynecology

Sakala

$18.95   Review/500 q

Lippincott Williams & Wilkins, 1997, 1st edition, 389 pages, ISBN 1683074989

General review text with questions at the ends of the chapters and a comprehensive exam at the end of the book. **Pros:** Appropriate content for boards and wards study. **Cons:** Some sections are overly detailed with few diagrams. Slow reading. Questions are brief with few clinical vignettes. **Summary:** Appropriate content review, but more helpful for wards than for boards preparation.

B– Obstetrics and Gynecology Recall

Bourgeois

$28.00   Review/350 q

Lippincott Williams & Wilkins, 1997, 1st edition, 528 pages, ISBN 0683182145

Recall series style question–answer style. **Pros:** Two-column format makes it useful for self-quizzing. Reviews many high-yield concepts and facts. **Cons:** Questions emphasize individual facts but do not integrate concepts. No vignettes or images. Spotty coverage of some topics. **Summary:** Useful for review of selected concepts but not a comprehensive source for USMLE preparation.

B– Obstetrics and Gynecology: Review for the New National Boards

Kramer

$25.00   Test/530 q

J&S, 1996, 1st edition, 190 pages, ISBN 0963287397

General review of OB/GYN in question-and-answer format. **Pros:** Good ultrasounds and fetal heart tracings. Appropriate depth of coverage. **Cons:** As many as 40 questions per vignette stem with corresponding multiple-page explanations. Focuses on some low-yield topics. **Summary:** Below-average source of questions. Does not reflect Step 2 format or style.

B– Obstetrics and Gynecology Secrets

Frederickson

$39.00   Review

Lippincott Williams & Wilkins, 1997, 2nd edition, 380 pages, ISBN 156053205X

Secrets series question-and-answer format, organized by topics within OB/GYN. **Pros:** Good coverage of many high-yield clinically relevant topics. **Cons:** Detailed, not useful for rapid review. No vignettes, or images. **Summary:** Good clinical context but does not serve as a formal topic review.

A&L's Review of Obstetrics and Gynecology   **$34.95**   Test/1600+ q

Vontver

McGraw-Hill, 2000, 6th edition, 400 pages, ISBN 0838503233

Detailed review of OB/GYN in question-and-answer format. **Pros:** Some high-yield sections such as clinical endocrinology. **Cons:** Overall emphasis is not appropriate for Step 2 preparation. May be more appropriate for specialty preparation. **Summary:** Far more detailed than required for Step 2. New edition not yet reviewed.

 MEPC Obstetrics and Gynecology   **$19.95**   Test/765 q

Ross

McGraw-Hill, 1997, 411 pages, ISBN 0838563287

Question-and-answer format with explanation. **Pros:** Another source of questions that may be quickly reviewed. Content of questions is appropriate for Step 2. Most explanations are thorough and well written. **Cons:** Very few vignette-based style questions. Few illustrations. **Summary:** Average source of additional questions that may be read quickly. Appropriate content emphasis, but questions do not reflect boards-style format.

 Oklahoma Notes Obstetrics and Gynecology   **$19.95**   Review/104 q

Miles, Oklahoma Notes

Springer-Verlag, 1996, 2nd edition, 218 pages, ISBN 0387946322

General text review of OB/GYN. **Pros:** Relatively inexpensive. **Cons:** Low emphasis on high-yield topics (e.g., risk factors, management). Very few diagrams or tables. Questions lack clinical vignettes or discussions. **Summary:** Limited review of OB/GYN that does not reflect Step 2 content.

 Clinical Obstetrics and Gynecology: A Problem-Based Approach   **$32.95**   Review

Burnett

Blackwell Science, 2000, 1st edition, 450 pages, ISBN 0632043539

Not yet reviewed or rated.

A&L's Review of Pediatrics $34.95   Test/1000+ q
Lorin

McGraw-Hill, 1997, 5th edition, 222 pages, ISBN 0838503039

Question-and-answer review of pediatrics with detailed explanations.
Pros: Questions are focused on boards-relevant content. One hundred
twenty excellent vignette-based questions in last chapter. Thorough, well-
written explanations. Nice primer on test-taking strategies. **Cons:** Non-
vignette-based questions are shorter and more straightforward than those
on Step 2. Needs more vignette-style questions. Some questions may be
too detailed for Step 2 preparation. Poorly illustrated. **Summary:** Excellent, concise review with appropriate content and good discussions, although the majority of questions do not reflect Step 2 style. New edition
not yet reviewed.

PreTest Pediatrics $21.95   Test/500 q
Yetman

McGraw-Hill, 2001, 9th edition, 295 pages, ISBN 0071359559

Question-and-answer review with detailed discussion. **Pros:** Organization
by organ system is useful for pinpointing weaknesses. Strong, thorough explanations. Fair number of vignettes-style questions. Well illustrated.
Cons: Some questions are too detailed, or emphasize low-yield topics.
Summary: Good source of questions and review for pediatrics. Appropriate content with good illustrations, though not entirely in Step 2 format.

Underground Clinical Vignettes: Pediatrics $18.95   Review
Bhushan

Blackwell Science, 1999, 1st edition, 100 pages, ISBN 1890061212

Clinical vignette review of frequently tested topics in pediatrics. **Pros:**
Well organized by focus points: pathogenesis, epidemiology, management,
complications, and associated diseases. Well illustrated. **Cons:** Not comprehensive, use as a supplement to text review. **Summary:** Well organized
and easy to read. New fully revised editions expected in late 2001 with
links to a color atlas supplement, new "mini-cases" and updated treatments.

Pediatrics: Review for USMLE Step 2 $25.00   Test/545 q
Paulson

J&S, 2000, 1st edition, 273 pages, ISBN 1888308087

Test booklet with many clinical vignettes covering a broad range of topics
within pediatrics. **Pros:** Organized by topics, informative answer explanations. Not too dense for last-minute review. **Cons:** Few images, includes
non–boards-type questions ("except" and K-type answers). **Summary:**
Good content review; does not replicate boards style.

B Blueprints in Pediatrics $29.95   Review/1269
Marino

Blackwell Science, 2000, 2nd edition, 246 pages, ISBN 0632044861

Text review of pediatrics with tables and diagrams. Question-and-answer section with explanations included. **Pros:** Appropriate focus on high-yield topics. **Cons:** Relatively dense text with few illustrations. Overly detailed. **Summary:** Good for the motivated student.

B Pediatrics Recall $28.00   Review
McGahren

Lippincott Williams & Wilkins, 1997, 1st edition, 459 pages, ISBN 068305855X

Concise question-and-answer format typical of *Recall* series. **Pros:** Two-column format makes self-quizzing easy. Emphasizes diagnosis and management. **Cons:** Requires a time commitment. Not all topics are covered thoroughly. No vignettes. **Summary:** Useful material, but does not provide a systematic review or substitute for practice tests.

B⁻ MEPC Pediatrics $19.95   Test/700 q
Hansbarger

McGraw-Hill, 1995, 9th edition, 248 pages, ISBN 083856223X

Question-and-answer format with brief discussion. **Pros:** Appropriate content emphasis. Quick read. **Cons:** Few vignette questions. Scanty explanations. Poor illustrations. **Summary:** Below-average source of questions with poor discussion of answers.

B⁻ NMS Pediatrics $33.00   Review/166+ q
Dworkin

Lippincott Williams & Wilkins, 2000, 4th edition,
ISBN 0683306375

General review of pediatrics in outline format. Questions at the end of each chapter. **Pros:** Very thorough, detailed review of pediatrics. Boldfacing highlights key points. Case studies and comprehensive exam (also provided on CD-ROM) at end of book are helpful. Good discussion. **Cons:** Dense, lengthy text. Lacks good illustrations of any kind. **Summary:** Thorough review but more appropriate for clerkships than for Step 2 review.

B⁻ Oklahoma Notes Pediatrics $19.95   Review/126 q
Puls

Springer-Verlag, 1996, 2nd edition, 390 pages, ISBN 0387946349

General outline format of pediatrics. **Pros:** Well organized by system. Good tables. **Cons:** Poorly illustrated. Incomplete explanations. Focuses on some low-yield topics. Questions lack clinical vignettes or explanations. **Summary:** Well-organized review of pediatrics with incomplete text. Above average for series.

B– **Pediatric Secrets** $39.00 Review

Polin

Lippincott Williams & Wilkins, 1997, 2nd edition, 575 pages, ISBN 1560531711

Question–answer format typical of *Secrets* series, organized by pediatric subspecialty. **Pros:** Thorough discussion of a wide variety of clinical topics. **Cons:** Detailed content geared for the wards, requires a large time investment. **Summary:** Too detailed for USMLE review.

C **STARS Pediatrics: A Primary Care Approach** $35.00 Text

Berkowitz

Saunders, 2000, 2nd edition, 579 pages, ISBN 0721656234

Text review of pediatrics. **Pros:** Comprehensive review. Has illustrative case vignettes and questions that relate to each disorder discussed. **Cons:** Dense and overly detailed text and tables. Covers many low-yield topics. Poorly illustrated. **Summary:** Very detailed and difficult to read.

PreTest Preventive Medicine and Public Health

B+

$21.95   Test/500 q

Ratelle

McGraw-Hill, 2001, 9th edition, 238 pages, ISBN 0071359621

Question-and-answer review of epidemiology, biostatistics, and preventive medicine. **Pros:** Majority of test questions appropriately simulate boards content and difficulty. Good explanations. **Cons:** Some questions are too heavy on calculations. Biostatistics chapter is too detailed. Very few vignettes. **Summary:** Good question-and-answer review for a low-yield topic.

MEPC Preventive Medicine and Public Health

B−

$21.95   Review/700 q

Hart

McGraw-Hill, 1996, 265 pages, ISBN 0838563198

Question-and-answer review with discussions. **Pros:** Appropriate level of biostatistics review. **Cons:** Few clinical vignettes. Many questions are too picky. Brief explanations with poor detail. **Summary:** Adequate content review, but questions do not follow boards format and explanations are poor.

NMS Clinical Epidemiology and Biostatistics

C+

$28.00   Review/300 q

Knapp

Lippincott Williams & Wilkins, 1992, 435 pages, ISBN 0683062069

Detailed outline review of epidemiology and biostatistics. **Pros:** Exhaustive coverage. **Cons:** Too much detail for a small subject area. Very slow read. Questions focus on low-yield topics. **Summary:** Inappropriate for Step 2 review. Better suited for an epidemiology student.

STARS Epidemiology, Biostatistics, and Preventive Medicine Review

C+

$21.95   Review/350 q

Katz

Saunders, 1997, 249 pages, ISBN 0721640842

Detailed text review of epidemiology and biostatistics. **Pros:** Good tables and diagrams. **Cons:** Small print makes for difficult reading. Text too detailed for quick review. Questions do not reflect boards style and format. Discussions of questions are too detailed. Requires time commitment. **Summary:** Too detailed for Step 2 review.

NMS Preventive Medicine and Public Health

C

$28.00   Review/450 q

Cassens

Lippincott Williams & Wilkins, 1992, 2nd edition, 497 pages, ISBN 068306262X

Detailed review of preventive medicine and public health. **Pros:** Very comprehensive review. Questions have thorough explanations. **Cons:** Too long and detailed for boards review. Too much low-yield material. **Summary:** Not ideal for Step 2 review. Better suited for a public health student.

REVIEW RESOURCES

Preventive Medicine

Blueprints in Psychiatry

Murphy

$26.95   Review/74 q

Blackwell Science, 2000, 2nd edition, 128 pages, ISBN 0632044888

Brief text review of psychiatry with DSM-IV criteria. Brief question-and-answer section at end of book. **Pros:** Clear, concise review of psychiatry with helpful tables. Good coverage of high-yield topics. Quick read. **Cons:** Relatively expensive for amount of material. **Summary:** Rapid review with appropriate coverage of high-yield topics.

High-Yield Psychiatry

Fadem

$18.95   Review

Lippincott Williams & Wilkins, 1998, 1st edition, 151 pages, ISBN 0683302035

Brief outline-format review of psychiatry. **Pros:** Quick read with clinical vignettes scattered throughout. Concise tables. **Cons:** Not enough detail for in-depth review. **Summary:** Excellent, quick review of psychiatry, may lack depth.

PreTest Psychiatry

Mezzacappa

$21.95   Test/500 q

McGraw-Hill, 2001, 9th edition, 255 pages, ISBN 0071361553

Question-and-answer review of topics in psychiatry. **Pros:** Questions are well written and organized. Most questions have appropriate content level. Good explanations. **Cons:** Too few vignette-type questions. Some questions are too detailed. **Summary:** Good source of questions and review for psychiatry, though format may not reflect the actual test.

Underground Clinical Vignettes: Psychiatry

Bhushan

$18.95   Review

Blackwell Science, 1999, 1st edition, 100 pages, ISBN 1890061247

Clinical vignette review of frequently tested topics in psychiatry. **Pros:** Well organized by focus points: pathogenesis, epidemiology, management, associated diseases. Well illustrated. **Cons:** Not comprehensive; use as a supplement to review. **Summary:** Well organized and easy-to-read practice vignettes. New fully revised editions expected in late 2001 with links to a color atlas supplement, new "mini-cases" and updated treatments.

NMS Psychiatry

Scully

$30.00   Review/400 q

Lippincott Williams & Wilkins, 1996, 3rd edition, 318 pages, ISBN 0683062638

General review of topics in outline format with questions at end of each chapter and a comprehensive final exam. **Pros:** Well-written text with concise disease discussions. Questions test appropriate content and have complete explanations. Good companion text for clerkship. **Cons:** Not enough vignette-style questions. Lengthy for purposes of board review. **Summary:** Detailed review that requires time commitment. Good single choice for clerkship study and boards review.

B | **A&L's Review of Psychiatry** | $34.95 | Test/900+ q

Oransky

McGraw-Hill, 2001, 6th edition, 306 pages, ISBN 0838503705

General review of psychiatry with questions and answers. **Pros:** Includes 114 vignette-style questions appropriate for boards review. Appropriate content emphasis. Thorough explanations. **Cons:** Questions are shorter and more straightforward than those of boards. **Summary:** Decent boards review for psychiatry, although does not reflect boards format.

B | **Behavioral Science/Psychiatry: Review for the New National Boards** | $25.00 | Test/521 q

Frank

J&S, 1998, 1st edition, 248 pages, ISBN 1888308001

General review of psychiatry in question-and-answer format. **Pros:** Includes some vignette-based questions with complete explanations. **Cons:** Does not emphasize high-yield topics. Does not follow boards format or style. Some questions are too short and easy. **Summary:** Mixed-quality questions with generally complete explanations.

B | **BRS Psychiatry** | $26.95 | Review/400 q

Shaner

Lippincott Williams & Wilkins, 2000, 2nd edition, 448 pages, ISBN 0863307665

Comprehensive review of psychiatry in outline format. Vignette-style questions follow each chapter. **Pros:** Thorough, systematic review of clinical psychiatry. Clear, concise definitions provided. **Cons:** A great deal of information for single-topic review. **Summary:** Good material but requires a large time investment; not for last-minute review of all topics.

B | **Psychiatry Recall** | $28.00 | Review

Fadem

Lippincott Williams & Wilkins, 1997, 1st edition, 250 pages, ISBN 0683180045

Quick question-and-answer format of *Recall* series. **Pros:** Two-column format is conducive to self-quizzing. Covers many high-yield facts and concepts necessary for the USMLE. **Cons:** Lacks vignettes so does not substitute for practice tests. **Summary:** Requires a time commitment. Some topics glossed over. Use as a supplement to other resources.

B⁻ | **MEPC Psychiatry** | $19.95 | Test/700 q

Chan

McGraw-Hill, 1995, 10th edition, 259 pages, ISBN 0838557805

Question-and-answer format organized by topics in psychiatry. **Pros:** Last chapter has many good clinical vignette questions. **Cons:** Most questions are not vignette-based. Some questions are picky and focus on low-yield topics. Many explanations are brief. **Summary:** Below-average source of review questions.

B⁻ **Psychiatric Secrets** — $39.00 — Review

Jacobson

Lippincott Williams & Wilkins, 2000, 2nd edition, 500 pages, ISBN
1560534184

Question–discussion format of *Secrets* series, organized by topic. **Pros:**
Clear explanations of important concepts in psychiatry. Good wards read-
ing. **Cons:** Too detailed and lengthy for review purposes. Lacks vignettes.
Summary: Requires a significant time to read; not for rapid, focused review.

C⁺ **Oklahoma Notes Psychiatry** — $19.95 — Review/103 q

Shaffer

Springer-Verlag, 1996, 2nd edition (revised), 247 pages, ISBN
0387946330

Outline-format review of clinical psychiatry. **Pros:** Inexpensive, quick
read. **Cons:** Haphazard text lacks tables and details. Matching-style questions do not reflect Step 2 format or content. **Summary:** Below-average
review of psychiatry.

C⁺ **Psychiatry at a Glance** — $19.95 — Review

Katona

Blackwell Science, 2000, 2nd edition, 96 pages, ISBN 0632055545

A discussion of some common psychiatric and neuropsychiatric conditions,
with multiple choice questions. **Pros:** Easy to read. Most important psychiatric conditions covered. **Cons:** Text is written to be an introduction of the
topics, so simplistic or generalized at times. Lacks emphasis on high-yield
facts or concepts. No vignettes. No explanations of questions. **Summary:**
More useful for overview or introduction than for focused USMLE review.

C **NMS Behavioral Sciences in Psychiatry** — $30.00 — Review/300 q

Wiener

Lippincott Williams & Wilkins, 1995, 3rd edition, 375 pages, ISBN
0683062034

Outline review of behavioral science in psychiatry. **Pros:** Clear outline
format. Case studies highlight differential diagnosis and management.
Cons: Focuses on many low-yield topics with little emphasis on clinical
syndromes. **Summary:** Poor choice for Psychiatry Step 2 review. Lacks adequate clinical emphasis for wards.

 Psychiatry Made Ridiculously Simple — $12.95 — Review

Good

MedMaster, 1999, 3rd edition, 93 pages, ISBN 0940780224
Not yet reviewed or rated.

 Saint-Frances Guide to Psychiatry — Review

McCarthy

Lippincott Williams & Wilkins, 2001, 1st edition, 279 pages,
ISBN 0683306618
Not yet reviewed or rated.

Blueprints in Surgery   **$26.95**   Review/62 q
Karp

Blackwell Science, 2000, 2nd edition, 160 pages, ISBN 063204487X

Short text review of general surgery with tables and diagrams. Brief question-and-answer section included. **Pros:** Well organized. Easy to read with strong focus on high-yield topics. Clear diagrams. **Cons:** Some sections are overly detailed (e.g., anatomy). Some information simplistic. Relatively expensive. **Summary:** Concise review of surgery with appropriate emphasis on high-yield topics.

 BRS General Surgery   **$28.95**   Review/375 q
Crabtree

Lippincott Williams & Wilkins, 2000, 1st edition, 564 pages, ISBN 0683306367

Comprehensive review in outline format, organized by topic or organ. **Pros:** Appropriate clinical emphasis for boards and wards. Vignette-style review questions at end of each chapter. **Cons:** Lengthy for single-topic review. Some information is not specific enough to be useful. Few images or illustrations. **Summary:** Overall, a strong review resource. Requires a time commitment, so may not be suited for rapid review.

B⁺ A&L's Review of Surgery   **$34.95**   Test/950+ q
Wapnick

McGraw-Hill, 1998, 3rd edition, 280 pages, ISBN 0838502458

General review of surgery with questions and answers. **Pros:** Good clinical emphasis. Many vignette-style questions. Explanations are thorough. **Cons:** Questions are shorter and style does not reflect that of the Step 2 exam. Questions are highly variable in difficulty. Few illustrations. **Summary:** Good content review for exam, although some questions are too picky.

B⁺ High-Yield Surgery   **$18.95**   Review
Nirula

Lippincott Williams & Wilkins, 2000, 1st edition, 160 pages, ISBN 068330691X

Outline review of most common general surgery topics. **Pros:** Concise, useful for quick topic review. Well-organized. **Cons:** Information can be superficial. Some topics omitted. No practice questions. **Summary:** Lean text for rapid review.

B⁺ Surgery 1   **$32.00**   Review/120 q
Lavelle-Jones

Saunders, 1997, 1st edition, 207 pages, ISBN 0443051720

Text review of general surgery with illustrations and questions. **Pros:** Concise, well-organized text. Excellent illustrations and radiographs. Illustrative case vignettes. **Cons:** Need *Surgery 2* to complete review of surgery. Questions are not boards style. **Summary:** Excellent review with classic illustrations, but incomplete without *Surgery 2* title.

B⁺   **Surgery: Review for the New National Boards**   **$25.00**   Test/562 q

Geelhoed

J&S, 1995, 1st edition, 246 pages, ISBN 0963287354

Question-and-answer review of surgery. **Pros:** Good focus on high-yield topics. Very good explanations. Classic illustrations. **Cons:** Lacks the lengthy clinical vignette style typical of Step 2. **Summary:** Appropriate review of Step 2–relevant content, but questions do not reflect current USMLE format.

B⁺   **Underground Clinical Vignettes: Surgery**   **$18.95**   Review

Bhushan

Blackwell Science, 1999, 1st edition, 100 pages, ISBN 1890061220

Clinical vignette review of frequently tested surgical topics. **Pros:** Well organized by focus points: pathogenesis, epidemiology, management, complications, and associated diseases. Well illustrated. **Cons:** Not comprehensive; use as a supplement to review. **Summary:** Well organized and easy-to-read practice vignettes. New fully revised editions expected in late 2001 with links to a color atlas supplement, new "mini-cases" and updated treatments.

B   **Abernathy's Surgical Secrets**   **$39.00**   Review

Harken

Lippincott Williams & Wilkins, 2000, 4th edition, 300 pages, ISBN 1560533633

Question-and-answer *Secrets* series format. **Pros:** Discussions are up-to-date and thorough. **Cons:** Too detailed for purposes of the USMLE, yet also not comprehensive. **Summary:** Not a well-organized review.

B   **BRS Surgical Specialties**   **$25.95**   Review/150 q

Crabtree

Lippincott Williams & Wilkins, 2000, 1st edition, 288 pages, ISBN 0781727715

Focused review of topics in the surgical subspecialties in outline format. **Pros:** Good emphasis for boards and wards. Good use of illustrations. Vignette-style review questions. **Cons:** Some information may be redundant from review of other topics. Some information may be beyond the scope of the Step 2 exam. **Summary:** For the advanced surgery student.

B   **NMS Surgery**   **$31.95**   Review/350 q

Jarrell

Lippincott Williams & Wilkins, 2000, 4th edition, 720 pages, ISBN 0683306154

Outline review of general surgery and surgical subspecialties. **Pros:** Well-organized, thorough. Vignette-style questions after each chapter, with good explanations. **Cons:** Dense, detailed text. Few tables or illustrations. **Summary:** Comprehensive surgery review, but very time consuming.

B | **PreTest Surgery** | **$21.95** | Test/500 q

Geller

McGraw-Hill, 2001, 9th edition, 328 pages, ISBN 0070525331

Question-and-answer format review of topics in general surgery. **Pros:** Predominantly case-based. Well organized by subspecialty. **Cons:** Many questions are too detailed or esoteric and do not reflect boards style. Some explanations are overly detailed. **Summary:** Thorough review, but questions may be beyond the level needed for Step 2 preparation.

B | **Surgical Recall** | **$28.00** | Review

Blackbourne

Lippincott Williams & Wilkins, 1997, 2nd edition, 751 pages, ISBN 0683301020

Question-and-answer format as with other *Recall* series books. **Pros:** Questions emphasize important, high-yield clinical concepts. Columns allow self-testing. **Cons:** Not boards-type questions. Poorly organized. Spotty coverage of some topics. **Summary:** A useful adjunct to a more organized topic review.

B− | **MEPC Surgery** | **$21.95** | Test/700 q

Metzler

McGraw-Hill, 1995, 11th edition, 317 pages, ISBN 0838561950

Question-and-answer self-examination for surgery. **Pros:** Questions have appropriate focus. Good explanations. Well illustrated. **Cons:** Questions do not reflect current boards format. **Summary:** Adequate source of questions for review, although it does not follow boards format.

B− | **Oklahoma Notes General Surgery** | **$19.95** | Review/168 q

Jacocks

Springer-Verlag, 1996, 2nd edition, 189 pages, ISBN 0387946373

Outline format for surgery. **Pros:** Inexpensive, quick read. **Cons:** Text lacks high-yield details and illustrations. Questions lack vignettes and explanations. **Summary:** Below average resource for this subject.

B− | **Sabiston's Review of Surgery** | **$41.00** | Test/900+ q

Sabiston

Saunders, 1997, 2nd edition, 280 pages, ISBN 0721686710

Question-and-answer review of surgery. **Pros:** Thorough discussion immediately follows questions, promoting retention. **Cons:** Questions do not reflect boards style or format. Poorly illustrated. Few clinical vignettes. **Summary:** Overly detailed, non–Step 2-specific review of surgery.

Surgery at a Glance   **$24.95**   Review

Grace

Blackwell Science, 1999, 1st edition, 176 pages, ISBN 0362049588

Overview of a variety of surgically correctable conditions. **Pros:** Individual entries are concise and well organized. **Cons:** Information frequently sparse or vague. No vignettes or illustrations. **Summary:** Not a comprehensive review resource.

Dermatology for Boards and Wards

$25.00   Review

Ayala

Blackwell Science, 2001, 96 pages, ISBN 0632045728

Not yet reviewed or rated.

Immunology for Boards and Wards

$15.00   Review

Ayala

Blackwell Science, 2001, 80 pages, ISBN 0632045744

Not yet reviewed or rated.

The IMG's Guide to Mastering the USMLE & Residency

$29.95   Test/500 q

Chander

McGraw-Hill, 2000, 1st edition, 310 pages, ISBN 007134724

Comprehensive guide for IMGs that navigates the complicated process of training in the U.S. Includes information on VISAs, USMLE and TOEFL exams, the Clinical Skills Assessment exam, applying to residencies, with emphasis on overcoming the many obstacles that IMGs face along the way. Also provides practical advice about establishing a home in the U.S., residency survival skills, and finding a job. Not yet rated.

Commercial Review Courses

Compass Medical Education Network

Kaplan Medical/National Medical School Review

Northwestern Learning Center

Postgraduate Medical Review Education

The Princeton Review

Youel's Prep, Inc.

Commercial preparation courses can be helpful for some students, but these courses are expensive and require significant time commitment. They are usually effective in organizing study material for students who feel overwhelmed by the volume of material. Note that the multiweek courses may be quite intense and may thus leave limited time for independent study. Also note that some commercial courses are designed for first-time test takers while others focus on students who are repeating the examination. Some courses focus on foreign medical graduates who want to take all three steps in a limited amount of time. Student experience and satisfaction with review courses are highly variable. We suggest that you discuss options with recent graduates of the review courses you are considering. Course content and structure can change rapidly. Some student opinions can be found in discussion groups on the World Wide Web. Below is contact information for some Step 2 commercial review courses.

Kaplan Medical
888 7th Avenue
New York, NY 10106
1-800-KAP-TEST (1-800-527-8378)
1-800-533-8850
www.kaplanmedical.com/usmle

Northwestern Medical Review
P.O. Box 22174
East Lansing, MI 48909-2174
800-837-7737
testbuster@aol.com
www.northwesternlearningcenter.com/nw

Postgraduate Medical Review Education
407 Lincoln Road, Suite 12E
Miami Beach, FL 33139
800-ECFMG-30 (800-323-6430)
PMRE@aol.com
www.PMRE.com

The Princeton Review
St. Leonard's Court
39th and Chestnut, Suite 317
Philadelphia, PA 19107
800-USMLE84
www.review.com

Youel's Prep, Inc.
701 Cypress Green Circle
Wellington, FL 33414
800-645-3985
561-795-0169 (Fax)
Fax: 561-795-0169
YouelsPrep@aol.com
www.youelsprep.com

Publisher Contacts

If you do not have convenient access to a medical bookstore, consider ordering directly from the publisher.

Appleton & Lange
Products are now sold by McGraw-Hill

Alert & Oriented
13025 Candela Place
San Diego, CA 92130–1866
(888) 253-7844
joel@alertandonline.com
www.alertandonline.com

Blackwell Science
350 Main Street
Malden, MA 02148
(800) 759-6102
(781) 388-8250
Fax: (781) 388-8255
www.blacksci.com

Churchill Livingstone
Products are now sold by Harcourt Health
 Sciences

FMSG Publishing Co.
35 Hollow Pine Dr.
DeBary, FL 32713
(904) 774-5277
Fax: (904) 774-5563
fmsgco@n-jcenter.com

Gold Standard Board Preparation Systems
6374 Long Run Road
Athens, OH 45701
(740) 592-4124
Fax: (740) 592-4045

Harcourt Health Sciences
11830 Westline Industrial Drive
St. Louis, MO 63146
(800) 325-4177
www.harcourthealth.com

J&S Publishing
1300 Bishop Lane
Alexandria, VA 22302
(703) 823-9833
Fax: (703) 823-9834
jandspub@ix.netcom.com
www.jandspub.com

Lippincott Williams & Wilkins
P.O. Box 1580
Hagerstown, MD 21741
(800) 777-2295
Fax: (301) 824-7390
www.lww.com

Maval Publishing, Inc.
567 Harrison St.
Denver, CO 80206

McGraw-Hill Customer Service
P.O. Box 545
Blacklick, OH 43004
(800) 262-4729
Fax: (614) 759-3644
www.mghmedical.com

MedMaster, Inc.
P.O. Box 640028
Miami, FL 33164
(800) 335-3480
(305) 653-3480
Fax: (954) 962-4508
mmbks@aol.com

Mosby–Year Book
Products are now sold by Harcourt Health
 Sciences

Springer-Verlag, NY Inc.
PO Box 2485
Secaucus, NJ 07096
(800) 777-4643
Fax: (201) 348-5405
www.Springer-NY.com
orders@Springer-NY.com

W.B. Saunders
Products are now sold by Harcourt Health
 Sciences

Abbreviations and Symbols

Abbreviation	Meaning
Ab	antibody
ABCs	airway, breathing, circulation
ABG	arterial blood gas
ACE	angiotensin-converting enzyme
ACh	acetylcholine
ACTH	adrenocorticotropic hormone
AD	autosomal dominant
ADH	antidiuretic hormone (vasopressin)
ADHD	attention-deficit hyperactivity disorder
AFP	alpha-fetoprotein
Ag	antigen
AIDS	acquired immunodeficiency syndrome
ALL	acute lymphocytic leukemia
ALS	amyotrophic lateral sclerosis
ALT	alanine aminotransaminase
AML	acute myelogenous leukemia
ANA	antinuclear antibody
ARDS	acute respiratory distress syndrome
ASD	atrial septal defect
ASO	antistreptolysin O
AST	aspartate aminotransaminase
AV	atrioventricular
AVM	arteriovenous malformation
AXR	abdominal x-ray
AZT	azidothymidine
β-HCG	β-human chorionic gonadotropin
BAL	British anti-Lewisite (dimercaprol)
BP	blood pressure
BPH	benign prostatic hyperplasia
BPPV	benign paroxysmal positional vertigo
BUN	blood urea nitrogen
CABG	coronary artery bypass grafting
CAD	coronary artery disease
CAST	computer-adaptive sequential testing
CBC	complete blood count
CBT	computer-based testing
CD	cluster of differentiation
CDC	Centers for Disease Control
CEA	carcinoembryonic antigen
CF	cystic fibrosis
CFTR	cystic fibrosis transmembrane regulator
CHF	congestive heart failure
CIN	cervical intraepithelial neoplasia
CIS	carcinoma in situ
CJD	Creutzfeldt–Jakob disease
CK	creatine phosphokinase
CLL	chronic lymphocytic leukemia
CML	chronic myelogenous leukemia
CMT	Computerized Mastery Test
CMV	cytomegalovirus
CN	cranial nerve
CNS	central nervous system

Abbreviation	Meaning
COPD	chronic obstructive pulmonary disease
CP	cerebral palsy
CPK-MB	creatine phosphokinase, MB fraction
Cr	creatinine
CSA	Clinical Skills Assessment (exam)
CSF	cerebrospinal fluid
CT	computed tomography
CV	cardiovascular
CXR	chest x-ray
D&C	dilation and curettage
DCIS	ductal carcinoma in situ
ddC	dideoxycytidine
DEA	Drug Enforcement Agency
DES	diethylstilbestrol
DI	diabetes insipidus
DIC	disseminated intravascular coagulation
DIP	distal interphalangeal
DKA	diabetic ketoacidosis
DMD	Duchenne muscular dystrophy
DNI	do not intubate
DNR	do not resuscitate
DPOA	durable power of attorney
DSM	Diagnostic and Statistical Manual
DTP	diphtheria–tetanus–pertussis
DTR	deep tendon reflex
DTs	delirium tremens
DVT	deep venous thrombosis
EBV	Epstein–Barr virus
ECFMG	Educational Commission for Foreign Medical Graduates
ECT	electroconvulsive therapy
EEG	electroencephalogram
EKG	electrocardiogram
ELISA	enzyme-linked immunosorbent assay
EMG	electromyogram
EPS	extrapyramidal symptoms
ER	emergency room
ERCP	endoscopic retrograde cholangiopancreatography
ESR	erythrocyte sedimentation rate
EtOH	ethanol
FAP	familial adenomatous polyposis
FDA	Food and Drug Administration
FEV	forced expiratory volume
FFP	fresh frozen plasma
FLEX	Federal Licensing Examination
FMG	foreign medical graduate
FOBT	fecal occult blood test
FSH	follicle-stimulating hormone
FSMB	Federation of State Medical Boards
FTA-ABS	fluorescent treponemal antibody—absorbed

Abbreviation	Meaning	Abbreviation	Meaning
5-FU	5-fluorouracil	MAC	*Mycobacterium avium–intracellulare* complex
FUO	fever of unknown origin		
FVC	forced vital capacity	MAOI	monoamine oxidase inhibitor
GBS	Guillain-Barré Syndrome	MCA	middle cerebral artery
GERD	gastroesophageal reflux disease	MCV	mean corpuscular volume
GFR	glomerular filtration rate	MD	muscular dystrophy
GI	gastrointestinal	MEN	multiple endocrine neoplasia
GnRH	gonadotropin-releasing hormone	MGUS	monoclonal gammopathy of unknown significance
HAV	hepatitis A virus		
Hb	hemoglobin	MHC	major histocompatibility complex
HBsAG	hepatitis B surface antigen	MI	myocardial infarction
HBV	hepatitis B virus	MMPI	Minnesota Multiphasic Personality Inventory
HCG	human chorionic gonadotropin		
HCV	hepatitis C virus	MMR	measles, mumps, rubella
HDL	high-density lipoprotein	MRI	magnetic resonance imaging
HDV	hepatitis D virus	MS	multiple sclerosis
HEV	hepatitis E virus	MTP	metatarsophalangeal
HHS	Department of Health and Human Services	NBME	National Board of Medical Examiners
		NCHS	National Center for Health Statistics
HHV	human herpesvirus	NG	nasogastric
HIDA	hepato-iminodiacetic acid	NIDA	National Institute on Drug Abuse
HIV	human immunodeficiency virus	NIDDM	non–insulin-dependent diabetes mellitus
HLA	human leukocyte antigen	NPO	nil per os (nothing by mouth)
HMG-CoA	hydroxymethylglutaryl-CoA	NPV	negative predictive value
HNPCC	hereditary nonpolyposis colorectal cancer	NSAID	nonsteroidal anti-inflammatory drug
HPV	human papillomavirus	OCP	oral contraceptive pill
HR	heart rate	OPV	oral polio vaccine
HRT	hormone replacement therapy	PAN	polyarteritis nodosa
HSV	herpes simplex virus	PCP	*Pneumocystis carinii* pneumonia; phencyclidine hydrochloride
5-HT	5-hydroxytryptamine (serotonin)		
HTN	hypertension	PCR	polymerase chain reaction
IBD	inflammatory bowel disease	PDA	patent ductus arteriosus
ICP	intracranial pressure	PFTs	pulmonary function tests
ICU	intensive care unit	PG	prostaglandin
IDDM	insulin-dependent diabetes mellitus	PID	pelvic inflammatory disease
IFN	interferon	PIH	pregnancy-induced hypertension
Ig	immunoglobulin	PIP	proximal interphalangeal
IL-1, -2, -3, -4, -5	interleukin-1, 2, 3, 4, 5	PML	progressive multifocal leukoencephalopathy
IM	intramuscular		
IMG	international medical graduate	PMN	polymorphonuclear leukocyte
INH	isonicotine hydrazine (isoniazid)	PMR	polymyalgia rheumatica
INS	Immigration and Naturalization Service	PO	by mouth
IPV	inactivated polio vaccine	PPD	purified protein derivative (of tuberculin)
ITP	idiopathic thrombocytopenic purpura		
IUD	intrauterine device	PPV	positive predictive value
IUGR	intrauterine growth retardation	prn	as needed
IV	intravenous	PSA	prostate-specific antigen
JRA	juvenile rheumatoid arthritis	PT	prothrombin time
LAD	left anterior descending	PTCA	percutaneous transluminal coronary angioplasty
LBO	large bowel obstruction		
LCA	left coronary artery	PTH	parathyroid hormone
LCIS	lobular carcinoma in situ	PTSD	post-traumatic stress disorder
LCME	Liaison Committee on Medical Education	PTT	partial thromboplastin time
		PUD	peptic ulcer disease
LDH	lactate dehydrogenase	RBC	red blood cell
LDL	low-density lipoprotein	RDS	respiratory distress syndrome
LES	lower esophageal sphincter	RLQ	right lower quadrant
LFT	liver function test	RPR	rapid plasma reagin
LH	luteinizing hormone	RR	respiratory rate
LLQ	left lower quadrant	RSV	respiratory syncytial virus
LP	lumbar puncture	RTA	renal tubular acidosis
LPS	lipopolysaccharide	RUQ	right upper quadrant
LUQ	left upper quadrant	RV	residual volume; right ventricle; right ventricular
LV	left ventricle; left ventricular		
LVH	left ventricular hypertrophy	RVH	right ventricular hypertrophy

Abbreviation	Meaning
RVRR	renal vein renin ratio
SA	sinoatrial
SAH	subarachnoid hemorrhage
SBO	small bowel obstruction
SC	sickle cell, subcutaneous
SCFE	slipped capital femoral epiphysis
SCID	severe combined immunodeficiency disease
SIRS	systemic inflammatory response syndrome
SLC	Sylvan Learning Center
SLE	systemic lupus erythematosus
SRP	sponsoring residency program
SRS-A	slow-reacting substance of anaphylaxis
SSRI	selective serotonin reuptake inhibitors
STC	Sylvan Testing Center
STD	sexually transmitted disease
SVC	superior vena cava
SVT	supraventricular tachycardia
TAT	thematic apperception test
TB	tuberculosis
TCA	tricyclic antidepressant
TGV	transposition of great vessels
TIBC	total iron binding capacity
TIPS	transjugular intrahepatic portosystemic shunt
TM	tympanic membrane
TMP-SMX	trimethoprim–sulfamethoxazole
TNM	tumor, node, metastasis
ToRCHeS	toxoplasmosis, rubella, CMV, herpes, syphilis
tPA	tissue plasminogen activator

Abbreviation	Meaning
TSH	thyroid-stimulating hormone
TTN	transcient tachypnea of the newborn
TTP	thrombotic thrombocytopenic purpura
TV	tidal volumeTXA thromboxane
UA	urinalysis
UMN	upper motor neuron
URI	upper respiratory infection
USMLE	United States Medical Licensing Examination
UTI	urinary tract infection
VDRL	Venereal Disease Research Laboratory
VMA	vanillylmandelic acid
V/Q	ratio of ventilation to perfusion
VSD	ventricular septal defect
VWF	von Willebrand factor
VZV	varicella-zoster virus
WBC	white blood cell

Symbol	Meaning
$\uparrow$	increase(s)
$\downarrow$	decrease(s)
$\rightarrow$	leads to
1°	primary
2°	secondary
3°	tertiary
$\approx$	approximately; homologous

Index

Pages followed by f indicate figure. Pages followed by t indicate table.

Bronchitis, chronic, 408
Bronchodilators
  asthma, 407–408
  cystic fibrosis, 401
Budd–Chiari syndrome, 160
Bulimia, 386, 394
Bullous impetigo, 93

C

Caffeine, 388t
Calcium channel blockers, 60, 64, 70t, 278, 447t
Calcium phosphate, nephrolithiasis, 434t
Calcium supplements, 244, 332, 427
  hypercalcemia, 427
  menopause, 332
  osteoporosis, 244
Calymmatobacterium granulomatis, 230t
Campylobacter jejuni, 234t
Cancer
  acoustic neuroma, 282t
  adenocarcinoma, 342
    pancreatic, 148
  adnexal mass, 342–343
  astrocytoma, 282t
  basal cell carcinoma, 88–89, 89f
  bladder, 439
  breast, 339–341
  carcinoma
    basal cell, 88–89, 89f
    cervical, 341
    hepatic, 213
    hepatocellular, 147, 226
    renal cell, 213
    squamous cell, 87–88, 88f, 223
  cervical, 341
  colorectal, 172–173, 172f
  endometrial, 342
  ependymoma, 282t
  esophageal, 150
  glioblastoma multiforme, 282t
  hepatocellular carcinoma, 147
  lung, 413–415
  medulloblastoma, 282t
  melanoma, 89–90, 90f
  meningioma, 282t
  myeloma, multiple, 195–196
  neuroblastoma, 370
  osteosarcoma, 259–260, 260f
  ovarian, 343
  pancreatic, 148, 158t
  pancreatic adenocarcinoma, 148
  prostate, 438–439
  schwannoma, 282t
  skin, 86–90

squamous cell carcinoma, 87–88, 88f
  Wilms' tumor, 369–370
Cancer screening, 131t
Candidal intertrigo, 101
Candidal vaginitis, 334–335, 334f
Carbamazepine, 268t, 272, 273, 315t, 379, 446t
Carbon anhydrase inhibitors, glaucoma, 292
Carbon monoxide poisoning, 451
Carcinoma in situ (CIS), 340
Carcinomas
  basal cell, 88–89, 89f
  cervical, 341
  hepatic, 213
  hepatocellular, 226
  renal cell, 213
  squamous cell, 87–88, 88f, 223
Cardiac cycle, 49f
Cardiac output (CO), 50f
  variables, 51f
Cardiac stress testing, 72
Cardiac tamponade, 77
Cardiomyopathies, 63–65
  hypertrophic, 64
  primary dilated, 63–64
  restrictive, 64–65
Cardiovascular medicine, 47–80
  anti-anginal therapy, 52f
  aortic aneurysm, 73–74
  aortic dissection, 74–75
  arrhythmias, 56–58
  cardiac cycle, 49f
  cardiac output, 50f
    variables, 51f
  cardiac stress testing, 72
  cardiac tamponade, 77
  cardiomyopathies, 63–65
  congestive heart failure, 62–63
  coronary artery anatomy, 48f
  electrocardiogram, 52f
  endocarditis, 65, 66f
  heart block, 56f
  heart murmurs, 50f
  hypercholesterolemia, 72–73
  hypertension
    primary, 68–69, 70t
    secondary, 71
  hypertensive urgency and emergency, 71–72
  ischemic heart disease, 59
  lipid-lowering agents, 54f
  myocardial action potential, 51f
  myocardial infarction, 48f, 60–62, 61f
  pericarditis, 65, 66f
  peripheral vascular disease, 76
  rheumatic heart disease, 68

temporal arteries, 75
  valvular disease, 55t
Cardiovascular system, during pregnancy, 302t
Carpal tunnel syndrome, 243–244
Case control study, 128
CAST (computer-adaptive sequential testing), 11–12, 13f
Cataracts, 293
Cefotaxime, 216t
Ceftriaxone, 216t, 233, 336
Celecoxib, 240t
Cellulitis, 94–95
Cerebral palsy (CP), 354–355
Cervical intraepithelial neoplasia (CIN), 341
Cervicitis, 335–336
Cervix, during pregnancy, 301t
Cesarean section, 317, 318
Chancroid, 230t
Charcot's triad, 158
Chédiak-Higashi, 353t
Chemotherapy
  bladder cancer, 439
  brain tumors, 282
  breast cancer, 340
  endometrial cancer, 342
  leukemias, 198
  melanoma, 90
  multiple myeloma, 196
  neuroblastoma, 370
  osteosarcoma, 260
  ovarian cancer, 343
  prostate cancer, 438
  Wilms' tumor, 369–370
Childhood vaccinations, 350t
Children. *See also* Pediatrics
  abuse of, 353–354
  asthma, 407
  congenital hip dislocation, 257–258
  congenital infections, 214–215
  developmental milestones, 350t
  diarrhea, 165
  herpes, 214
  leukemias, 196–198
  orthopedic injuries, 255t
  rubella, 214–215
  sepsis, 212, 213t
  syphilis, 214–215
  vaccinations, 350t
Chlamydia trachomatis, 228–229, 335–336
Chloramphenicol, 446t
Cholangitis, 157–158
Cholecystitis, acute, 155, 156f, 157
Cholelithiasis, 154–155
Cholesterol, preventative measures, 132–133
Cholestyramine, 54f, 73